1

BEST *of* SLEEP MEDICINE 2011

Edited by
Teofilo Lee-Chiong
Professor of Medicine and Chief
Division of Sleep Medicine
National Jewish Health
Denver, Colorado

Professor of Medicine
Division of Pulmonary
and Critical Care Medicine
University of Colorado Denver
School of Medicine

Disclaimer

Every effort has been made to verify the accuracy of the facts in this book. The editor cannot accept any legal responsibility for any errors or omissions that may be made, and cannot make any warranty related to the material contained in this book. Medication usage should be confirmed with current reference materials and medical textbooks.

Lee-Chiong, Teofilo. Best of Sleep Medicine 2011.
ISBN-13: 978-1460993859
ISBN-10: 1460993853

Information Overload 2011

Increasingly, sleep clinicians, researchers and technologists are being asked to assume new responsibilities in the sleep laboratories and clinics – i.e., as care providers, researchers, managers, educators, mentors and community leaders. Furthermore, advances in science and technology will continue to radically transform the way we evaluate and treat individuals with sleep disorders. Our understanding of sleep medicine is changing each day, and the rate of growth in knowledge will only accelerate along with our inability to keep up with new research findings. For many, the easiest solution to this *information overload* is reading a review article. However, unlike published clinical trials that can be graded and, therefore, compared to each other, review articles often do not follow strict guidelines of disclosure and methodology. Among several review articles on a topic of interest, which should one choose?

I am proposing a criteria for grading medical review articles for your consideration. I hope you find this useful.

Criteria for Grading of Medical Review Articles

1. *Disclosure*: Was there full disclosure by author/s of potential conflicts of interests?
2. *Methodology*: Did the author/s provide method/s for selection of references and was it systematic and comprehensive? Did the author/s discuss the limitations of their method/s?
3. *Use of Original References*: Did the author/s include original research publications? Was the percentage of original references (vs. review articles) greater than 70%?
   a. Number of original research publications ÷ Total number of references: > 70%
4. *Use of Recent References*: Did the authors include recent publications? Was the percentage of recent references (within 5 years) greater than 70%?
   a. Number of references within last 5 years ÷ Total number of references: > 70%

Grading: 0-4 (1 point for every positive response)

I am indebted to the many authors for the excellent commentaries they have generously provided. This book is dedicated to Dolores Grace Zamudio and Zoe Lee-Chiong.

Teofilo Lee-Chiong MD

Editor

Teofilo Lee-Chiong
Division of Sleep Medicine
National Jewish Health
Denver, Colorado

Contributors

Gail K Adler
Harvard Medical School
Division of Endocrinology, Diabetes and
Hypertension
Department of Medicine
Brigham and Women's Hospital

Offer Amir
WideMed Ltd.

Sonia Ancoli-Israel
Gillin Sleep and Chronomedicine Research
Center
Department of Psychiatry
University of California San Diego

Antonio Antón
Respiratory Medicine Dept.
Hospital de la Santa Creu i Sant Pau
Barcelona, Spain

Chun T Au
Department of Pediatrics
Prince of Wales Hospital
The Chinese University of Hong Kong

M. Safwan Badr
John D Dingell VA Medical Center
Wayne State University

Dennis Bailey
Dental Sleep Medicine Mini-Residency
School of Dentistry
University of California Los Angeles
Los Angeles, California

Jessie P. Bakker
WellSleep Sleep Investigation Centre
Department of Medicine
University of Otago

Deganit Barak-Shinar
WideMed Ltd.

Ferran Barbé
IRB Lleida, Lleida and CIBERes, Madrid

Jean Claude Barthélémy
Department of Clinical Physiology
Department of Neurology
University of Lyon

Olivier Beauchet
Department of Clinical Physiology
Department of Neurology
University of Lyon

Rakesh Bhattacharjee
Department of Pediatrics
Comer Children's Hospital
The University of Chicago

Konrad E. Bloch
Pulmonary Divisions
University Hospital of Zurich

Richard K. Bogan
University of South Carolina
School of Medicine
SleepMed Incorporated

Ricardo Vieira Botelho
Disciplina de Medicina e Biologia do Sono
Departamento de Psicobiologia
Universidade Federal de São Paulo
Hospital do Servidor Público do Estado de
São Paulo

T. Douglas Bradley
Sleep Research Laboratory of Toronto
Rehab Institute
Centre for Sleep Health and Research
Toronto General Hospital of the University
Health Network

Serge Brand
Sleep and Depression Research Unit
Psychiatric Hospital of the University of
Basel

Dawn M. Bravata
VA Stroke Quality Enhancement Research
Initiative (QUERI)
Indiana University School of Medicine
VA HSR&D Center of Excellence on
Implementing Evidence-Based Practice
Richard L. Roudebush VA Medical Center

Laurent Brondel
Centre Européen des Sciences du Goût
Univ. Dijon

Richard A. Bryant
School of Psychology
University of New South Wales

Casey Burg
Division of Sleep Medicine
National Jewish Health

Orfeu M. Buxton
Division of Sleep Medicine
Harvard Medical School
Department of Medicine
Brigham and Women's Hospital

Sébastien Celle
Department of Clinical Physiology
Department of Neurology
University of Lyon

Andrew S. L. Chan
Centre for Sleep Health and Research
Department of Respiratory Medicine
Royal North Shore Hospital

Susmita Chowdhuri
John D Dingell VA Medical Center
Wayne State University

Peter A. Cistulli
Woolcock Institute of Medical Research
University of Sydney

Stephanie Connors
Center for Women's Mental Health
Massachusetts General Hospital
Harvard Medical School

Aisha Cortoos
Research Unit Biological Psychology
Vrije Universiteit Brussel

Christopher C. Cranston
Department of Psychology
University of Tulsa

Damien Davenne
INSERM ERI27, Univ. Caen

Joanne L. Davis
Department of Psychology
University of Tulsa

Michael Deuschle
Central Institute of Mental Health,
Mannheim, Germany

Charmane I. Eastman
Biological Rhythms Research Lab
Behavioral Sciences Department
Rush University Medical Center

Margherita Fabbri
Department of Neurological Sciences
University of Bologna

Marcello Ferrari
Department of Medicine
University of Verona

Raffaele Ferri
Sleep Research Centre
Department of Neurology IC
Oasi Institute for Research on Mental
Retardation and Brain Aging IRCCS, Troina

Mariana G. Figueiro
Lighting Research Center
Rensselaer Polytechnic Institute

Michael Friedman
Section of Otolaryngology
Advocate Illinois Masonic Medical Center,
Chicago
Department of Otolaryngology – Head and
Neck Surgery
Section of Sleep Surgery
Rush University Medical Center

Barbara C Galland
Department of Women's & Children's
Health
University of Otago

Robert N. Glidewell
Lynn Institute for Healthcare Research

David Gozal
Department of Pediatrics
Comer Children's Hospital
The University of Chicago

María Rosa Güell
Respiratory Medicine Dept.
Hospital de la Santa Creu i Sant Pau
Barcelona, Spain

Erik Hemmingsson
Department of Medicine
Karolinska Institutet, Stockholm

Max Hirshkowitz
Department of Medicine & Menninger
Department of Psychiatry
Baylor College of Medicine
Sleep Disorders & Research Center
VA Medical Center, Houston

Imran Iftikhar
Division of Pulmonary, Allergy, Critical
Care, and Sleep Medicine
The Ohio State University Medical Center

Alex Iranzo
Neurology Service
Hospital Clinic of Barcelona
University of Barcelona Medical School

Shahrokh Javaheri
University of Cincinnati
Sleepcare Diagnostics

Sanja Jelic
Division of Pulmonary, Allergy, and Critical
Care Medicine
Columbia University College of P&S

Poul Jennum
Danish Center for Sleep Medicine
Department of Clinical Neurophysiology
University of Copenhagen
Glostrup Hospital

Hadine Joffe
Center for Women's Mental Health
Massachusetts General Hospital
Harvard Medical School

Kari Johansson
Department of Medicine
Karolinska Institutet, Stockholm

Shuji Joho
Second Department of Internal Medicine
Toyama University Hospital

Carla Jungquist
University of Rochester

Takatoshi Kasai
Sleep Center
Toranomon Hospital, Tokyo
Department of Cardiology
Juntendo University
School of Medicine, Tokyo

Kanwar Kelley
Section of Otolaryngology
Advocate Illinois Masonic Medical Center,
Chicago

Judith Kerleroux
Department of Clinical Physiology
Department of Neurology
University of Lyon

Meena Khan
Division of Pulmonary, Sleep, Critical Care,
and Allergy
Division of Neurology
The Ohio State University Medical Center

Leila Kheirandish-Gozal
Department of Pediatrics
Comer Children's Hospital
The University of Chicago

William D. S. Killgore
Harvard Medical School
Neuroimaging Center
McLean Hospital

Michael Kluge
Klinik und Poliklinik für Psychiatrie
Universitätsklinikum Leipzig AöR

Samuel Krachman
Division of Pulmonary and Critical Care
Temple University School of Medicine

Samuel T. Kuna
Philadelphia Veterans Affairs Medical
Center and
University of Pennsylvania

Daniela Lanza
Department of Medicine
University of Verona

Bernard Laurent
Department of Clinical Physiology
Department of Neurology
University of Lyon

Albert M. Li
Department of Pediatrics
Prince of Wales Hospital
The Chinese University of Hong Kong

Franco Lumachi
Department of Surgical &
Gastroenterological Sciences
School of Medicine
University of Padua

Enrico A. Marcelli
Department of Sociology
San Diego State University

Roser Masa-Font
Servicio de Atención Primaria Litoral
Institut Català de Salut, Barcelona

Delphine Maudoux
Department of Clinical Physiology
Department of Neurology
University of Lyon

Mercedes Mayos
Respiratory Medicine Dept.
Hospital de la Santa Creu i Sant Pau
Barcelona, Spain

Walter McNicholas
Respiratory Sleep Disorders Unit
Department of Respiratory Medicine
St. Vincent's University Hospital

Reena Mehra
Division of Pulmonary, Critical Care and
Sleep Medicine
University Hospitals Case Medical Center
Case School of Medicine

Eli O. Meltzer
Allergy & Asthma Medical Group &
Research Center

Robert L. Merrill
School of Dentistry
University of California, Los Angeles

Taku Miyagawa
Department of Human Genetics
Graduate School of Medicine
The University of Tokyo

Peter T. Morgan
Department of Psychiatry
Yale University

Dominic A. Munafo
Sleep Data, Inc.

Alan Mulgrew
Bon Secours Hospital, Tralee

Carlos E. Negrão
Heart Institute (InCor)
University of São Paulo Medical School
School of Physical Education and Sports
University of São Paulo

Evangelia Nena
Medical School
Democritus University of Thrace

Martin Neovius
Department of Medicine
Karolinska Institutet, Stockholm

Tore Nielsen
Université de Montréal
Dream & Nightmare Laboratory
Hopital du Sacre-Coeur

William G Ondo
Baylor College of Medicine

Laura Palacios-Soler
Consorci d'Atenció Primària de
Salut de l'Eixample, Barcelona

Giselle Soares Passos
Exercise and Psychobiology Research
Center (CEPE)
Departament of Psychobiology
Universidade Federal de São Paulo

Michel A. Paul
Performance Group
Individual Readiness Section
Defence R&D Canada

Milena Pavlova
Harvard Medical School
Division of Epilepsy, Neurophysiology and
Sleep
Department of Neurology
Brigham and Women's Hospital

Michael L. Perlis
University of Pennsylvania

Barbara Phillips
Division of Pulmonary, Critical Care and
Sleep Medicine
Department of Internal Medicine
University of Kentucky College of Medicine

Vincent Pichot
Department of Clinical Physiology
Department of Neurology
University of Lyon

Wilfred R. Pigeon
Sleep & Neurophysiology Research Lab
University of Rochester Medical Center
Canandaigua VA Medical Center
Center for Integrated Healthcare
Syracuse VA Medical Center

Manju Pillai
National Jewish Health
University of Colorado Denver School of
Medicine

Fabio Pizza
Department of Neurological Sciences
University of Bologna

Sukanya Pranathiageswaran
Wayne State University

Lisa Rafalson
D'Youville College
State University of New York
University at Buffalo

Jamie L. Rhudy
Department of Psychology
University of Tulsa

Frédéric Roche
Department of Clinical Physiology
Department of Neurology
University of Lyon

George W. Rodway
University of Utah College of Nursing

Russell P. Rosenberg
NeuroTrials Research and Atlanta School of
Sleep Medicine

Leon Rosenthal, MD
Sleep Medicine Associates of Texas
Dallas, TX

Thomas Roth
Sleep Disorders Center
Henry Ford Hospital

Gregory A. Ruff
Pulmonary Associates, Colorado Springs

Clodagh Ryan
University of Toronto
Toronto General Hospital

Frank Ryan
Respiratory Division
Department of Medicine
University of British Columbia

Silke Ryan
Respiratory Sleep Disorders Unit
St. Vincent's University Hospital

Daniel Samolski
Respiratory Medicine Dept.
Hospital de la Santa Creu i Sant Pau
Barcelona, Spain

Manuel Sánchez de la Torre
IRB Lleida, Lleida and CIBERes, Madrid

Gemma Sansa
Neurology Service
Corporació Sanitària Parc Taulí, Sabadell
Susumu Tanaka
Tokyo Institute of Psychiatry

Joan Santamaria
Neurology Service
Hospital Clinic of Barcelona
University of Barcelona Medical School

Otto D. Schoch
Pulmonary Divisions
Cantonal Hospital St. Gallen

Emilia Sforza
Department of Clinical Physiology
Department of Neurology
University of Lyon

Hideto Shinno
Department of Neuropsychiatry
Kagawa University

Robert Skomro
Division of Respiratory, Critical Care and
Sleep Medicine
Department of Medicine
University of Saskatchewan

Mark R. Smith
Biological Rhythms Research Lab
Behavioral Sciences Department
Rush University Medical Center

Virend K. Somers
Division of Cardiovascular Diseases
Department of Internal Medicine
Mayo Clinic and Foundation

Paschalis Steiropoulos
Medical School
Democritus University of Thrace

Mariana Szklo-Coxe
School of Community and Environmental
Health
College of Health Sciences
Old Dominion University
Division of Sleep Medicine
Department of Internal Medicine
Eastern Virginia Medical School

Susumu Tanaka
Tokyo Institute of Psychiatry

Catherine Thomas-Anterion
Department of Clinical Physiology
Department of Neurology
University of Lyon

Georgia Trakada
Medical School
Democritus University of Thrace

Katsushi Tokunaga
Department of Human Genetics
Graduate School of Medicine
The University of Tokyo

Luca Tomaello
Department of Medicine
University of Verona

Thanh G.N. Ton
Department of Neurology
University of Washington

Hiromi Toyoda
Department of Human Genetics
Graduate School of Medicine
The University of Tokyo
The Sleep Disorders Research Project
Tokyo Institute of Psychiatry

Ivani C. Trombetta
Heart Institute (InCor)
University of São Paulo Medical School

Adrienne M. Tucker
Columbia University

Sergio Tufik
Exercise and Psychobiology Research
Center (CEPE)
Departament of Psychobiology
Universidade Federal de São Paulo

Marco Túlio de Mello
Exercise and Psychobiology Research
Center (CEPE)
Departament of Psychobiology
Universidade Federal de São Paulo

Marjorie Vennelle
Department of Sleep Medicine
Royal Infirmary of Edinburgh
University of Edinburgh

Nathaniel F. Watson
UW Medicine Sleep Center
University of Washington

Terri E. Weaver
University of Illinois at Chicago College of
Nursing

Lichuan Ye
Boston College
William F. Connell School of Nursing

Dai Yumino
Department of Cardiology
Tokyo Women's Medical University

Luisa Zanolla
Department of Medicine
University of Verona

Contents

Sleep Deprivation

Hypersomnia

Insomnia

58 A 12-week, randomized, double-blind, placebo-controlled study evaluating the effect of eszopiclone 2 mg on sleep/wake function in older adults with primary and comorbid insomnia. Ancoli-Israel S, Krystal AD, McCall WV, Schaefer K, Wilson A, Claus R, Rubens R, Roth T. *Sleep. 2010 Feb 1;33(2):225-34.*

60 An exploratory study on the effects of tele-neurofeedback and tele-biofeedback on objective and subjective sleep in patients with primary insomnia. Cortoos A, De Valck E, Arns M, Breteler MH, Cluydts R. *Appl Psychophysiol Biofeedback. 2010 Jun;35(2):125-34.*

63 Association between a serotonin transporter length polymorphism and primary insomnia. Deuschle M, Schredl M, Schilling C, Wüst S, Frank J, Witt SH, Rietschel M, Buckert M, Meyer-Lindenberg A, Schulze TG. *Sleep. 2010 Mar 1;33(3):343-7.*

65 Effect of acute physical exercise on patients with chronic primary insomnia. Passos GS, Poyares D, Santana MG, Garbuio SA, Tufik S, Mello MT. *J Clin Sleep Med. 2010 Jun 15;6(3):270-5.*

68 Effectiveness of Valerian on insomnia: a meta-analysis of randomized placebo-controlled trials. Fernández-San-Martín MI, Masa-Font R, Palacios-Soler L, Sancho-Gómez P, Calbó-Caldentey C, Flores-Mateo G. *Sleep Med. 2010 Jun;11(6):505-11.*

70 Habitual sleep duration and insomnia and the risk of cardiovascular events and all-cause death: report from a community-based cohort. Chien KL, Chen PC, Hsu HC, Su TC, Sung FC, Chen MF, Lee YT. *Sleep. 2010 Feb 1;33(2):177-84.*

74 Prospective associations of insomnia markers and symptoms with depression. Szklo-Coxe M, Young T, Peppard PE, Finn LA, Benca RM. *Am J Epidemiol. 2010 Mar 15;171(6):709-20.*

80 The efficacy of cognitive-behavioral therapy for insomnia in patients with chronic pain. Jungquist CR, O'Brien C, Matteson-Rusby S, Smith MT, Pigeon WR, Xia Y, Lu N, Perlis ML. *Sleep Med. 2010 Mar;11(3):302-9.*

82 Treatment effects of gabapentin for primary insomnia. Lo HS, Yang CM, Lo HG, Lee CY, Ting H, Tzang BS. *Clin Neuropharmacol. 2010 Mar-Apr;33(2):84-90.*

Sleep-Related Breathing Disorders

85 A multicenter, prospective study of a novel nasal EPAP device in the treatment of obstructive sleep apnea: efficacy and 30-day adherence. Rosenthal L, Massie CA, Dolan DC, Loomas B, Kram J, Hart RW. *J Clin Sleep Med. 2009 Dec 15;5(6):532-7.*

88 Adenotonsillectomy outcomes in treatment of obstructive sleep apnea in children: a multicenter retrospective study. Bhattacharjee R, Kheirandish-Gozal L, Spruyt K, Mitchell RB, Promchiarak J, Simakajornboon N, Kaditis AG, Splaingard D, Splaingard M, Brooks LJ, Marcus CL, Sin S, Arens R, Verhulst SL, Gozal D. *Am J Respir Crit Care Med. 2010 Sep 1;182(5):676-83.*

91 Automatic slow eye movement (SEM) detection of sleep onset in patients with obstructive sleep apnea syndrome (OSAS): comparison between multiple sleep latency test (MSLT) and maintenance of wakefulness test (MWT). Fabbri M, Pizza F, Magosso E, Ursino M, Contardi S, Cirignotta F, Provini F, Montagna P. *Sleep Med. 2010 Mar;11(3):253-7.*

94 Auto-titrating continuous positive airway pressure for patients with acute transient ischemic attack: a randomized feasibility trial. Bravata DM, Concato J, Fried T, Ranjbar N, Sadarangani T, McClain V, Struve F, Zygmunt L, Knight HJ, Lo A, Richerson GB, Gorman M, Williams LS, Brass LM, Agostini J, Mohsenin V, Roux F, Yaggi HK. *Stroke. 2010 Jul;41(7):1464-70.*

97 Beneficial effects of adaptive servo ventilation in patients with chronic heart failure. Koyama T, Watanabe H, Kobukai Y, Makabe S, Munehisa Y, Iino K, Kosaka T, Ito H. *Circ J. 2010 Oct;74(10):2118-24.*

103 Cheyne-Stokes respiration and obstructive sleep apnoea are independent risk factors for malignant ventricular arrhythmias requiring appropriate cardioverter-defibrillator therapies in patients with congestive heart failure. Bitter T, Westerheide N, Prinz C, Hossain MS, Vogt J, Langer C, Horstkotte D, Oldenburg O. *Eur Heart J. 2010 Sep 16.*

106 Cognitive function and sleep related breathing disorders in a healthy elderly population: the SYNAPSE study. Sforza E, Roche F, Thomas-Anterion C, Kerleroux J, Beauchet O, Celle S, Maudoux D, Pichot V, Laurent B, Barthélémy JC. *Sleep. 2010 Apr 1;33(4):515-21.*

109 Comparison of positional therapy to CPAP in patients with positional obstructive sleep apnea. Permut I, Diaz-Abad M, Chatila W, Crocetti J, Gaughan JP, D'Alonzo GE, Krachman SL. *J Clin Sleep Med. 2010 Jun 15;6(3):238-43.*

112 Consequences of comorbid sleep apnea in the metabolic syndrome--implications for cardiovascular risk. Trombetta IC, Somers VK, Maki-Nunes C, Drager LF, Toschi-Dias E, Alves MJ, Fraga RF, Rondon MU, Bechara MG, Lorenzi-Filho G, Negrão CE. *Sleep. 2010 Sep 1;33(9):1193-9.*

115 Continuous positive airway pressure deepens sleep in patients with Alzheimer's disease and obstructive sleep apnea. Cooke JR, Ancoli-Israel S, Liu L, Loredo JS, Natarajan L, Palmer BS, He F, Corey-Bloom J. *Sleep Med. 2009 Dec;10(10):1101-6.*

118 Craniofacial Changes After 2 Years of Nasal Continuous Positive Airway Pressure Use in Patients With Obstructive Sleep Apnea. Tsuda H, Almeida FR, Tsuda T, Moritsuchi Y, Lowe AA. *Chest. 2010; 138;870-874.*

121 Effect of a very low energy diet on moderate and severe obstructive sleep apnoea in obese men: a randomised controlled trial. Johansson K, Neovius M, Lagerros YT, Harlid R, Rössner S, Granath F, Hemmingsson E. *BMJ. 2009 Dec 3;339:b4609.*

124 Effect of episodic hypoxia on the susceptibility to hypocapnic central apnea during NREM sleep. Chowdhuri S, Shanidze I, Pierchala L, Belen D, Mateika JH, Badr MS. *J Appl Physiol. 2010 Feb;108(2):369-77.*

127 Effect of flow-triggered adaptive servo-ventilation compared with continuous positive airway pressure in patients with chronic heart failure with coexisting obstructive sleep apnea and Cheyne-Stokes respiration. Kasai T, Usui Y, Yoshioka T, Yanagisawa N, Takata Y, Narui K, Yamaguchi T, Yamashina A, Momomura SI; JASV Investigators. *Circ Heart Fail. 2010 Jan;3(1):140-8.*

129 Endothelial repair capacity and apoptosis are inversely related in obstructive sleep apnea. Jelic S, Lederer DJ, Adams T, Padeletti M, Colombo PC, Factor P, Le Jemtel TH. *Vasc Health Risk Manag. 2009;5:909-20.*

131 Evaluation of sham-CPAP as a placebo in CPAP intervention studies. Rodway GW, Weaver TE, Mancini C, Cater J, Maislin G, Staley B, Ferguson KA, George CF, Schulman DA, Greenberg H, Rapoport DM, Walsleben JA, Lee-Chiong T, Kuna ST. *Sleep. 2010 Feb 1;33(2):260-6.*

135 Gender differences in obstructive sleep apnea and treatment response to continuous positive airway pressure. Ye L, Pien GW, Ratcliffe SJ, Weaver TE. *J Clin Sleep Med. 2009 Dec 15;5(6):512-8.*

138 Impact of sleeping position on central sleep apnea/Cheyne-Stokes respiration in patients with heart failure. Joho S, Oda Y, Hirai T, Inoue H. *Sleep Med. 2010 Feb;11(2):143-8.*

141 Long-term effect of continuous positive airway pressure in hypertensive patients with sleep apnea. Barbé F, Durán-Cantolla J, Capote F, de la Peña M, Chiner E, Masa JF, Gonzalez M, Marín JM, Garcia-Rio F, de Atauri JD, Terán J, Mayos M, Monasterio C, del Campo F, Gomez S, de la Torre MS, Martinez M, Montserrat JM; Spanish Sleep and Breathing Group. *Am J Respir Crit Care Med. 2010 Apr 1;181(7):718-26.*

144 Nasopharyngoscopic evaluation of oral appliance therapy for obstructive sleep apnoea. Chan AS, Lee RW, Srinivasan VK, Darendeliler MA, Grunstein RR, Cistulli PA. *Eur Respir J. 2010 Apr;35(4):836-42.*

148 Natural history and predictors for progression of mild childhood obstructive sleep apnoea. Li AM, Au CT, Ng SK, Abdullah VJ, Ho C, Fok TF, Ng PC, Wing YK. *Thorax. 2010 Jan;65(1):27-31.*

152 Nocturnal rostral fluid shift: a unifying concept for the pathogenesis of obstructive and central sleep apnea in men with heart failure. Yumino D, Redolfi S, Ruttanaumpawan P, Su MC, Smith S, Newton GE, Mak S, Bradley TD. *Circulation. 2010 Apr 13;121(14):1598-605.*

155 Obstructive sleep apnea and risk of motor vehicle crash: systematic review and meta-analysis. Tregear S, Reston J, Schoelles K, Phillips B. *J Clin Sleep Med. 2009 Dec 15;5(6):573-81.*

157 Otolaryngology office-based treatment of obstructive sleep apnea-hypopnea syndrome with titratable and nontitratable thermoplastic mandibular advancement devices. Friedman M, Pulver T, Wilson MN, Golbin D, Leesman C, Lee G, Joseph NJ. *Otolaryngol Head Neck Surg. 2010 Jul;143(1):78-84.*

160 Outcomes of home-based diagnosis and treatment of obstructive sleep apnea. Skomro RP, Gjevre J, Reid J, McNab B, Ghosh S, Stiles M, Jokic R, Ward H, Cotton D. *Chest. 2010 Aug;138(2):257-63.*

163 Plasma levels of MCP-1 and adiponectin in obstructive sleep apnea syndrome. Kim J, Lee CH, Park CS, Kim BG, Kim SW, Cho JH. *Arch Otolaryngol Head Neck Surg. 2010 Sep;136(9):896-9.*

166 Prevalence and clinical characteristics of obesity hypoventilation syndrome among individuals reporting sleep-related breathing symptoms in northern Greece. Trakada GP, Steiropoulos P, Nena E, Constandinidis TC, Bouros D. *Sleep Breath. 2010; 14(4):381-6.*

169 Randomized controlled trial comparing flexible and continuous positive airway pressure delivery: effects on compliance, objective and subjective sleepiness and vigilance. Bakker J, Campbell A, Neill A. *Sleep. 2010 Apr 1;33(4):523-9.*

172 Randomized controlled trial of variable-pressure versus fixed-pressure continuous positive airway pressure (CPAP) treatment for patients with obstructive sleep apnea/hypopnea syndrome (OSAHS). Vennelle M, White S, Riha RL, Mackay TW, Engleman HM, Douglas NJ. *Sleep. 2010 Feb 1;33(2):267-71.*

175 Residual sleep apnea on polysomnography after 3 months of CPAP therapy: clinical implications, predictors and patterns. Mulgrew AT, Lawati NA, Ayas NT, Fox N, Hamilton P, Cortes L, Ryan CF. *Sleep Med. 2010 Feb;11(2):119-25.*

179 Shift in sleep apnoea type in heart failure patients in the CANPAP trial. Ryan CM, Floras JS, Logan AG, Kimoff RJ, Series F, Morrison D, Ferguson KA, Belenkie I, Pfeifer M, Fleetham J, Hanly PJ, Smilovitch M, Arzt M, Bradley TD; CANPAP Investigators. *Eur Respir J. 2010 Mar;35(3):592-7.*

182 Sleep disordered breathing is associated with appropriate implantable cardioverter defibrillator therapy in congestive heart failure patients. Tomaello L, Zanolla L, Vassanelli C, LoCascio V, Ferrari M. *Clin Cardiol. 2010 Feb;33(2):E27-30.*

186 Sustained hyperoxia stabilizes breathing in healthy individuals during NREM sleep. Chowdhuri S, Sinha P, Pranathiageswaran S, Safwan Badr M. *J Appl Physiol. 2010 Nov;109(5):1378-83.*

190 The effects of posterior fossa decompressive surgery in adult patients with Chiari malformation and sleep apnea. Botelho RV, Bittencourt LR, Rotta JM, Tufik S. *J Neurosurg. 2010 Apr;112(4):800-7.*

Circadian Neurobiology and Circadian Rhythm Sleep Disorders

193 A compromise circadian phase position for permanent night work improves mood, fatigue, and performance. Smith MR, Fogg LF, Eastman CI. *Sleep. 2009 Nov 1;32(11):1481-9.*

196 A phase 3, double-blind, randomized, placebo-controlled study of armodafinil for excessive sleepiness associated with jet lag disorder. Rosenberg RP, Bogan RK, Tiller JM, Yang R, Youakim JM, Earl CQ, Roth T. *Mayo Clin Proc. 2010 Jul;85(7):630-8.*

199 Caffeine for the prevention of injuries and errors in shift workers. Ker K, Edwards PJ, Felix LM, Blackhall K, Roberts I. *Cochrane Database Syst Rev. 2010 May 12;5:CD008508.*

210 Lack of short-wavelength light during the school day delays dim light melatonin onset (DLMO) in middle school students. Figueiro MG, Rea MS. *Neuro Endocrinol Lett. 2010;31(1):92-6.*

204 Melatonin treatment for eastward and westward travel preparation. Paul MA, Miller JC, Gray GW, Love RJ, Lieberman HR, Arendt J. *Psychopharmacology (Berl). 2010 Feb;208(3):377-86.*

Movement Disorders

207 Acute dopamine-agonist treatment in restless legs syndrome: effects on sleep architecture and NREM sleep instability. Ferri R, Manconi M, Aricò D, Sagrada C, Zucconi M, Bruni O, Oldani A, Ferini-Strambi L. *Sleep. 2010 Jun 1;33(6):793-800.*

211 Intravenous iron dextran for severe refractory restless legs syndrome. Ondo WG. *Sleep Med. 2010 May;11(5):494-6.*

214 Long-term maintenance treatment of restless legs syndrome with gabapentin enacarbil: a randomized controlled study. Bogan RK, Bornemann MA, Kushida CA, Trân PV, Barrett RW; XP060 Study Group. *Mayo Clin Proc. 2010 Jun;85(6):512-21.*

217 Proposed dose equivalence between clonazepam and pramipexole in patients with restless legs syndrome. Shinno H, Oka Y, Otsuki M, Tsuchiya S, Mizuno S, Kawada S, Innami T, Sasaki A, Hineno T, Sakamoto T, Inami Y, Nakamura Y, Horiguchi J. *Prog Neuropsychopharmacol Biol Psychiatry. 2010 Apr 16;34(3):522-6.*

Parasomnias

221 Cognitive-behavioral treatment for chronic nightmares in trauma-exposed persons: assessing physiological reactions to nightmare-related fear. Rhudy JL, Davis JL, Williams AE, McCabe KM, Bartley EJ, Byrd PM, Pruiksma KE. *J Clin Psychol. 2010 Apr;66(4):365-82.*

224 Controlled clinical, polysomnographic and psychometric studies on differences between sleep bruxers and controls and acute effects of clonazepam as compared with placebo. Saletu A, Parapatics S, Anderer P, Matejka M, Saletu B. *Eur Arch Psychiatry Clin Neurosci. 2010 Mar;260(2):163-74.*

226 Effect of botulinum toxin injection on nocturnal bruxism: a randomized controlled trial. Lee SJ, McCall WD Jr, Kim YK, Chung SC, Chung JW. *Am J Phys Med Rehabil. 2010 Jan;89(1):16-23.*

Medical, Neurological and Psychiatric Disorders

228 Effects of salmeterol on sleeping oxygen saturation in chronic obstructive pulmonary disease. Ryan S, Doherty LS, Rock C, Nolan GM, McNicholas WT. *Respiration. 2010;79(6):475-81.*

231 Intranasal mometasone furoate therapy for allergic rhinitis symptoms and rhinitis-disturbed sleep. Meltzer EO, Munafo DA, Chung W, Gopalan G, Varghese ST. *Ann Allergy Asthma Immunol. 2010 Jul;105(1):65-74.*

234 Nocturnal periodic breathing during acclimatization at very high altitude at Mount Muztagh Ata (7,546 m). Bloch KE, Latshang TD, Turk AJ, Hess T, Hefti U, Merz TM, Bosch MM, Barthelmes D, Hefti JP, Maggiorini M, Schoch OD. *Am J Respir Crit Care Med. 2010 Aug 15;182(4):562-8.*

237 Short and long sleep are positively associated with obesity, diabetes, hypertension, and cardiovascular disease among adults in the United States. Buxton OM, Marcelli E. *Soc Sci Med. 2010 Sep;71(5):1027-36.*

239 Sleep disturbance immediately prior to trauma predicts subsequent psychiatric disorder. Bryant RA, Creamer M, O'Donnell M, Silove D, McFarlane AC. *Sleep. 2010 Jan 1;33(1):69-74.*

242 Sleep hypoventilation due to increased nocturnal oxygen flow in hypercapnic COPD patients. Samolski D, Tárrega J, Antón A, Mayos M, Martí S, Farrero E, Güell R. *Respirology. 2010 Feb;15(2):283-8.*

246 The effect of pregabalin on pain-related sleep interference in diabetic peripheral neuropathy or postherpetic neuralgia: a review of nine clinical trials. Roth T, van Seventer R, Murphy TK. *Curr Med Res Opin. 2010; 26(10):2411-9.*

Pediatric Sleep Medicine

249 Caffeine for Apnea of Prematurity trial: benefits may vary in subgroups. Davis PG, Schmidt B, Roberts RS, Doyle LW, Asztalos E, Haslam R, Sinha S, Tin W; Caffeine for Apnea of Prematurity Trial Group. *J Pediatr. 2010 Mar;156(3):382-7.*

253 High exercise levels are related to favorable sleep patterns and psychological functioning in adolescents: a comparison of athletes and controls. Brand S, Gerber M, Beck J, Hatzinger M, Pühse U, Holsboer-Trachsler E. *J Adolesc Health. 2010 Feb;46(2):133-41.*

255 Sleep quality and motor vehicle crashes in adolescents. Pizza F, Contardi S, Antognini AB, Zagoraiou M, Borrotti M, Mostacci B, Mondini S, Cirignotta F. *J Clin Sleep Med. 2010 Feb 15;6(1):41-5.*

258 The sleep of children with attention deficit hyperactivity disorder on and off methylphenidate: a matched case-control study. Galland BC, Tripp EG, Taylor BJ. *J Sleep Res. 2010 Jun;19(2):366-73.*

Aging

261 Ghrelin increases slow wave sleep and stage 2 sleep and decreases stage 1 sleep and REM sleep in elderly men but does not affect sleep in elderly women. Kluge M, Gazea M, Schüssler P, Genzel L, Dresler M, Kleyer S, Uhr M, Yassouridis A, Steiger A. *Psychoneuroendocrinology. 2010 Feb;35(2):297-304.*

Sleep Among Women

264 Eszopiclone improves insomnia and depressive and anxious symptoms in perimenopausal and postmenopausal women with hot flashes: a randomized, double-blinded, placebo-controlled crossover trial. Joffe H, Petrillo L, Viguera A, Koukopoulos A, Silver-Heilman K, Farrell A, Yu G, Silver M, Cohen LS. *Am J Obstet Gynecol. 2010 Feb;202(2):171.e1-171.e11.*

Miscellaneous

268 An automated sleep-analysis system operated through a standard hospital monitor. Amir O, Barak-Shinar D, Amos Y, MacDonald M, Pittman S, White DP. *J Clin Sleep Med. 2010 Feb 15;6(1):59-63.*

270 Hypoxemia and hypoventilation syndrome improvement after laparoscopic bariatric surgery in patients with morbid obesity. Lumachi F, Marzano B, Fanti G, Basso SM, Mazza F, Chiara GB. *In Vivo. 2010 May-Jun;24(3):329-31.*

273 Normalizing effects of modafinil on sleep in chronic cocaine users. Morgan PT, Pace-Schott E, Pittman B, Stickgold R, Malison RT. *Am J Psychiatry. 2010 Mar;167(3):331-40.*

Sleep Deprivation

Acute partial sleep deprivation increases food intake in healthy men. Brondel L, Romer MA, Nougues PM, Touyarou P, Davenne D. *Am J Clin Nutr. 2010 Jun;91(6):1550-9.*

Does acute partial sleep deprivation modify subsequent physical activity and energy intake?

Subjects	Methods	Outcomes
12 male subjects • Age: 22 ± 3 yrs • BMI: 22.30 ± 1.83	Randomized 2-condition crossover study Protocol for each 48-hr session: • During the first night, subjects were randomized to either: 1. 8 hrs of sleep (from 0000-0800) 2. 4 hrs of sleep (from 0200-0600) • Subsequently, all foods were eaten ad libitum Assessments • Physical activity (by actimetry) • Subjective sensations of hunger, pleasantness of foods, desire to eat, and sleepiness	Compared to 8-hr sleep durations, sleep restriction was associated with: • Greater energy consumption (22% or 559 ± 617 kcal) on the day after sleep* • Higher hunger before breakfast** and dinner*** • Higher physical activity (from 1215 to 2015)[#] • Greater sleepiness[##] • No difference in sensation of food pleasantness or desire to eat

BMI: body mass index; *$P < 0.01$; **$P < 0.001$; ***$P < 0.05$; [#]$P < 0.01$; [##]$P < 0.01$

Conclusion
One night of partial sleep deprivation was associated with greater physical activity and higher food intake.

Commentary
During the last decade obesity became a worldwide public health.[1] Obesity has been proven to be behind a number of debilitating health problems including diabetes, cardiovascular disease, stroke, infertility, depression and neurological disease.[2,3] Attempts to understand the causes of this phenomenon and develop new therapeutic strategies have mostly focused on calorific intake, dietary choices, and exercise. Recent human studies linked the increase in obesity with the general reduction in sleep duration observed in most of the industrialized countries, such as France[4], Spain[5], Japan[6] and the United States.[7] For example, in the United States, the duration

of sleep, which averaged 8-9 h/night in 1960[8], fell to less than 7 hours in 1995.[9] This drastic reduction in sleep coincides with increasing rates of obesity and metabolic disorders in this country.

The mechanisms by which sleep restriction may affect the energy balance and lead to obesity are unknown but three main mechanisms have been put forward.[10] First, an increase in free time to eat, which assumes that food is easily available and that subjects have a sedentary lifestyle.[11] Second, an increase in appetite; in keeping with this hypothesis, it has been noted that habitual short-sleepers ate proportionally more often (i.e. more than three meals per day) than longer sleepers.[12] Recently, it was also observed that sleep restriction increases hunger/appetite[13] and plasma concentrations of ghrelin (a "hunger" hormone), and that it causes decreases in leptin concentrations (a "satiety" hormone).[14,15]

In order to explore whether or not sleep deprivation leads to weight gain because people who are sleep deprived eat more, 12 men (mean age 22+3 years) with a body mass index of 22.3+1.8 kg/m^2, completed a randomized two-condition crossover study where the conditions involved sleeping for 8 hours or sleeping for 4 hours. Two days served as a control period, during which the study participants stuck to their normal routines but kept track of their sleep, eating and activities in a diary. During the second two-day period, the participants went to bed at midnight and woke up at 8 a.m. 'on one day, went to bed at 2 a.m. on the next day and woke up at 6 a.m. on the following day. These two periods of sleep were centred on 2 a.m. in order to minimize the change in circadian rhythms[16] and centre the sleep from food intakes.[17] Participants were allowed to eat as much as they liked during breakfast (from 8 to 8.30 a.m.), lunch (from 12 to 12.30 a.m.) and dinner (from 8 to 8.30 p.m.). They wore actimeters to measure physical activity and the men were also surveyed to discover their feelings of hunger, the pleasantness of food, their cravings and their sensation of sleepiness.

As expected, the total duration of sleep was shorter (3 h 46 min ± 0 h 14 min) during the short night than during the normal night (7 h 14 min ± 0 h 40 min) and the participants found the duration of their sleep insufficient during the short night. But sleep was judged satisfactory in terms of quality during both types of night. In the morning, physical activity was the same whether sleep deprived or not, but it was a little bit greater during the rest of day in the sleep deprived state. There was no difference in feelings of hunger, perceived pleasantness of food, or cravings. The main result was that the sleep deprived people ate 22% more calories (plus 559 ± 617 kcal) the day after a poor night's sleep than the day after a good night's sleep. The increase in energy intake and duration of food intake were observed during breakfast and dinner, while no difference was observed during lunch.

The main results of this study, conducted on normal weight men who spent 31 h during 48 h of measurement in free-living conditions, indicate that only one night of sleep restriction subsequently increased food intake and the estimated physically "related" energy expenditure during the following day. These results are consistent with previous studies on humans which supported the theory that acute sleep deprivation leads to an increase in hunger and in the desire to eat calorie-dense foods, an increase in the orexigenic factor ghrelin and a decrease in the anorexigenic hormone leptin.[14,15,18]

After sleep deprivation, the increase in energy intake was quantitatively higher than the estimated energy expenditure related to physical activity. As control of mammalian sleep is closely integrated within the mechanisms that support overall energy balance[17,19,20], and since it has been reported that one of the functions of sleep is to conserve energy[21] or, conversely, that the availability of metabolic fuel influences the duration of subsequent sleep[22], we can hypothesize that perhaps a heightened drive to eat following sleep deprivation would reflect the aim to store more calories in the longer days of summer where the nights are shorter and food more plentiful prior to winter, when the days are shorter, sleep duration longer, and food is hardly available.

The findings also suggest that sleeping better may help with weight management efforts and, more generally, that people need to do their best to get an adequate amount of sleep so their body can function properly.

Damien Davenne
INSERM ERI27, Univ. Caen

Laurent Brondel
Centre Européen des Sciences du Goût
Univ. Dijon

References

1. World Health Organization. Obesity and overweight. Fact sheet N°311 September 2006. internet: http://www.who.int/mediacentre/factsheets/fs311/en/index.html (accessed April 2009).
2. Kopelman PG. Obesity as a medical problem. Nature. 2000; 404:635-43.
3. Fabricatore AN et al. Obesity. Annu Rev Clin Psychol. 2006; 2:357-77.
4. Cournot M et al. Environmental factors associated with body mass index in a population of Southern France. Eur J Cardiovasc Prev Rehabil. 2004; 11:291-7.
5. Vioque J et al. Time spent watching television, sleep duration and obesity in adults living in Valencia, Spain. Int J Obes Relat Metab Disord. 2000; 24:1683-8.
6. Shigeta H et al. Lifestyle, obesity, and insulin resistance. Diabetes Care. 2001; 24:608.
7. Gangwisch JE et al. Inadequate sleep as a risk factor for obesity: analyses of the NHANES I. Sleep. 2005 ;28:1289-96.
8. Kripke DF et al. Short and long sleep and sleeping pills. Is increased mortality associated? Arch Gen Psychiatry. 1979; 36:103-16.
9. Gallup. Sleep In America. The Gallup Organization. Princeton, NJ, National Sleep Foundation. 1995: 1–78.
10. Knutson KL et al. The metabolic consequences of sleep deprivation. Sleep Med Rev. 2007 ;11:163-78.
11. Sivak M. Sleeping more as a way to lose weight. Obes Rev. 2006; 7:295-6.
12. Hicks RA et al. Sleep duration and eating behaviors of college students. Percept Mot Skills. 1986; 62:25-6.
13. Spiegel K et al. Brief communication: Sleep curtailment in healthy young men is associated with decreased leptin levels, elevated ghrelin levels, and increased hunger and appetite. Ann Intern Med. 2004; 141:846-50.

14. Chaput JP et al. Short sleep duration is associated with reduced leptin levels and increased adiposity: Results from the Quebec family study. Obesity (Silver Spring). 2007 ;15:253-61.
15. Spiegel K et al. Leptin levels are dependent on sleep duration: relationships with sympathovagal balance, carbohydrate regulation, cortisol, and thyrotropin. J Clin Endocrinol Metab. 2004; 89:5762-71.
16. Laposky AD et al. Sleep and circadian rhythms: key components in the regulation of energy metabolism. FEBS Lett. 2008; 582:142-51.
17. Pardini L et al. Feeding and circadian clocks. Reprod Nutr Dev. 2006; 46:463-80.
18. Shi Z et al. Dietary fat and sleep duration in Chinese men and women. Int J Obes (Lond). 2008; 32:1835-40.
19. Nicolaidis S. Metabolic mechanism of wakefulness (and hunger) and sleep (and satiety): Role of adenosine triphosphate and hypocretin and other peptides. Metabolism. 2006; 55:S24-9.
20. Sakurai T. The neural circuit of orexin (hypocretin): maintaining sleep and wakefulness. Nat Rev Neurosci. 2007; 8:171-81.
21. Siegel JM. Clues to the functions of mammalian sleep. Nature. 2005; 437:1264-71.
22. Jenkins JB et al. Sleep is increased in mice with obesity induced by high-fat food. Physiol Behav. 2006; 87:255-62.

Effects of sleep deprivation on dissociated components of executive functioning. Tucker AM, Whitney P, Belenky G, Hinson JM, Van Dongen HP. *Sleep. 2010 Jan 1;33(1):47-57.*

Does sleep deprivation involve a selective deficit in higher level executive cognitive processes?

Subjects	Methods	Outcomes
23 healthy subjects • Age: 22-38 yrs • Gender: 52% men	Subjects were randomized to either total SD protocol (n =12) or control (n = 11) for 6 consecutive days and nights Subjects were continuously monitored in the laboratory across 7 days and nights • SD subjects had 2 baseline nights, then were kept awake for 2 days and nights, and then had 2 recovery nights • Control subjects were given time in bed for sleep every night Assessments: • Executive functions 1. Modified Sternberg task 2. Phonemic verbal fluency task 3. Probed recall task • Control task battery Assessments were performed thrice at 1100: • At baseline • After 51 hrs of total SD (or after no SD among controls) • After 2 nights of recovery sleep	Several components of executive function were selectively preserved after 2 days and nights of total sleep loss Compared to controls, sleep deprivation was associated with the following changes in performance: • Impaired control task battery • Impaired modified Sternberg task (except for 2 components, namely working memory scanning efficiency and resistance to proactive interference) • Preserved resistance to proactive interference on the probed recall task • Enhanced phonemic verbal fluency task

SD: sleep deprivation

Conclusion

Sleep deprivation resulted in differential impairments of specific components of executive cognitive processing, and several key components of executive functioning were preserved after two days and nights of total sleep loss.

Commentary

As formalized in the prefrontal model, it was commonly believed that prefrontal, executive functions tasks were especially impaired by sleep deprivation.[1] Executive functions is an umbrella term that refers to a number of loosely related higher level cognitive processes that allow one to initiate, monitor, and stop actions in order to achieve goals; these functions are supported by neural networks that often involve various subregions of the prefrontal cortex working in concert with other brain regions.[2] There were some reasons to be skeptical of the prefrontal model, as executive functions deficits were not uniformly observed after sleep deprivation.[3-8] Additionally, one test highly sensitive to sleep deprivation is a simple reaction time test which requires relatively little executive functioning.[9] Finally, the sleep research had relied heavily on global scores and one area where this is especially problematic is in assessing executive functioning. Since executive functions operate on and through other cognitive processes, any task that taps executive functions taps other more basic processes as well (i.e., the task impurity problem).[10] Thus, it is possible that some of the low scores previously observed on executive functions tasks during sleep deprivation were not due to deficits in executive functioning but instead to deficits in other non-executive components of task performance.

Indeed, a dirty secret of executive functions tests is that the majority of variance in performance is not explained by executive functioning. To give a sense of the scope of this task impurity problem, let us consider our Sternberg working memory task. Variance on this task is classically subdivided into the slope, representing the executive functions component of working memory scanning efficiency, and the intercept, representing non-executive components of task performance. A stepwise regression predicting global RTs from dissociated component scores at baseline reveals that the non-executive intercept component is the dominant source of attributable variance – explaining 50% of the global score – while the slope, representing the executive functions component, explains a mere 31% of global score variance. Because the non-executive component predicts the lion's share of the variance in global scores in this and other executive functions tasks, a careful parcellation of global scores into executive and non-executive components is critical for a valid categorization of any deficits observed.

In this study, we took this novel approach of dissociating global scores into executive and non-executive components of performance. In other words, we moved beyond looking at tasks to looking at cognitive processes. When we did this, we were able to ascertain that although global scores on executive functions tasks were often changed, this was due to deficits in non-executive components of performance. For example, on a modified Sternberg working memory task, the intercept representing non-executive processing was impaired but the slope representing executive processing was spared. These results indicate that sleep deprivation-induced deficits in basic non-executive cognitive processes were responsible for the changes observed in the global scores on executive functions tasks. In contrast to conventional wisdom then, executive components were selectively preserved after two days and night of total sleep loss.

In this article, a use-dependent explanation of the deficits of sleep deprivation is put forward for the first time. This theory builds upon the preceding state-instability and local sleep theories to posit that it is those cognitive processes that are used more heavily and continuously that will be the ones to suffer the effects of fatigue during sleep loss. Sustained processes involve networks of brain regions that sometimes include prefrontal regions and sometimes do not[11, 12]; additionally, some sustained processes represent executive functions and some do not.[13, 14] Thus, use-dependency represents a paradigm shift and implies that the key distinction in determining which cognitive processes will be impacted is not whether they are executive versus non-executive or prefrontal versus non-prefrontal but instead whether they are sustained versus transient. Importantly, executive and prefrontal components can be either sustained or transient. Thus an important implication of use-dependency theory is that there are some executive and prefrontal components that will be impaired and some non-prefrontal non-executive components that will not. Use-dependency theory generates straightforward predictions that can be empirically tested.

This work was supported by USAMRMC award W81XWH-05-1-0099 and DURIP grant FA9550-06-1-0281.

Adrienne M. Tucker
Columbia University

References

1. Harrison Y et al. Prefrontal neuropsychological effects of sleep deprivation in young adults—A model for healthy aging? Sleep. 2000; 23(8):1-7.
2. Collette F et al. Exploration of the neural substrates of executive functioning by functional neuroimaging. Neuroscience. 2006; 139:209-21.
3. Pace-Schott EF et al. Failure to find executive function deficits following one night's total sleep deprivation in university students under naturalistic conditions. Behavioral Sleep Medicine. 2009; 7(3):136-63.
4. Binks PG et al. Short-term total sleep deprivations does not selectively impair higher cortical functioning. Sleep. 1999; 22(3):328-34.
5. Habeck C et al. An event-related fMRI study of the neurobehavioral impact of sleep deprivation on performance of a delayed-match-to-sample task. Cognitive Brain Research. 2004; 18:306-21.
6. Sagaspe P et al. Effects of sleep deprivation on Color-Word, Emotional, and Specific Stroop interference and on self-reported anxiety. Brain Cogn. 2006; 60:76-87.
7. Venkatraman V et al. Sleep deprivation elevates expectation of gains and attenuates responses to losses following risky decisions. Sleep. 2007; 30(5):603-9.
8. Verstraeten E et al. Executive function in sleep apnea: controlling for attentional capacity in assessing executive attention. Sleep. 2004; 27(4):685.
9. Dorrian J et al. Psychomotor vigilance performance: Neurocognitive assay sensitive to sleep loss. In: Kushida CA, ed. Sleep Deprivation: Clinical Issues, Pharmacology and Sleep Loss Effects. New York: Marcel Dekker, Inc., 2005.
10. Phillips LH. Do 'frontal tests' measure executive functions? Issues of assessment and evidence from fluency tests. In: Rabbitt P, ed. Methodology of Frontal and Executive Function. Hove: Psychology Press. 1997; 191-213.

11. Courtney SM et al. Transient and sustained activity in a distributed neural system for human working memory. Nature. 1997; 386(6625):608-11.

12. Axmacher N et al. Sustained Neural Activity Patterns during Working Memory in the Human Medial Temporal Lobe. J. Neurosci. 2007; 27(29):7807-16.

13. Braver TS et al. Neural Mechanisms of Transient and Sustained Cognitive Control during Task Switching. Neuron. 2003; 39(4):713-26.

14. Burgund ED et al. Sustained and transient activity during an object-naming task: a mixed blocked and event-related fMRI study. Neuroimage. 2003; 19(1):29-41.

Odor identification ability predicts executive function deficits following sleep deprivation.
Killgore WD, Killgore DB, Grugle NL, Balkin TJ. *Int J Neurosci. 2010 May;120(5):328-34.*

Does odor identification ability, which is sensitive to dysfunction of the prefrontal lobe, decline after sleep deprivation, and, if so, does it predict associated deficits in executive functioning?

Subjects	Methods	Outcomes
54 healthy adult subjects	Assessments: • Test of odor identification using SIT after 24-hr SD • WCST after 45-hr of wakefulness	Reduction in odor identification (SIT) predicted deficits in executive functioning (WCST) after an additional night of SD

SD: sleep deprivation; SIT: University of Pennsylvania Smell Identification Test; WCST: Wisconsin Card Sorting Test

Conclusion
Sleep deprivation was associated with a decline in odor identification, the latter predicting executive function deficits.

Commentary
Sleep deprivation reliably produces significant declines in alertness and psychomotor vigilance performance.[1] Interestingly some individuals are particularly vulnerable to the effects of sleep deprivation on these elementary aspects of cognitive performance while others appear to be quite resistant. Moreover, the degree to which an individual shows vulnerability or resistance to sleep loss appears to be a stable trait-like phenomenon that is reproducible across sessions.[2] While some evidence suggests that these individual differences may have genetic underpinnings[3], most attempts to identify behavioral or physiological markers that identify vulnerability to sleep loss have met with only limited success.[4]

In contrast to the consistent declines in simple alertness and vigilance that emerge during sleep loss, research on the effects of sleep deprivation on higher-level cognitive abilities such as executive functions has been rife with inconsistencies.[5] Some studies find that sleep deprivation impairs executive functions[6], while others fail to observe such effects.[7] One possibility is that there are also individual differences in the degree to which executive functions are degraded by sleep loss and these differences may obscure the group level effects. It would, therefore, be useful to identify behavioral or cognitive markers that predict declines in executive functions during sleep deprivation.

Odor identification ability has been suggested to be a crude index of prefrontal cortex integrity and is correlated with executive function ability in healthy normal individuals.[8] Our prior work had shown that the ability to identify odors, a measure of the functional integrity of the ventral regions of the prefrontal cortex, declines with 24 to 48 hours of sleep deprivation[9, 10], consistent with neuroimaging evidence that the prefrontal cortex shows significant declines in metabolic activity during prolonged wakefulness.[11] Therefore, we tested the possibility that small changes in the ability to identify odors on a simple "scratch & sniff" test during one night of sleep deprivation would be predictive of subsequent executive function performance following another night of sleep deprivation.

Subjects completed a short version of the Smell Identification Test, a standardized index of odor identification ability, when normally rested and again following 24-hours of sleep deprivation.[12] After an additional night of sleep loss, participants also completed the Wisconsin Card Sorting Test (WCST), widely considered to be the "gold standard" measure of executive functioning. As predicted, the magnitude of decline in odor identification accuracy following 24 hours of sleep loss significantly ($P < .05$) predicted executive function performance on several indices of the WCST after 45 hours of wakefulness, even after controlling for stimulant medications taken an hour before assessment of executive functions. Declines in odor identification were associated with fewer correctly answered items, fewer completed categories, fewer conceptual level responses, and more non-perseverative errors.

The findings suggest that changes in performance on a simple test of odor identification accuracy following sleep deprivation are reflective of altered functioning within prefrontal systems that also mediate higher-level executive functioning. Furthermore, these findings suggest that individual differences in trait-like vulnerability to the effects of sleep loss may extend beyond simple alertness and vigilance and may also involve higher-level executive functions. Thus, with further validation, assessment of odor identification may provide a simple but crude index of the effects of sleep loss on prefrontal functioning.

William D. S. Killgore
Harvard Medical School
Neuroimaging Center
McLean Hospital

References
1. Doran SM et al. Sustained attention performance during sleep deprivation: evidence of state instability. Archives Italiennes de Biologie (Pisa). 2001; 139(3):253-67.
2. Van Dongen HP et al. Systematic interindividual differences in neurobehavioral impairment from sleep loss: evidence of trait-like differential vulnerability. Sleep. 2004; 27(3):423-33.
3. von Schantz M. Phenotypic effects of genetic variability in human clock genes on circadian and sleep parameters. Journal of Genetics. 2008; 87(5):513-9.
4. Van Dongen HP et al. Individual differences in vulnerability to sleep loss in the work environment. Ind Health. 2009; 47(5):518-26.
5. Killgore WD. Effects of sleep deprivation on cognition. Prog Brain Res. 2010; 185:105-29.
6. Jones K et al. Frontal lobe function, sleep loss and fragmented sleep. Sleep Med Rev. 2001; 5(6):463-75.
7. Pace-Schott EF et al. Failure to find executive function deficits following one night's total sleep deprivation in university students under naturalistic conditions. Behav Sleep Med. 2009; 7(3):136-63.
8. Seidman LJ et al. Neuropsychological probes of fronto-limbic system dysfunction in schizophrenia. Olfactory identification and Wisconsin Card Sorting performance. Schizophr Res. 1991; 6(1):55-65.

9. Killgore WDS et al. Odor identification accuracy declines following 24 h of sleep deprivation. J Sleep Res. 2006; 15:111-6.

10. McBride SA et al. Olfactory decrements as a function of two nights of sleep deprivation. Journal of Sensory Studies. 2006; 21:456-63.

11. Thomas M et al. Neural basis of alertness and cognitive performance impairments during sleepiness. I. Effects of 24 h of sleep deprivation on waking human regional brain activity. J Sleep Res. 2000; 9(4):335-52.

12. Killgore WD et al. Odor identification ability predicts executive function deficits following sleep deprivation. Int J Neurosci. 2010; 120(5):328-34.

REM sleep characteristics of nightmare sufferers before and after REM sleep deprivation.
Nielsen TA, Paquette T, Solomonova E, Lara-Carrasco J, Popova A, Levrier K. *Sleep Med. 2010 Feb;11(2):172-9.*

Do changes in REM sleep propensity play a role in nightmares?

Subjects	Methods	Outcomes
14 subjects with frequent nightmares • Age: 27.6 ± 9.9 yrs • Nightmare episodes: ≥ 1 per week 11 healthy controls • Age: 24.3 ± 5.3 yrs • Nightmare episodes: < 1 per month	Assessments: • Sleep and dream logs • 3 PSG nights (REM SD on night 2) • Battery of REM sleep and dream measures (on nights 1 and 3)	Subjects with frequent nightmares had abnormally low REM sleep propensity as measured by: • % REM (late night) • Dream vividness • Number of skipped early-night REM periods • REM density (early/late) • REM latency • REM rebound • REM/NREM cycle length

NREM: non-rapid eye movment; PSG: polysomnography; REM: rapid eye movement; SD: sleep deprivation

Conclusion
Abnormally low rapid eye movement (REM) sleep propensity was noted in persons with frequent nightmares.

Commentary
One commonsense explanation of recurring nightmares is that abnormally increased REM sleep propensity is sporadically released during REM sleep, producing dreaming that is dramatically more vivid, dysphoric and accompanied by intense autonomic activation. This explanation has defied scientific assessment, however, because nightmare sufferers under observation in the sleep laboratory only rarely exhibit nightmares.[1,2] Systematically increasing REM sleep propensity using a REM deprivation procedure would seem to be an appropriate challenge procedure for overcoming the latter problem and possibly evoking nightmares that may be studied more closely in the laboratory.

Application of a partial REM sleep deprivation procedure in the present study was successful in moderately reducing the amount of REM sleep on Night 2 and in increasing REM sleep propensity on Night 3, as evidenced by a REM sleep rebound effect. However, contrary to expectations, nightmare sufferers exhibited *reduced* REM sleep propensity at baseline and after REM sleep deprivation. A marked illustration of reduced REM sleep propensity at baseline was the occurrence of more early-night skipped REM periods among the nightmare sufferers; of the 14 initial REM periods expected for this group on Night 1, fully 50% did not occur at the expected times. For the control group only 1 (9%) was skipped in this manner (p=.042, Fisher exact test, 2-tailed). Three of 7 nightmare sufferers also skipped their 2nd expected REM period.

These novel observations suggest that skipped early-night REM periods may be a useful indicator of REM sleep pathophysiology for protocols that use only a single night of PSG recording.

Beyond baseline differences, on Night 3 nightmare sufferers exhibited a lower than average visual intensity of dream imagery than did control subjects and they appeared to recover more quickly from REM sleep deprivation. These findings, too, are consistent with the view that nightmare sufferers had abnormally low REM sleep propensity during the 3 days of the protocol.

The unexpected findings are not necessarily incompatible with the commonsense explanation of nightmares as due to *higher* than normal REM sleep propensity. One possibility, entirely consistent with the ubiquitous lack of nightmares in the sleep laboratory, is that nightmare pathophysiology results from disruption of the regulation of REM sleep propensity such that it fluctuates more widely or erratically over time among nightmare sufferers. Such disruption might be due to perturbation of the circadian, ultradian or sleep-dependent factors underlying REM propensity.[3] Consistent with this possibility is our recent observation that, among women, nightmare frequency and distress are associated with the eveningness chronotype.[4] Another possible explanation is that REM sleep propensity among nightmare sufferers is more easily suppressed by situational factors such as the pre-sleep stress engendered by staying in a sleep laboratory than it is among control subjects[5] Yet another possibility is that nightmare sufferers have a profile of disturbed autonomic functioning similar to that of other anxiety disorders patients.[6] We recently supported this possibility in observing that heart rate variability (HRV) following REM sleep deprivation is abnormally reduced among nightmare sufferers.[7]

Tore Nielsen
Université de Montréal
Dream & Nightmare Laboratory
Hopital du Sacre-Coeur

References
1. Hartmann E. Sleep and Dreaming. Boston: Little, Brown and Co, 1970.
2. Woodward SH et al. Laboratory sleep correlates of nightmare complaint in PTSD inpatients. Biol Psychiatry. 2000; 48:1081-1087.
3. Nielsen TA. Ultradian, circadian, and sleep-dependent features of dreaming. In Kryger M et al (eds.). Principles and Practice of Sleep Medicine, 5th. New York: Elsevier, 2010; pp 576-584.
4. Nielsen T. Nightmares associated with the eveningness chronotype. J Biol Rhythms. 2010; 25:53-62.
5. Germain A et al. Psychophysiological reactivity and coping styles influence the effects of acute stress exposure on rapid eye movement sleep. Psychosom Med. 2003; 65:857-864.
6. Piccirillo G et al. Abnormal passive head-up tilt test in subjects with symptoms of anxiety power spectral analysis study of heart rate and blood pressure. Int J Cardiol 1997; 60:121-131.
7. Nielsen TA et al. Changes in cardiac variability after REM sleep deprivation in recurrent nightmares. Sleep. 2010; 33:123-129.

Short sleep duration is associated with the development of impaired fasting glucose: The Western New York Health Study. Rafalson L, Donahue RP, Stranges S, Lamonte MJ, Dmochowski J, Dorn J, Trevisan M. *Ann Epidemiol. 2010 Jul 9.*

Is sleep duration associated with incident-impaired fasting glucose?

Subjects	Methods	Outcomes
1455 subjects without DM and known CVD at baseline (1996-2001) • 91 cases • 272 controls FPG levels: • Subjects 1. Baseline: < 100 mg/dL 2. Follow-up: 100-125 mg/dL • Controls 1. Baseline: < 100 mg/dL 2. Follow-up: < 100 mg/dL	Case control study (Western New York Health Study) Subjects were reexamined in 2003-2004 Definitions of average sleep duration: • Short: < 6 hrs • Mid-range: 6-8 hrs • Long: > 8 hrs	In multivariate logistic regression, after adjustment for DM risk factors, OR of IFG among short sleepers was 3.0* compared to mid-range sleepers • Association for short sleepers was attenuated after adjustment for insulin resistance (OR 2.5**) No association was noted between long sleep and IFG (OR 1.6***)

CVD: cardiovascular disease; DM: type 2 diabetes mellitus; FPG: fasting plasma glucose; IPG: impaired fasting glucose; OR: odds ratio; *95% confidence limit [CL]: 1.05, 8.59; **95% CL: 0.83, 7.46; ***95% CL: 0.45, 5.42

Conclusion
Short, but not long, sleep duration was associated with increased risk of impaired fasting glucose.

Commentary
Sleep is a restorative process required for normal metabolic homeostasis.[1] In the United States, the average number of hours of sleep for adults has declined since the mid 1900s from about 9 hours a night to current estimates of 7 hours a night.[2-4] Observational epidemiologic studies have shown that inadequate sleep is associated with obesity[5], hypertension[6], coronary heart disease[7], and overall mortality.[8,9]

Prospective studies have demonstrated a U or J-shaped association between sleep duration and incident type 2 diabetes mellitus (T2DM). For example, after 12 years of follow-up of 1,100 men (40-70 years) short sleepers (6h) and long sleepers (> 8h) were respectively two and three times more likely to develop T2DM compared to people who slept 7h a night.[10] Among nurses (n= 70,000 females, age 30-55 years) long sleepers (≥ 9h) had a RR 1.29 (95% CI: 1.05-1.59) of T2DM compared to 8h night, but no association was noted among short sleepers.[11] After 12 years of follow-up of 1,187 middle-aged Swedish residents, ≤5h sleep was associated with a three-fold increased risk of T2DM among men only (P < 0.005).[12] In a multiethnic cohort, Non-

Hispanic Whites, and Hispanics who slept ≤7h compared to 8h were 2.5 times more likely to develop T2DM: Long sleepers also had twice the risk, but this was not statistically significant. No associations were noted among African-American subjects.[13]

The few studies that have specifically examined the sleep-impaired glucose tolerance (IGT) association have been limited by their cross-sectional design. For example, among 223 Canadian families (n=740) the odds of developing IGT and T2DM combined, were twice as high among short sleepers, and 58% greater among long sleepers compared to mid-range sleepers ($P < 0.05$ for both).[14] The Sleep Heart Health Study[15] reported the odds of IGT was 33% and 80% higher among short (≤ 5h) and long sleepers (≥ 9h), respectively vs. 7-8h ($P < 0.001$).

The Western New York Health Study was the first to prospectively examine the association between sleep duration and incident impaired fasting glucose (IFG), a predecessor to T2DM. Over six years of follow-up 91 cases of incident IFG were identified and matched to 272 normoglycemic controls. At baseline, the average weekday sleep duration was 6.8 h among cases and 7.1h among controls ($P = 0.019$). Compared to controls, cases were older (58 years vs. 54 years, $P = 0.005$), had a larger abdominal height (21.3 vs. 20.1 cm, $P = 0.005$), higher mean fasting glucose (94.3 mg/dL vs. 90.5 mg/dL, $P < 0.001$) and insulin (15.0 µU/mL vs.13.3 µU/ml, $P = 0.04$). Cases were more insulin resistant than controls: HOMA-IR 3.5 vs. 3.0, respectively; $P = 0.01$. Cases were less educated, more likely to have a positive family history of T2DM, currently smoke, and have hypertension ($P < 0.05$ for all). No differences were noted with respect to physical activity, alcohol consumption, or resting heart rate. Short and long sleep, were each noted among 6.6% of the sample. Only age significantly differed by sleep category, with short sleep being associated with younger age.

In multivariate modeling compared to 6-8h sleep, short sleepers were 3.0 times more likely to develop IFG (95%CI:1.05-8.59) after adjusting for sex, race, year of baseline interview, age, abdominal height, weight change, baseline weight, family history of diabetes, smoking, hypertension and depression. When insulin resistance was additionally added to the model the OR of IFG among short sleepers was 2.5 (95%CI: 0.83-7.46), suggesting that insulin resistance explains some, but not all of the observed association. Long sleep duration was associated with a 60% increased, but not significant, risk of IFG in both models.

Alterations in the neurohormonal regulation of feeding behaviors is one plausible biologic pathways through which sleep loss can lead to disordered glucose metabolism. Experimentally, sleep curtailment has been associated with significant increases in ghrelin, an appetite stimulating hormone, and decreases in the anorexigenic hormone leptin. Sleep curtailment was also significantly associated with self-reported increased hunger and appetite, especially for calorie dense foods, despite normalizing caloric intake via a continuous glucose infusion.[16]

Another possible pathway is through the activation of the sympathetic nervous system which increases secretion of epinephrine, norepinephrine, cortisol, growth hormone and glucagon, and decreases insulin secretion. These neuroendocrine changes interfere with mechanisms regulating plasma glucose, resulting in a higher steady state plasma glucose concentration.[17-19]

The activation of inflammatory pathways may also play a role in the observed association between short sleep duration and impaired glucose metabolism. Experimental studies have shown that reduced sleep is associated with increased TNFα, IL-6 and CRP.[20,21] Moreover, it is well established that inflammation predicts subsequent T2DM.[22,23]

Finally, short sleep duration may represent a risk marker rather than a causal risk factor. In fact, short sleepers are likely to be characterized by a distinctive pattern of socio-demographic, lifestyle, and co-morbid medical conditions that may confound the observed associations.[24]

In summary, persons who self-reported short sleep duration were three times more likely to develop IFG compared to those whose average sleep was 6-8 hrs a night. The importance of this finding is that IFG is a predecessor to T2DM, and any modifiable risk factors should be addressed as possible targets of intervention with the intent of delaying or preventing overt disease.

Lisa Rafalson
D'Youville College
State University of New York
University at Buffalo

References

1. Penev PD. Sleep deprivation and energy metabolism: to sleep, perchance to eat? Curr Opin Endocrinol Diabetes Obes. 2007, 14(5):374-81.
2. National Sleep Foundation "Sleep in America" Poll. 2005, National Sleep Foundation 2005: Washington DC.
3. Krueger PM, Friedman EM. Sleep duration in the United States: a cross-sectional population-based study. Am J Epidemiol. 2009, 169(9):1052-63.
4. Broman JE et al. Insufficient sleep in the general population. Neurophysiologie Clinique. 1996, 26(1):30-9.
5. Knutson KL. Associations between sleep loss and increased risk of obesity and diabetes. Annals of the New York Academy of Sciences. 2008: 1129:287-304.
6. Gangwisch JE et al. Short sleep duration as a risk factor for hypertension: analyses of the first National Health and Nutrition Examination Survey. Hypertension. 2006, 47(5):833-9.
7. Ayas NT et al. A prospective study of sleep duration and coronary heart disease in women. Archives of Internal Medicine. 2003, 163(2):205-9.
8. Kripke DF et al. Short and long sleep and sleeping pills. Is increased mortality associated? Archives of General Psychiatry. 1979, 36(1):103-16.
9. Ferrie JE et al. A prospective study of change in sleep duration: associations with mortality in the Whitehall II cohort. Sleep. 2007, 30(12):1659-66.
10. Duckworth W et al. Glucose Control and Vascular Complications in Veterans with Type 2 Diabetes. N Engl J Med. 2008: p. NEJMoa0808431.
11. Ayas NT et al. A prospective study of self-reported sleep duration and incident diabetes in women. Diabetes Care. 2003, 26(2):380-4.
12. Mallon L. et al. High Incidence of Diabetes in Men with Sleep Complaints or Short Sleep Duration A 12-year follow-up study of a middle-aged population. Diabetes Care. 2005, 28:2762-2767.
13. Beihl DA et al. Sleep Duration as a Risk Factor for Incident Type 2 Diabetes in a Multiethnic Cohort. Ann Epidemiol. 2009, 19:351-357.

14. Chaput JP et al. Association of sleep duration with type 2 diabetes and impaired glucose tolerance. Diabetologia. 2007, 50(11):2298-304.

15. Gottlieb DJ et al. Association of sleep time with diabetes mellitus and impaired glucose tolerance. Archives of Internal Medicine. 2005, 165(8):863-7.

16. Spiegel K et al. Brief communication: Sleep curtailment in healthy young men is associated with decreased leptin levels, elevated ghrelin levels, and increased hunger and appetite. Ann Intern Med. 2004, 141(11):846-50.

17. Havel P et al. Stress-induced activation of the neuroendocrine system and Its effects on carboydrate metabolism. In Ellenberg & Rifkin's Diabetes Mellitus, D.J. Porte, R.S. Sherwin, and A. Baron, Editors. 2003, McGraw Hill, 127.

18. Leproult R et al. Sleep loss results in an elevation of cortisol levels the next evening. Sleep. 1997, 20(10):865-70.

19. Spiegel K et al. Impact of sleep debt on metabolic and endocrine function. Lancet. 1999, 354(9188):1435-9.

20. Irwin MR et al. Sleep deprivation and activation of morning levels of cellular and genomic markers of inflammation. Arch Intern Med. 2006, 166(16):1756-62.

21. Meier-Ewert HK et al. Effect of sleep loss on C-reactive protein, an inflammatory marker of cardiovascular risk. J Am Coll Cardiol. 2004, 43(4): 678-83.

22. Hu FB et al. Inflammatory markers and risk of developing type 2 diabetes in women. Diabetes. 2004, 53(3):693-700.

23. Pradhan AD et al. C-reactive protein, interleukin 6, and risk of developing type 2 diabetes mellitus. JAMA. 2001, 286(3):327-34.

24. Stranges S et al. Correlates of short and long sleep duration: a cross-cultural comparison between the United Kingdom and the United States: the Whitehall II Study and the Western New York Health Study. Am J Epidemiol. 2008, 168(12):1353-64.

Sleep restriction for 1 week reduces insulin sensitivity in healthy men. Buxton OM, Pavlova M, Reid EW, Wang W, Simonson DC, Adler GK. *Diabetes. 2010 Sep;59(9):2126-33.*

Does sleep restriction alter insulin sensitivity, and, if so, does modafinil affect these changes in glucose metabolism?

Subjects	Methods	Outcomes
20 healthy subjects • Age: 20-35 yrs • Gender: 100% men • BMI: 20-30	Components of 12-day protocol: • Sleep-replete condition: 10 hrs per night in bed for ≥ 8 nights • Sleep-restricted condition: 5 hrs per night in bed for 7 nights • Diet and activity were controlled Subjects were randomized to the following during SR: • Modafinil: 300 mg/day • Placebo Assessments on the last 2 days of each condition: • 24-h urine catecholamines • Glucose metabolism (IVGTT and EHC) • Neurobehavioral performance • Salivary cortisol	SR was associated with (results were not affected by modafinil administration): • Reduction in insulin sensitivity 1. By 20 ± 24%* (IVGTT technique) 2. By 11 ± 5.5%** (clamp technique) 3. No correlation with changes in salivary cortisol (increase of 51 ± 8% with SR***), SWS or urinary catecholamines • Decreased glucose tolerance and disposition index • No significant change in insulin secretory response

BMI: body mass index; EHC: euglycemic-hyperinsulinemic clamp; IVGTT: intravenous glucose tolerance test; SR: sleep restriction; SWS: slow wave sleep; *P = 0.001; **P < 0.04; ***P < 0.02

Conclusion
Sleep restriction reduced insulin sensitivity, and the latter was unaffected by modafinil administration.

Commentary
Sleep deficiency has been linked to an increased risk of chronic disease[1] and early mortality.[2-8] This risk is likely causal, as insufficient sleep is associated with adverse metabolic changes[4,5], obesity[6], and type 2 diabetes mellitus.[7,8] A recent IOM report "Sleep Disorders and Sleep Deprivation: an Unmet Public Health Problem" highlighted the critical need to improve sleep health in the US.[9] For these reasons and others, increasing the proportion of US adults who

obtain adequate sleep has been included as a federal priority, for the first time. The latest *Healthy People 2020*[10] proposes as a goal increasing the proportion of Americans obtaining adequate sleep (≥ 7 hrs /night).

In a study of healthy adult men, we demonstrated that sleep restriction to 5 hours per night of time in bed for one week leads to elevations of afternoon and evening cortisol, no change in resting metabolic rate, and a specific pattern of changes to glucose metabolism: reduced insulin sensitivity. This measurement was confirmed by both intravenous glucose tolerance tests and euglycemic hyperinsulinemic clamp procedures. Of particular note, behavioral sleep restriction[2] or slow wave sleep suppression by acoustic tones[11] has now been linked in several studies in healthy individuals to a reduction in insulin sensitivity without a compensatory change in the insulin secretory response. Insufficient sleep duration of moderate severity (5hrs/night) for just one week thereby increases diabetes risk (as quantified by the Disposition Index).

We also observed other notable features of sleep restriction. Sleep-restricted subjects reported sleepiness on the Karolinska Sleepiness Scale (KSS) that was elevated after just a single night and then sustained at that level for the rest of the week. Similarly, objective levels of vigilance on a computerized Psychomotor Vigilance Task (PVT) demonstrated an immediate increase in lapses of attention that was maintained at that level over the week. These data are in contrast to other studies of sleep restriction and vigilance showing a progressive decrement in vigilance but subjective sleepiness that appears to plateau.[12] Further studies are needed to better understand the impact, time-course, and dose response relationships of chronic sleep restriction, and recovery, on cognitive function.

Unexpectedly, the efficacy of modafinil (a wake-promoting agent) to ameliorate these effects on sleepiness and vigilance was limited: sleepiness with modafinil administration was reduced relative to the placebo group for only the first day of sleep restriction for subjective sleepiness, and reduced lapses of attention for only the first 3 days of sleep restriction. Thereafter the effects were no longer present.

Modafinil activates central dopaminergic and noradrenergic mechanisms promoting wakefulness. The effects of sleep deprivation on alertness and performance have been linked to reduced brain glucose utilization.[13] Thus, in this study we tested the hypothesis that the metabolic effects of sleep restriction could be reversed by this medication, which reverses the subjective sleepiness associated with sleep restriction. However, improved subjective sleepiness from use of modafinil did not translate to reversal of the metabolic consequences of sleep restriction. The lack of effectiveness of modafinil on sleepiness and vigilance over the course of a week may have limited the possibility of finding a relationship between sleepiness, brain glucose utilization and changes in measures peripheral metabolism such as insulin sensitivity.

Orfeu M. Buxton
Division of Sleep Medicine
Harvard Medical School
Department of Medicine
Brigham and Women's Hospital

Milena Pavlova
Harvard Medical School
Division of Epilepsy, Neurophysiology and Sleep
Department of Neurology
Brigham and Women's Hospital

Gail K Adler
Harvard Medical School
Division of Endocrinology, Diabetes and Hypertension
Department of Medicine
Brigham and Women's Hospital

References

1. Buxton OM et al. Short and Long Sleep Are Positively Associated with Obesity, Diabetes, Hypertension, and Cardiovascular Disease among Adults in the United States. Social Science & Medicine. 2010; 71(5):1027-36.
2. Wingard DL et al. Mortality risk associated with sleeping patterns among adults. Sleep. 1983; 6(2):102-7
3. Grandner MA et al. Mortality associated with short sleep duration: The evidence, the possible mechanisms, and the future. Sleep Med Rev. 2010; 14(3):191-203.
4. Spiegel K et al. Impact of sleep debt on metabolic and endocrine function. Lancet. 1999; 354:1435-9
5. Nedeltcheva AV et al. Exposure to recurrent sleep restriction in the setting of high caloric intake and physical inactivity results in increased insulin resistance and reduced glucose tolerance. J Clin Endocrinol Metab. 2009; Sep; 9:3242-50.
6. Cappuccio FP et al. Meta-analysis of short sleep duration and obesity in children and adults. Sleep. 2008; 31(5):619-26.
7. Knutson KL et al. Associations between sleep loss and increased risk of obesity and diabetes. Annals of the NY Academy of Science. 2008; 1129:287-304.
8. Cappuccio FP et al. Quantity and quality of sleep and incidence of type 2 diabetes: a systematic review and meta-analysis. Diabetes Care. 2010; 33(2):414-20.
9. Institute of Medicine. Sleep disorders and sleep deprivation: An unmet public health problem. Washington, D.C.: National Academies Press; 2006. Report No.: ISBN:0-309-66012-2.
10. Department of Health and Human Services. Healthy People 2020 Objective Topic Areas and Page Numbers 2010 [cited 2011 Jan 4]:300-1.
11. Tasali E et al. Slow-wave sleep and the risk of type 2 diabetes in humans. Proc Natl Acad Sci USA 105:1044-1049, 2008
12. Van Dongen HPA et al. The cumulative cost of additional wakefulness: Dose-response effects on neurobehavioral functions and sleep physiology from chronic sleep restriction and total sleep deprivation. Sleep. 2003; 26:117-126.
13. Drummond SPA et al. Sleep deprivation-induced reduction in cortical functional response to serial subtraction. Neuroreport. 1999; 10:3745-3748.

Hypersomnia

Anti-Tribbles homolog 2 autoantibodies in Japanese patients with narcolepsy. Toyoda H, Tanaka S, Miyagawa T, Honda Y, Tokunaga K, Honda M. *Sleep. 2010 Jul 1;33(7):875-8.*

How prevalent are autoantibodies against Tribbles homolog 2 in Japanese patients with narcolepsy?

Subjects	Methods	Outcomes
Japanese subjects with narcolepsy or IH, and controls • 88 NC+ • 18 NC- • 11 IH • 87 healthy controls • 37 healthy controls were + for HLA-DRB1*1501-DQB1*0602	Assessments: • Anti-TRIB2 autoantibodies • Anti-TRIB3 autoantibodies	Anti-TRIB2 autoantibodies were present in: • NC+: 26.1% • Healthy controls: 2.3% Anti-TRIB3 autoantibodies were rare in NC+

HLA: human leukocyte antigen; IH: idiopathic hypersomnia with long sleep time; NC+: narcolepsy with cataplexy; NC-: narcolepsy without cataplexy; TRIB2: Tribbles homolog 2

Conclusion
Autoantibodies against Tribbles homolog 2 were common and relatively specific in Japanese patients with narcolepsy-cataplexy.

Commentary
Narcolepsy with cataplexy has been hypothesized to be caused by an autoimmune-mediated process targeting hypocretin-producing neurons (HCRT neurons) in the hypothalamus. Several studies have found associations with HLA-DQB1*0602 [1-3], T-cell receptor alpha locus [4] and purinergic receptor subtype P2Y$_{11}$ [5] in narcolepsy with cataplexy, supporting this hypothesis. However, no definitive answers had been obtained for many years. A recent study reported an increased prevalence of autoantibodies against Tribbles homolog 2 (TRIB2) in Caucasian narcolepsy with cataplexy patients. [6] We evaluated the presence of anti-TRIB2 autoantibodies in Japanese narcolepsy with cataplexy patients and demonstrated that TRIB2 antibodies were found in 26% of the patients, a significantly higher prevalence than that in healthy controls (2%). [7] At the same time, Kawashima et al. also reported that 21% of Caucasian narcolepsy with cataplexy patients had elevated levels of TRIB2 antibodies compared to 4% in matched controls. [8] These suggest a subgroup within narcolepsy with cataplexy might be affected by a TRIB2 antibody-mediated autoimmune mechanism.

However, many questions remain to be solved. One fundamental question is that TRIB2 antibodies are the cause or the effect of narcolepsy with cataplexy? From the present results, both seem to be possible. If TRIB2 antibodies are causal autoantibodies, people with TRIB2 antibodies might have a higher risk of developing narcolepsy with cataplexy in near future. As for lower-TRIB2-antibody patients, other autoantibodies might have additive effects on developing the disease. Further functional studies are required to clarify whether TRIB2 antibodies are responsible for the disease or not.

Assuming that TRIB2 antibodies are the cause of narcolepsy with cataplexy, the question is how they cause the disease? In other words, how can they specifically attack HCRT neurons? *TRIB2* seems to be specifically expressed in HCRT neurons rather than other regions in the brain[6], however, it is known that *TRIB2* is widely expressed in other human tissues.[9] As one possible clue to the solution of this problem, there is an interesting report showing selective neuronal cytotoxicity.[10] Huntington's disease (HD) is caused by the abnormally expanded polyglutamine repeat in the protein huntingtin. The pathological change is restricted to striatum in the brain, although causal mutated huntingtin is expressed not only in striatum but throughout the tissues. This study demonstrated that the small guanine nucleotide-binding protein Rhes, which is localized very specifically to the striatum, binds to mutated huntingtin and this interaction can induce the neuronal death.[10] As for narcolepsy with cataplexy, Cvetkovic-Lopes et al. showed twenty-three genes were specifically expressed in mice Hcrt neurons.[6] Likewise, there might be additive factors possessing supportive roles which can explain the specific HCRT neuronal death.

In case that the effect of TRIB2 are not be limited to HCRT neurons, TRIB2 antibodies are expected to induce some symptoms in the peripheral tissues of narcolepsy with cataplexy patients. An *in vitro* functional study showed TRIB2 suppresses adipocyte differentiation through the inhibition of Akt activation and C/EBP degradation, suggesting TRIB2 is involved in energy metabolism.[11] If TRIB2 antibodies attack the peripheral tissues, it is possible that narcolepsy with cataplexy patients might develop metabolic disorders. Indeed, it is well known that some narcolepsy with cataplexy patients have the symptoms related to metabolic disorders, such as obesity and type II diabetes.[12-16] These symptoms would be relevant to the loss of HCRT neurons which regulate not only sleep but also feeding behavior. Besides, it could be that TRIB2 antibodies attack adipose tissues resulting in malfunction of energy metabolism. More clinical investigations must be helpful for understanding the role of TRIB2 antibodies.

The pathophysiology of narcolepsy still remains unclear. It is the most important that this study can incite discussion for the understanding of this disease.

Hiromi Toyoda
Department of Human Genetics
Graduate School of Medicine
The University of Tokyo
The Sleep Disorders Research Project
Tokyo Institute of Psychiatry

Taku Miyagawa
Department of Human Genetics
Graduate School of Medicine
The University of Tokyo

Katsushi Tokunaga
Department of Human Genetics
Graduate School of Medicine
The University of Tokyo

References

1. Juji T et al. HLA antigens in Japanese patients with narcolepsy. All the patients were DR2 positive. Tissue Antigens. 1984; 24:316-319.
2. Langdon N et al. Genetic markers in narcolepsy. Lancet. 1984; 2:1178-1180.
3. Mignot E et al. Complex HLA-DR and -DQ interactions confer risk of narcolepsy-cataplexy in three ethnic groups. Am J Hum Genet. 2001; 68:686-699.
4. Hallmayer J et al. Narcolepsy is strongly associated with the T-cell receptor alpha locus. Nat Genet. 2009; 41:708-711.
5. Kornum BR et al. Common variants in P2RY11 are associated with narcolepsy. Nat Genet. 2011; 43:66-71.
6. Cvetkovic-Lopes V et al. Elevated Tribbles homolog2-specific antibody levels in narcolepsy patients. J Clin Invest. 2010; 120:713-719.
7. Toyoda H et al. Anti-Tribbles homolog 2 autoantibodies in Japanese patients with narcolepsy. Sleep. 2010; 33:875-878.
8. Kawashima M et al. Anti-Tribbles homolog 2 (TRIB2) autoantibodies are associated with recent onset in human narcolepsy-cataplexy. Sleep. 2010; 33:869-874.
9. Wu C et al. BioGPS: an extensible and customizable portal for querying and organizing gene annotation resources. Genome Biol. 2009; 10:R130
10. Subramaniam S et al. Rhes, a Striatal Specific Protein, Mediates Mutant-Huntingtin Cytotoxicity. Science. 2009; 324:1327-1330.
11. Naiki T et al. TRB2, a Mouse Tribbles Ortholog, Suppresses Adipocyte Differentiation by Inhibiting AKT and C/EBP□□ J Biol Chem. 2007; 282:24075–24082.
12. Honda Y et al. Increased frequency of non-insulin-dependent diabetes mellitus among narcoleptic patients. Sleep. 1986; 9: 254-259.
13. Schuld A et al. Increased body-mass index in patients with narcolepsy. Lancet. 2000; 355:1274-1275.
14. Dahmen N et al. Increased prevalence of obesity in narcoleptic patients and relatives. Eur Arch Psychiatry Clin Neurosci. 2001; 251:85-89.
15. Kok SW et al. Hypocretin deficiency in narcoleptic humans is associated with abdominal obesity. Obes Res. 2003; 11:1147-1154.
16. Poli F et al. Body mass index-independent metabolic alterations in narcolepsy with cataplexy. Sleep. 2009; 32:1491-1497.

Does narcolepsy symptom severity vary according to HLA-DQB1*0602 allele status? Watson NF, Ton TG, Koepsell TD, Gersuk VH, Longstreth WT Jr. *Sleep. 2010 Jan 1;33(1):29-35.*

*What is the association, if any, between symptom severity in narcolepsy and HLA-DQB1*0602 allele status?*

Subjects	Methods	Outcomes
279 subjects with narcolepsy • Age: 47.6 ± 17.1 yrs • Gender: 37% males • Race: 82% Caucasian Number of HLA DQB1*0602 alleles: • None: 141 (51%) • One: 117 (42%) • Two: 21 (7%)	Cross-sectional population-based study Assessments: • Buccal genomic DNA analysis • Chart review • Clinical sleep parameters • Diagnostic sleep study • ESS • Subjective SL and sleep duration • UNS	After adjustment for African American race, HLA-DQB1*0602 frequency was linearly correlated with: • Sleepiness (ESS)* • Narcolepsy severity (UNS)** • Age of symptom onset*** • SL[#] In univariate analyses, HLA-DQB1*0602 frequency was associated with: • Napping[#] • Increased car and work accidents[###] • Near accidents[###] HLA status was not associated with habitual sleep duration

ESS: Epworth sleepiness scale; HLA: human leukocyte antige; SL: sleep latency; UNS: Ullanlinna narcolepsy scale; *$P < 0.01$; **$P < 0.001$; ***$P < 0.05$; [#]$P < 0.001$; [##]$P < 0.05$; [###]$P < 0.01$

Conclusion
There was a linear correlation between HLA-DQB1*0602 allele frequency and symptom severity in persons with narcolepsy.

Commentary
The HLA-DQB1*0602 allele is associated with narcolepsy, particularly narcolepsy with cataplexy, but has never been shown to modify aspects of disease expression. This paper demonstrated variation in the symptomatic components of narcolepsy based on the number of HLA-DQB1*0602 alleles. Because the HLA system is tightly linked to immunity and numerous autoimmune diseases, the results provide further evidence supporting narcolepsy as an autoimmune disease.

Although narcolepsy has long been suspected to have an immunologic basis, its classification as an autoimmune disease has been more apparent in recent studies. Specifically, narcolepsy with cataplexy is associated with polymorphisms of the T-cell receptor alpha locus encoding for the major receptor for HLA-peptide presentation.[1] Higher titers of antibodies for Tribbles homolog 2, a known autoantigen in an autoimmune disease, were also observed among patients with narcolepsy with cataplexy relative to their controls.[2] Furthermore, because Group A *Streptococcus* can induce autoimmune disease involving the central nervous system[3] such as in the case of Sydenham's Chorea and Pediatric Autoimmune Disorders Associated with Streptococcal Infections (PANDAS)[3,4], associations of narcolepsy with streptococcal infections provide further evidence that narcolepsy has an autoimmune basis. Early reports have been inconsistent in observing an association between streptococcal infections and narcolepsy[5-7], but recent studies have brought this association back into the spotlight. Elevated anti-streptococcal antibodies among patients with narcolepsy with cataplexy was reported in one study[8] and replicated in another.[9] Our population-based case-control study also reported strong associations of narcolepsy with a history of streptococcal infections[10] as well as with passive smoke exposure before age 21.[11] Possibly, exposure to passive smoke in infancy or childhood predisposes children to bacterial infections such as Group A *Streptococcus*, which might then trigger an autoimmune response causing selective destruction of orexin cells in the dorsolateral hypothalamus.[12] Interestingly, the HLA-DQB1*0602 allele is part of a haplotype that confers a different immunologic response to streptococcal infections.[13] However, streptococcal infections may not be the only factor involved in inducing an immunologic response that can lead to an increased risk of narcolepsy. A recent case report suggests that narcolepsy may be a side effect of H1N1 vaccinations or infections. All post-H1N1 narcolepsy cases in this report carried HLA-DQB1*0602; interestingly, 69% were also exposed to vaccines that contained antistreptolysin O as an adjuvant.[14] Whether streptococcal or H1N1, these and perhaps other types of infections or environmental insults may set in to motion a series of immunologic reactions that push individuals who are already genetically susceptible to narcolepsy towards developing the disease.

Ours and other recent studies highlighting the relationships between HLA-DQB1*0602, phenotype severity, streptococcal infections, passive smoking, and H1N1 vaccinations provide support for the notion of narcolepsy as an autoimmune disease with an etiology rooted in a complex interplay between genetic and environmental factors - a concept noted by Guilleminault over 15 years ago.[15] Today, we are closer to understanding a little more about the etiology of narcolepsy in hopes of preventing the disease tomorrow.

Thanh G.N. Ton
Department of Neurology
Harborview Medical Center
University of Washington

Nathaniel F. Watson
UW Medicine Sleep Center
Department of Neurology
University of Washington

References

1. Hallmayer J et al. Narcolepsy is strongly associated with the T-cell receptor alpha locus. Nat Genet. 2009; 41(6):708-711.
2. Cvetkovic-Lopes V et al. Elevated Tribbles homolog 2-specific antibody levels in narcolepsy patients. J Clin Invest. 2010; 120(3):713-719.
3. Dale RC. Post-streptococcal autoimmune disorders of the central nervous system. Dev Med Child Neurol. 2005; 47(11):785-791.
4. Snider LA et al. Post-streptococcal autoimmune disorders of the central nervous system. Curr Opin Neurol. 2003; 16(3):359-365.
5. Billiard M et al. Elevated antibodies to streptococcal antigens in narcoleptic subjects. Sleep Res. 1989; 18:201.
6. Montplaisir J et al. Streptococcal antibodies in narcolepsy and idiopathic hypersomnia. Sleep Res. 1989; 18:271.
7. Mueller-Eckhardt G et al. Is there an infectious origin of narcolepsy (letter)? Lancet. 1990; 335:424.
8. Aran A et al. Elevated anti-streptococcal antibodies in patients with recent narcolepsy onset. Sleep. 2009; 32(8):979-983.
9. Thorpy M. Antistreptococcal antibodies found in patients with narcolepsy. Curr Neurol Neurosci Rep. 2010. Feb 24.
10. Koepsell TD et al. Medical exposures in youth and the frequency of narcolepsy with cataplexy: a population-based case-control study in genetically predisposed people. J Sleep Res. 2010; 19(1):80-86.
11. Ton TG et al. Active and passive smoking and risk of narcolepsy in people with HLA DQB1*0602: a population-based case-control study. Neuroepidemiology. 2009; 32(2):114-121.
12. Longstreth WT Jr et al. Narcolepsy and streptococcal infections. Sleep. 2009; 32(12):1548.
13. Kotb M et al. An immunogenetic and molecular basis for differences in outcomes of invasive group A streptococcal infections. Nat Med. 2002; 8(12):1398-1404.
14. Dauvilliers Y et al. Post-H1N1 narcolepsy-cataplexy. Sleep. 2010; 33(11):1428-1430.
15. Guilleminault C. Narcolepsy. In: Chokroverty S, ed. Sleep Disorders Medicine: Basic Science, Technical Considerations, and Clinical Aspects. Boston: Butterworth-Heinemann; 1994:241-254.

IgG abnormality in narcolepsy and idiopathic hypersomnia. Tanaka S, Honda M. *PLoS One. 2010 Mar 5;5(3):e9555.*

Are narcolepsy and idiopathic hypersomnia associated with abnormalities in IgG?

Subjects	Methods	Outcomes
159 subjects with NC+ and HLA-DQB1*0602 allele+ 28 subjects with IH (long sleep time) 123 healthy controls • 45 with HLA-DQB1*0602 allele+	Assessments: • Serum IgG levels: total and subclass	Serum IgG levels (mg/ml) were: • NC+: 9.67 ± 3.38 • IH: 13.81 ± 3.80 • Controls without HLA-DQB1*0602 allele: 11.66 ± 3.55 • Controls with HLA-DQB1*0602 allele: 11.45 ± 3.43 None of the following factors were associated with IgG levels in NC+ or IH: • Age • BMI • Disease duration • ESS • Smoking habit Changes in IgG subclass in NC+ with low IgG levels included: • Decrease in IgG1 and IgG2 levels • Stable IgG3 levels • Increase in proportion of IgG4 • (also present in NC+ with normal total IgG) Changes in IgG subclass in IH included: • High IgG3 and IgG4 levels • Low IgG2 level • Imbalance of IgG1/IgG2

BMI: body mass index; ESS: Epworth sleepiness scale; HLA: human leukocyte antigen; IH: idiopathic hypersomnia with long sleep time; NC+: narcolepsy with cataplexy

Conclusion

Abnormalities in total IgG levels and IgG subclasses were noted in persons with narcolepsy-cataplexy and idiopathic hypersomnia.

Commentary

The involvement of the immune system and/or an autoimmune processes underlies the pathophysiology of narcolepsy has been suggested.[1] Moreover, the challenge of High-dose intravenous immunoglobulins success to decrease the frequency and severity of cataplexy in narcolepsy.[2] To evidence the autoimmune background on narcolepsy, the candidate autoantibody screenings (against orexin, orexin receptors[3], AQP4[4], and unpublished antigens) were conducted. The autoantibody indices with narcolepsy patients on these candidate autoantibody screenings were generally low contrary to expectations as compared with that in healthy subjects. These findings are in line with one possibility as low levels of initial total IgG level in the narcolepsy serum. In this study, IgG abnormalities in a large number of Japanese hypersomnia patients were determined.

In narcolepsy patients, total IgG levels decreased, while the IgG3 subclass level stayed unchanged; thus, the proportion of IgG3 relatively increased in narcolepsy patients. IgG3 production and B cell maturation for the IgG3 subclass might be unaffected in narcolepsy patients despite the decrease in the total IgG levels. IgG3 antibodies appear first in the course of infection before IgG1, IgG2 and IgG4 subclasses, reflecting the genomic position of gamma genes for the constant region in the immunoglobulin heavy chain (IGH) locus. I hypothesize that the class switch from IgG3 to other IgG subclass in somatic rearrangement of the IGH gamma genes is dysregulated in narcolepsy. This dysregulation could also explain the decrease in IgG1 and IgG2 in narcolepsy with abnormally low total IgG levels (It would be worth referring to CD3 receptors in narcolepsy, because of the relationship with IgG2 deficiencies[5] and the association with T cell receptor-alpha locus in narcolepsy).[6] An immunoglobulin switch-like sequence was once reported as a tight linkage marker for canine narcolepsy gene 1.[7] At that time narcolepsy was reportedly not associated with the human IGH region including the *mu*-switch and gamma 1 genes by the comparison of restriction fragment length polymorphism (RFLP) pattern. Nevertheless, I insist that it would be worthwhile to reanalyze it in detail, since human IGH gamma 3 region corresponding to the IgG3 subclass is one of the most polymorphic regions and is difficult to examine completely by RFLP analysis

Elevated IgG4 ratio in narcolepsy patients regardless of the total IgG levels was found. IgG4 abnormalities could be detected more efficiently when the proportion of IgG4 was used. IgG4 responds to allergens but has no complement activation capacity. Measuring the IgE levels together with the Interleukin (IL)-4 and IL-13 levels might help to understand the reason of the abnormal increase of IgG4 in narcolepsy, since these cytokines are key factors that induces IgG4 and IgE synthesis in human B cells.[8]

Two narcolepsy patients showed low IgG4 levels along with a marked reduction in IgG1 and IgG2. General immune-suppression may have occurred in these patients, similar to that observed in the common variable immunodeficiency syndrome after the onset of narcolepsy.[9] However, these two patients took a typical clinical course of narcolepsy without severe immunological comorbid symptoms. Therefore any specific changes in these two patients have not been defined yet.

Idiopathic hypersomnia patients showed characteristically high total IgG, IgG1, IgG3, and IgG4 levels and low IgG2 levels. Upon antigenic stimulation, naive CD4(+) T cells activate and differentiate into T-helper (Th) subsets. Th1 cells secrete high levels of interferon-gamma, which strongly induces IgG1 production, and IL-2. Th2 cells predominantly secrete IL-4, which induces IgG2, IL-5, and IL-13 [10]; therefore, the IgG1/IgG2 ratio has been considered to reflect the Th1-Th2 balance. The IgG1/IgG2 ratio in narcolepsy patients showed large variance but did not change, which is consistent with previous reports.[11-13] On the other hand, a significant increase in the IgG1/IgG2 ratio in idiopathic hypersomnia patients was indicated, suggesting the Th1 predominance in idiopathic hypersomnia. A new Th subset, which produces IL-17, IL-17F, and IL-22 in preference to other cytokines, plays an important role in autoimmune inflammations.[14] Further studies are required to measure these cytokines together with Th17-specific transcription factors, interferon-gamma, and IL-2 in idiopathic hypersomnia.

Susumu Tanaka
Tokyo Institute of Psychiatry

References

1. Mignot E et al. Complex HLA-DR and -DQ interactions confer risk of narcolepsy-cataplexy in three ethnic groups. Am J Hum Genet. 2001; 68:686-99.
2. Dauvilliers Y. Follow-up of four narcolepsy patients treated with intravenous immunoglobulins. Ann Neurol. 2006; 60:153.
3. Tanaka S et al. Detection of autoantibodies against hypocretin, hcrtrl, and hcrtr2 in narcolepsy: anti-Hcrt system antibody in narcolepsy. Sleep. 2006; 29:633-8.
4. Tanaka S et al. Absence of Anti-aquaporin-4 Antibody in Narcolepsy. Sleep Biol Rhythms. 2009; 7:66-70.
5. Carbonari M et al. Relative increase of T cells expressing the gamma/delta rather than the alpha/beta receptor in ataxia-telangiectasia. N Engl J Med. 1990; 322:73-6.
6. Hallmayer J et al. Narcolepsy is strongly associated with the T-cell receptor alpha locus. Nat Genet. 2009; 41:708-11.
7. Mignot E et al. An immunoglobulin switchlike sequence is linked with canine narcolepsy. Sleep. 1994; 17:S68-76.
8. Punnonen J et al. Role of interleukin-4 and interleukin-13 in synthesis of IgE and expression of CD23 by human B cells. Allergy. 1994; 49:576-86.
9. Valko PO et al. No persistent effect of intravenous immunoglobulins in patients with narcolepsy with cataplexy. J Neurol. 2008; 255:1900-3.
10. Mosmann TR et al. TH1 and TH2 cells: different patterns of lymphokine secretion lead to different functional properties. Annu Rev Immunol. 1989; 7:145-73.
11. Matsuki K et al. Lymphocyte subsets in HLA-DR2-positive narcoleptic patients. Folia Psychiatr Neurol Jpn. 1985; 39:499-505.
12. Honda Y et al. HLA-DR2 and Dw2 in narcolepsy and in other disorders of excessive somnolence without cataplexy. Sleep. 1986; 9:133-42.
13. Hinze-Selch D et al. In vivo and in vitro immune variables in patients with narcolepsy and HLA-DR2 matched controls. Neurology. 1998; 50:1149-52.
14. Langrish CL et al. IL-23 drives a pathogenic T cell population that induces autoimmune inflammation. J Exp Med. 2005; 201:233-40.

Obstructive sleep apnea in narcolepsy. Sansa G, Iranzo A, Santamaria J. *Sleep Med. 2010 Jan;11(1):93-5.*

What is the prevalence of obstructive sleep apnea in persons with narcolepsy?

Subjects	Methods	Outcomes
133 subjects narcolepsy diagnosed with PSG and MSLT	Assessments: • Clinical interview for features of OSA and narcolepsy • Response to CPAP treatment	24.8% (n = 33) of subjects had AHI > 10 (mean 28.5 ± 15.7) Diagnosis of sleep disorder • 10 subjects were initially diagnosed only with OSA 1. Narcolepsy diagnosis was delayed by 6.1 ± 7.8 yrs • 23 subjects were diagnosed with both narcolepsy and OSA at the same time OSA diagnosis was associated with: • Male gender • Older age • Higher BMI

AHI: apnea hypopnea index; BMI: higher body mass index; CPAP: continuous positive airway pressure; EDS: excessive daytime sleepiness; MSLT: multiple sleep latency test; OSA: obstructive sleep apnea; PSG: nocturnal polysomnography

Conclusion
Nearly a quarter of persons with narcolepsy had concurrent obstructive sleep apnea.

Commentary
Patients with narcolepsy may have an abnormally high apnea hypopnea index (AHI). This may complicate their diagnosis, because both narcolepsy and OSAS cause EDS. Our study is the first evaluating the clinical significance of sleep apnea in a large series of patients with narcolepsy (n = 133) and the effect of CPAP therapy in narcoleptics with comorbid OSA.

Previous studies assessing the prevalence of OSA in narcolepsy are scarce and reported results ranging between 2% and 68%. Guilleminault et al[1] noted two patients with narcolepsy and central sleep apnea. Laffont et al[2] described the occurrence of sleep apnea in five patients. Kales et al[3] studied the prevalence of sleep apnea in a series of 50 narcoleptics with cataplexy and only one had sleep apnea on the polysomnogram (AHI of 67), and Chokroverty et al[4] reported the presence of apneic episodes, predominantly central, in 11 of 16 narcoleptic patients. A few additional isolated case reports of narcolepsy with OSA have been described.[5-7] Other studies have noted that the occurrence of AHI > 5 in 9.8 to 19% of narcoleptics undergoing polysomnography.[8-11] In none of these studies the effect of CPAP on EDS was assessed.

We found that 24.8% of 133 narcoleptics had an AHI ≥ 10. These patients had a higher BMI, male gender and older age than those with a normal AHI. Cataplexy, EDS, sleep efficiency, REM latency in multiple latency sleep test and number of sleep onset REM periods were not significantly different in patients with AHI ≥10 and AHI < 10.

Interestingly, 30% of narcoleptics with AHI ≥ 10 were initially diagnosed as having only OSA syndrome in other sleep centers. Eighty percent of them had cataplexy and this symptom was already present when patients first complained of EDS in the other sleep centers. Narcolepsy was not diagnosed because patients did not spontaneously report that they had cataplexy and because physicians did not ask for its presence. Underecognition of cataplexy and other narcoleptic symptoms delayed several years the diagnosis of narcolepsy. Rye et al reported that, the diagnosis of narcolepsy could be delayed because of 1) late-life expression of cataplexy after initial consultation, 2) mild disease, 3) narcolepsy lacking cataplexy with later-life onset of EDS, and, as in our series, 4) misdiagnosis.[12] Lack of diagnosis of narcolepsy delays a proper management of the disease. Moreover, in our study, CPAP did not improve sleepiness in most of our narcoleptics with OSA. This finding suggests that OSA does not play a major role in the pathophysiology and severity of EDS in narcolepsy.

We suggest that cataplexy should be always actively looked for 1) in patients referred to sleep centers with EDS attributed to OSAS, and 2) in patients with OSA and residual EDS despite the correct use of CPAP therapy.

Gemma Sansa
Neurology Service
Corporació Sanitària Parc Taulí, Sabadell

Joan Santamaria
Neurology Service
Hospital Clinic of Barcelona
University of Barcelona Medical School

Alex Iranzo
Neurology Service
Hospital Clinic of Barcelona
University of Barcelona Medical School

References
1. Guilleminault C et al. Insomnia, narcolepsy and sleep apnea. Bull Eur Physiopathol Respir. 1972; 8:1127–38.
2. Laffont F et al. Sleep respiratory arrhythmias in control subjects, narcoleptics and non-cataplectic hypersomniacs. Electroencephalogr Clin Neurophysiol. 1978; 44:697–705.
3. Kales A et al. Clinical and electrophysiologic characteristics. Arch Neurol. 1982; 39:164–8.

4. Chokroverty S. Sleep apnea in narcolepsy. Sleep. 1986; 9:250–3.
5. Carpio Muñoz V et al. Botebol Benhamou G, Cano Gómez S, Capote Gil F. Association of obstructive apnea syndrome during sleep and narcolepsy. Arch Bronconeumol. 1998; 34:310–1.
6. Zamarrón C et al. Obstructive sleep apnea syndrome and narcolepsy. A report of 2 cases. Arch Bronconeumol. 1998; 34:466.
7. Reimao R et al. Concomitant narcolepsy and sleep apnea: report of a case. Arq Neuropsiquiatr. 1986; 44:73–7.
8. Baker TL et al. Comparative polysomnographic study of narcolepsy and idiopathic central nervous system hypersomnia. Sleep. 1986; 9:232–42.
9. Harsh J et al. Night-time and daytime sleepiness in narcolepsy. J Sleep Res. 2000; 9:309–16.
10. Mosko SS et al. Nocturnal REM latency and sleep disturbance in narcolepsy. Sleep. 1984; 7:115–25.
11. Plazzi G et al. Nocturnal aspects of narcolepsy with cataplexy.Sleep Med Rev. 2008; 12:109–28.
12. Rye DB et al. Presentation of narcolepsy after 40. Neurology. 1998; 50:459–65.

The socio-economical burden of hypersomnia. Jennum P, Kjellberg J. *Acta Neurol Scand. 2010 Apr;121(4):265-70.*

What is the economic cost of hypersomnia on society?

Subjects	Methods	Outcomes
2208 subjects with hypersomnia • Identified using the Danish national patient registry (1998-2005)	Assessments: • Estimation of health costs based on the following sources of data: 1. Costs of discharges and outpatient use (data from Danish Ministry of Health) 2. Costs of drugs (data from Danish Medicines Agency) 3. Costs from primary sectors (data from National Health Security) 4. Indirect costs based on income data (data from coherent social statistics) 5. Each subject was compared with 4 age- and gender-matched controls (data from Civil Registration System Statistics)	Compared to controls, subjects with hypersomnia had: • Higher health-related contact rate, expenses and medication use • No differences in employment and income Annual total cost (including direct and indirect) were: • Hypersomnia: euro 3402 • Controls: euro 1212* • Note: Yearly excess costs related to hypersomnia: euro 2190

*P < 0.001

Conclusion
Hypersomnia was associated with a significant socio-economic burden.

Commentary
Sleep disorders are common, affect the population at different ages and often causes significant health related burden and reduced quality of life.

Hypersomnia is part of the international sleep disorders classification related to sleep disordered breathing or of non-respiratory causes like narcolepsy and other hypersomnias of central origins. Former studies have presented evidence that sleep disorders like insomnia, narcolepsy, restless legs and sleep apnea influence quality of life, social or economical aspects.[1-22] These studies were carried out in out-patient clinic in selected patients using questionnaire or telephone based information, model-based information or quality of life estimates and the economical burden was extracted from this information. Another limitation with these studies is the lack of controls. There are however limited or no information regarding the impact of hypersomnia on the socio-economical burden, including the factual indirect and direct costs. In order to evaluate the health related consequences for patients with hypersomnia the current study were conducted in order to evaluate the socio-economical consequences evaluated in a population-based study.

The current study was initiated to estimate the factual cost of sleep disorders on a national basis as compared to control subjects. In Denmark, it is possible to calculate direct and indirect costs related to diseases because information from public and private hospitals and clinics in the primary and secondary sector—including medication, social transfers, labor market income, and employment data from all patients—is registered in a central database for all Danes. All patient contacts with the healthcare system are recorded in the NPR at the time of contact and include the primary diagnosis. The NPR includes administrative information, diagnoses, and diagnostic and treatment procedures using several international classification systems, including the International Classification of Disorders (ICD-10). By reviewing NPR we identified all patients with a diagnosis of hypersomnia. Ascertainment of socioeconomic status was performed by selecting control subjects who resided in the same area of the country in which the patients lived. The ratio of control subjects to patients was 4:1.

In this study, the economic consequence of hypersomnia was estimated by determining the yearly cost of illness per patient diagnosed with hypersomnia and comparing that calculation with the cost of healthcare in a matched control group. The annual health cost was then divided into direct and indirect healthcare costs. Costs were measured on a yearly basis and adjusted to 2006 prices using the health sector price index for health sector costs; the general price index was applied to nonmedical costs.

The study shows that the patients show significant direct and indirect costs (especially due to reduced work ability and income). Furthermore, the study shows a significant increased transfer income.

An extension of the study including patients with narcolepsy[23] and snoring, sleep apnoea and obesity hyperventilation[24] shows that these disorders show and even higher socio-economical burden.

Poul Jennum
Danish Center for Sleep Medicine
Department of Clinical Neurophysiology
University of Copenhagen
Glostrup Hospital

References

1. Beusterien KM et al. Health-related quality of life effects of modafinil for treatment of narcolepsy. Sleep. 1999; 22(6):757-65.
2. Daniels E et al. Health-related quality of life in narcolepsy. J Sleep Res. 2001; 10(1):75-81.

3. Dodel R et al. Health-related quality of life in patients with narcolepsy. Sleep Med. 2007; 8(7-8):733-41.

4. Ervik S et al. Health-related quality of life in narcolepsy. Acta Neurol Scand. 2006; 114(3):198-204.

5. Reimer MA et al. Quality of life in sleep disorders. Sleep Med Rev. 2003; 7(4):335-49.

6. Stores G et al. The psychosocial problems of children with narcolepsy and those with excessive daytime sleepiness of uncertain origin. Pediatrics. 2006; 118(4):e1116-e1123.

7. Vignatelli L et al. Health-related quality of life in Italian patients with narcolepsy: the SF-36 health survey. Sleep Med. 2004; 5(5):467-75.

8. Gureje O et al. Insomnia and role impairment in the community : results from the Nigerian survey of mental health and wellbeing. Soc Psychiatry Psychiatr Epidemiol. 2007; 42(6):495-501.

9. Terzano MG et al. Studio Morfeo 2: survey on the management of insomnia by Italian general practitioners. Sleep Med. 2006; 7(8):599-606.

10. Metlaine A et al. Socioeconomic impact of insomnia in working populations. Ind Health. 2005; 43(1):11-9.

11. Gellis LA et al. Socioeconomic status and insomnia. J Abnorm Psychol. 2005; 114(1):111-8.

12. Souza JC et al. Insomnia and hypnotic use in Campo Grande general population, Brazil. Arq Neuropsiquiatr. 2002; 60(3-B):702-7.

13. Leger D et al. Medical and socio-professional impact of insomnia. Sleep. 2002; 15;25(6):625-9.

14. Chilcott LA et al. The socioeconomic impact of insomnia. An overview. Pharmacoeconomics. 1996; 10 Suppl 1:1-14.

15. Molnar MZ et al. Restless legs syndrome, insomnia, and quality of life after renal transplantation. J Psychosom Res. 2007; 63(6):591-7.

16. Kushida C et al. Burden of restless legs syndrome on health-related quality of life. Qual Life Res. 2007; 16(4):617-24.

17. Kushida CA. Clinical presentation, diagnosis, and quality of life issues in restless legs syndrome. Am J Med. 2007; 120(1 Suppl 1):S4-S12.

18. Abetz L et al. The reliability, validity and responsiveness of the Restless Legs Syndrome Quality of Life questionnaire (RLSQoL) in a trial population. Health Qual Life Outcomes. 2005; 3:79.

19. Hening W et al. Impact, diagnosis and treatment of restless legs syndrome (RLS) in a primary care population: the REST (RLS epidemiology, symptoms, and treatment) primary care study. Sleep Med. 2004; 5(3):237-46

20. Atkinson MJ et al. Validation of the Restless Legs Syndrome Quality of Life Instrument (RLS-QLI): findings of a consortium of national experts and the RLS Foundation. Qual Life Res. 2004; 13(3):679-93.

21. Sonka K et al. Socioeconomic aspects of sleep-related breathing disorders. Sb Lek. 2002; 103(1):59-63.

22. Ayas NT et al. Cost-effectiveness of continuous positive airway pressure therapy for moderate to severe obstructive sleep apnea/hypopnea. Arch Intern Med. 2006; 8; 166(9):977-84.

23. Jennum P et al. The economic consequences of narcolepsy. J Clin Sleep Med. 2009; 15; 5(3):240-5.

24. Jennum P et al. Health, social and economical consequences of sleep-disordered breathing: a controlled national study. Thorax. 2011; Jan 2.

Insomnia

A 12-week, randomized, double-blind, placebo-controlled study evaluating the effect of eszopiclone 2 mg on sleep/wake function in older adults with primary and comorbid insomnia. Ancoli-Israel S, Krystal AD, McCall WV, Schaefer K, Wilson A, Claus R, Rubens R, Roth T. *Sleep. 2010 Feb 1;33(2):225-34.*

How effective is long-term eszopiclone therapy for primary and comorbid insomnia in older adults?

Subjects	Methods	Outcomes
Outpatient subjects with insomnia • Age: 65-85 yrs • + DSM-IV-TR criteria for insomnia • TST ≤ 6 hrs • WASO ≥ 45 min	Subjects were randomized to either: • 12 weeks of eszopiclone 2 mg (n = 194) • Placebo (n = 194) • These were followed by a 2-week single-blind placebo run-out Assessments: • Subjective measures of sleep (TST, SL and WASO) • Daytime function (alertness, concentration, wellbeing, ability to function) • Adverse effects	Compared to placebo, administration of eszopiclone was associated with: • Longer subjective TST* (360.08 vs. 297.86 min at baseline; mean change of 63.24 min) • Greater subjective improvement in SL** (mean decrease of 24.62 vs. 19.92 min for placebo) • Greater subjective decrease in WASO*** (mean decrease of 36.4 vs. 14.8 min for placebo) • No rebound effects post-discontinuation vs. baseline[#] Common adverse effects (≥ 5%) included: • Headache (13.9% vs. 12.4% for placebo) • Unpleasant taste (12.4% vs. 1.5%) • Nasopharyngitis (5.7% vs. 6.2%)

SL: sleep latency; TST: total sleep time; WASO: wake time after sleep onset; *$P < 0.0001$; **$P = 0.0014$; [#]$P ≤ 0.01$

Conclusion
Improvements in nighttime sleep among older adults with insomnia with eszopiclone were maintained for 3 months with no rebound effects post-discontinuation.

Commentary

Chronic sleep disturbances in older adults are associated with poorer health outcomes, cognitive and functional impairments, and decreased quality of life. Poor sleep has also been shown to result in increased nursing home placements, increased risk of falls, and greater risk of mortality in older individuals. Although it is yet unknown if these relationships are casual or even bidirectional, it is clear that poor sleep is associated with poorer functional outcome.

It has been estimated that over half of older adults suffer from insomnia and therefore at risk for poor physical and cognitive health. Although behavioral treatments are the treatment of choice for insomnia, sedative hypnotics are used most often. And when sedative hypnotics are used, they are often used for long time periods as these problems are often chronic in this population. Yet, there have been few long-term pharmacologic studies for insomnia in older individuals.

This study evaluated the efficacy and safety of 12 weeks of nightly use of eszopiclone in elderly outpatients with chronic insomnia. Close to 400 participants were randomized to 12 weeks of eszopiclone 2 mg or placebo. Subjective reports of total sleep time, sleep latency, wake time and daytime function (alertness, concentration, well-being, ability to function) were all assessed. The results showed that those treated with eszopiclone 2 mg slept longer at every time point compared to baseline than the placebo group. Participants in the active drug group, compared to placebo, also fell asleep significantly faster and spent less time awake during the night.

This phase IV trial of older adults with insomnia therefore, showed that eszopiclone significantly improved patient-reported sleep and daytime function relative to placebo. Improvements occurred within the first week and were maintained for 3 months. Eszopiclone had already been approved by the FDA for the treatment of primary insomnia including chronic use where required. But chronic use had not yet been tested in older patients suffering from insomnia. The significance of this study is that a drug known to be safe and effective in older adults in short term use can also be used long term with continued safety and efficacy.

Another very important point is that Improvement was also seen in daytime function. A comprehensive assessment of daytime function showed that subjective reports of daytime alertness, ability to function, ability to concentrate, and sense of physical well-being were all significantly improved in the eszopiclone group compared with placebo. These findings are of particularly important in older adults as problems with daytime functioning and concentration are often misinterpreted as dementia, but may actually be a function of poor sleep. The impact of this study is that since many older adults suffer from insomnia, and not all are able to receive behavioral treatment, having a medication that is both safe and effective long term gives the health care professional more treatment options for improving sleep, and thus quality of life, in older adults.

Sonia Ancoli-Israel
Gillin Sleep and Chronomedicine Research Center
Department of Psychiatry
University of California San Diego

An exploratory study on the effects of tele-neurofeedback and tele-biofeedback on objective and subjective sleep in patients with primary insomnia. Cortoos A, De Valck E, Arns M, Breteler MH, Cluydts R. *Appl Psychophysiol Biofeedback. 2010 Jun;35(2):125-34.*

Are tele-neurofeedback and tele-biofeedback effective therapies for primary insomnia?

Subjects	Methods	Outcomes
17 subjects with insomnia 12 healthy controls	Subjects were randomized to either: • Tele-neurofeedback (n = 9) • EMG tele-biofeedback (n = 8) Assessment: • PSG before and after treatment	Results compared to baseline included: • Decrease in SL in both groups • Increased TST in the neurofeedback group • Improved home sleep logs in the neurofeedback group • No change in lab sleep logs

CNS: central nervous system; EMG: electromyography; PSG: polysomnography; SL: sleep latency; TST: total sleep time

Conclusion

In persons with insomnia, tele-neurofeedback improved sleep latency and total sleep time, and tele-biofeedback shortened sleep latency.

Commentary

Although for most people sleeping is a natural phenomenon, during life we will inevitably encounter situations that can result in occasional insomnia. When confronted with a few sleepless nights, most people won't really dwell upon this transient phenomenon and will quickly return to their usual sleeping pattern. However, sometimes these occasional sleepless nights might evolve into a constant event, re-occurring several nights per week during several months. As a result, people become worried and anxious, and feel like losing control of something that ought to be a natural process. It becomes more difficult to carry out the daily routines and the impairment in daytime functioning increases, ultimately resulting in a disruption of general wellbeing. The concomitant increase in arousal, specifically related to sleep environmental stimuli, will further disrupt the sleep pattern and a vicious cycle is set in motion.

The above described situation is a reflection of the behavioral model, which has been dominantly used as the theoretical framework to explain the onset and maintenance of insomnia.[1] The main focus is the presence of conditioned arousal, which is reflected by anxiety, muscle tension, increased cortisol levels at bedtime, destructive and obsessive cognitions related to the consequences of sleep shortage, etc... As such, conditioned arousal has been the starting point for treatment interventions in this patient population.

Nowadays, a specific and standardized treatment program called Cognitive Behavioral Therapy for Insomnia (CBT-I), is regarded as the gold standard of non-pharmacological treatment for insomnia. This training modality has been the topic of many international studies and has shown to be quite effective. However, a recent review[2] showed that the CBT-I effects in insomnia are consistently smaller compared to CBT effects in other psychological disorders. Furthermore, the change induced by CBT-I does not always result in a sleeping pattern that falls into the 'good sleeper range', which suggests that there is still some impairment after treatment. Finally, approximately 20% of all patients do not respond at all to CBT-I. This raises the question whether another factor is in play that is not taken into account in standard non-pharmacological approaches.[3]

A possible explanation might be found in the neurocognitive perspective[4], which adds a third arousal component to the concept of conditioned arousal, namely cortical arousal. This is reflected by the presence of increased high frequency EEG activity and is thought to result in increased information processing at a time and place - being nighttime and in the bedroom – were this is not appropriate and even disruptive for a good night sleep. This framework has important consequences for our view on treatment modalities, namely that an additional focus on information processes on the level of the central nervous system (CNS) might also be an interesting way to intervene in insomnia patients, specifically for those who do not benefit from the standard CBT-I training. Furthermore, an in depth analysis of the wake and sleep EEG profile of insomnia patients might clarify whether the cortical arousal component is a mediator in the CBT-I results.

In our study we used neurofeedback (NFB) or EEG biofeedback, which is a treatment modality targeting cortical processes and has been successfully applied to improve cognitive functioning in healthy volunteers, as well as children and adults with attention deficit disorder (ADD). Accordingly, we implemented a protocol targeting the improvement of cognitive functioning, as previous studies[5,6] showed that not all insomnia patients respond to a treatment mimicking sleep onset, e.g. increasing slow frequencies.

Additionally, by using an internet based protocol we were able to counter some usual difficulties when using NFB. Firstly, the relatively high frequency of sessions required, which is a minimum of 2 sessions a week for at least 8 weeks. Secondly, the reduced patient – therapist contact - a 5 minute phone call every session - might compensate for the lack of a double-blind methodology, and as such possibly reduce the effects of confounding variables typically of a single blind study.

Aisha Cortoos
Research Unit Biological Psychology
Vrije Universiteit Brussel

References

1. Spielman AJ et al. A behavioural perspective on insomnia treatment. Psychiatr Clin North Am. 1987; 10(4):541-53.
2. Harvey AG et al. Cognitive behaviour therapy for primary insomnia: Can we rest yet? Sleep Medicine Reviews. 2003; 7:237-262.

3. Cortoos A et al. Neurophysiological aspects of insomnia: implications for its treatment. Sleep Medicine Reviews. 2006; 10:255-266.
4. Perlis ML et al. Psychophysiological insomnia: the behavioural model and a neurocognitive perspective. Journal of Sleep Research. 1997; 6:179-188.
5. Hauri P. Treating psychophysiologic insomnia with biofeedback. Archives of General Psychiatry. 1981; 38:752-758.
6. Hauri P et al. The treatment of psychophysiological insomnia with biofeedback: a replication study. Biofeedback and Self-Regulation. 1982; 7:223-235.

Association between a serotonin transporter length polymorphism and primary insomnia.
Deuschle M, Schredl M, Schilling C, Wüst S, Frank J, Witt SH, Rietschel M, Buckert M, Meyer-Lindenberg A, Schulze TG. *Sleep. 2010 Mar 1;33(3):343-7.*

Is primary insomnia associated with a 44-base-pair insertion/deletion polymorphism in the 5' regulatory region of the serotonin transporter gene?

Subjects	Methods	Outcomes
157 subjects with primary insomnia (with PSG) 827 healthy controls (without PSG)	Association study Assessment: • Genotyping of 5-HTTLPR: presence of 44-base-pair insertion/deletion polymorphism in 5-HTTLPR	The s-allele of the 5-HTTLPR is significantly more frequent in patients with primary insomnia Prevalence of short (s-) allele of 5-HTTLPR: • Primary insomnia: 47.1% • Healthy controls: 39.9%*

5-HTTLPR: 5' regulatory region of the serotonin transporter gene; PSG: polysomnography; *OR = 1.34

Conclusion
Compared to healthy controls, primary insomnia was associated with a higher prevalence of a short (s-) allele of the 5' regulatory region of the serotonin transporter gene; this is the first association between a genetic variant and primary insomnia.

Commentary
Family and twin studies have shown that insomnia is under strong genetic influence. Also, stressful live events contribute to the onset of the disorder. Thus, primary insomnia may be regarded as a potential consequence of a gene-environment interaction. Moreover, primary insomnia is related to major depressive disorder.[1] Insomnia could be a risk factor for depression. Also, both disorders could share a common biological background as two conditions of a spectrum of stress-related disorders.

We found primary insomnia to be associated with the s-allele of the 5-HTTLPR (OR: 1.34; P = 0.018) and, of borderline significance on genotypic level (P = 0.052). After post hoc exclusion of 38 subjects with lifetime affective disorders, currently in full remission, the finding still remained significant (P = 0.032). Sleep apnea, known to be associated with the l-allele of the 5-HTTLPR, was controlled in patients, but not controls. Post hoc exclusion of 4 % of the control group in order to model the exclusion of sleep apnea led to minimal changes of the model, with the s-allele still being associated with primary insomnia (OR: 1.32; P = 0.024).

Earlier, the 5-HTTLPR has been found to be associated with stress-related psychiatric disorders, like trait anxiety or affective disorders, especially in interaction with environmental adversity. Also, the 5-HTTLPR is associated with processing style of negative information and emotion.[2] Thus, our finding implicates the 5-HTTLPR in the presence of stressful live events to be related to conditioning of sleeplessness with situational stimuli normally associated with sleep. These mechanisms may play a role in the pathogenesis of various sleep-related disorders ranging from insomnia to anxiety and affective disorders. The common sequence insomnia-depression may not only be explained by unspecific stress, but also common genetic factors.

Michael Deuschle
Central Institute of Mental Health, Mannheim, Germany

References
1. Riemann D et al. Primary insomnia: a risk factor to develop depression? J Affect Disord. 2003; 76:255-259.
2. Pezawas L et al. 5-HTTLPR polymorphism impacts human cingulated-amygdala interactions: a genetic susceptibility mechanism for depression. Nat Neurosci. 2005; 8:828-834

Effect of acute physical exercise on patients with chronic primary insomnia. Passos GS, Poyares D, Santana MG, Garbuio SA, Tufik S, Mello MT. *J Clin Sleep Med. 2010 Jun 15;6(3):270-5.*

What types of acute physical exercises best improve sleep of persons with chronic primary insomnia?

Subjects	Methods	Outcomes
48 subjects with chronic primary insomnia • Age (mean): 44.4 ± 8 yrs • Gender: 21% males	Subjects were randomized to 4 groups, namely: • Control: n = 12 • Moderate-intensity aerobic exercise: n = 12 • High-intensity aerobic exercise: n = 12 • Moderate-intensity resistance exercise: n = 12 Assessments before and after acute exercise: • PSG • Daily sleep log • Anxiety (STAI)	Compared to baseline, moderate-intensity aerobic exercise was associated with the following: • PSG: 1. Decrease in SOL: 55% 2. Decrease in TWT: 30% 3. Increase in TST: 18% 4. Increase in SE: 13% • Daily sleep log data 1. Increase in TST: 26% 2. Decrease in SOL: 39% • Anxiety scale 1. Decrease in anxiety: 15%

CTR: control; HAE: high-intensity aerobic exercise; MAE: moderate-intensity aerobic exercise; MRE: moderate-intensity resistance exercise; PSG: polysomnography; SE: sleep efficiency; SOL: sleep onset latency; TST: total sleep time; TWT: total wake time

Conclusion
Moderate-intensity aerobic exercise improved objective and subjective sleep parameters and reduced pre-sleep anxiety in persons with chronic primary insomnia.

Commentary
The prevalence of chronic insomnia in the general population is between 10 and 15%; it is common in adulthood and predominantly affects women.[1] Drug therapy is frequently prescribed for its treatment. However, sleeping pills have been associated with several side effects when used for extended periods.[2] Prolonged use of benzodiazepines has been associated with cognitive deficits[3] and also with an increase in mortality.[4] Recently, new hypnotic drugs have been approved by regulatory agencies for long-term use. However, there is lack of research examining the effects of these drugs on patients with primary insomnia.[5-7] Given the problems associated with the pharmacological treatment of insomnia, several non-pharmacological alternatives have been suggested in the literature.[8,10] Exercise has been proposed as a low cost and accessible alternative treatment.[11,12] This indication is based on epidemiological studies that have reported an association between exercise and a reduction in complaints of insomnia[13], as well as a relationship between low levels of physical activity and an increased incidence of insomnia.[14] However, there has been limited experimental investigation

of the effects of exercise on sleep in individuals with insomnia[15,16], beyond a few studies that examined older adults with sleep complaints[17, 18], and there is no consensus on the best type, intensity or duration of exercise required to produce significant benefits.

The purpose of this study was to evaluate the acute effects of three types of physical exercise: moderate-intensity aerobic exercise (walking), high-intensity aerobic exercise (running) and moderate-intensity resistance exercise (strength) on both pre-sleep anxiety and sleep in patients with chronic primary insomnia. We observed positive results only in the moderate-intensity aerobic exercise group. Improvements were observed for objective sleep (polysomnography), subjective sleep and pre-sleep anxiety.

To evaluate the chronic effects of aerobic exercise (and other modalities), it is necessary to confirm these positive findings. Additionally, studies comparing different times of day and various conventional non-pharmacological and pharmacological therapies on chronic primary insomnia are essential for the inclusion of exercise in the group of non-pharmacological therapies (co-adjuvant or not) that are prescribed to treat chronic insomnia.

Marco Túlio de Mello
Exercise and Psychobiology Research Center (CEPE)
Departament of Psychobiology
Universidade Federal de São Paulo

Giselle Soares Passos
Exercise and Psychobiology Research Center (CEPE)
Departament of Psychobiology
Universidade Federal de São Paulo

Sergio Tufik
Exercise and Psychobiology Research Center (CEPE)
Departament of Psychobiology
Universidade Federal de São Paulo

References
1. Ohayon MM. Epidemiology of insomnia: what we know and what we still need to learn. Sleep Med Rev. 2002; 6(2):97-111.
2. Ringdahl EN et al. Treatment of primary insomnia. J Am Board Fam Pract. 2004; 17(3):212-9.
3. Bierman EJ et al. The effect of chronic benzodiazepine use on cognitive functioning in older persons: good, bad or indifferent? Int J Geriatr Psychiatry. 2007; 22(12):1194-200.
4. Kripke DF et al. Mortality hazard associated with prescription hypnotics. Biol Psychiatry. 1998; 43(9):687-93.
5. Erman M et al. Zolpidem extended-release 12.5 mg associated with improvements in work performance in a 6-month randomized, placebo-controlled trial. Sleep. 2008; 31(10):1371-8.
6. Krystal AD et al. Long-term efficacy and safety of zolpidem extended-release 12.5 mg, administered 3 to 7 nights per week for 24 weeks, in patients with chronic primary

insomnia: a 6-month, randomized, double-blind, placebo-controlled, parallel-group, multicenter study. Sleep. 2008; 31(1):79-90.

7. Neubauer DN. Current and new thinking in the management of comorbid insomnia. Am J Manag Care. 2009; 15 Suppl:S24-32.

8. Morin CM et al. Nonpharmacological interventions for insomnia: a meta-analysis of treatment efficacy. Am J Psychiatry. 1994; 151(8):1172-80.

9. Passos GS et al. Nonpharmacologic treatment of chronic insomnia. Rev Bras Psiquiatr. 2007; 29(3):279-82.

10. Driver HS et al. Exercise and sleep. Sleep Med Rev. 2000; 4(4):387-402.

11. Youngstedt SD. Effects of exercise on sleep. Clin Sports Med. 2005; 24(2):355-65, xi.

12. Youngstedt SD et al. The effects of acute exercise on sleep: a quantitative synthesis. Sleep. 1997; 20(3):203-14.

13. De Mello MT et al. Levantamento Epidemiológico da prática de atividade física na cidade de São Paulo. Rev Bras Med Esporte. 2000; 6:119-24.

14. Morgan K. Daytime activity and risk factors for late-life insomnia. J Sleep Res. 2003; 12(3):231-8.

15. Guilleminault C et al. Nondrug treatment trials in psychophysiologic insomnia. Arch Intern Med. 1995; 155(8):838-44.

16. Reid KJ et al. Aerobic exercise improves self-reported sleep and quality of life in older adults with insomnia. Sleep Med. 2010; 11(9):934-40.

17. King AC et al. Moderate-intensity exercise and self-rated quality of sleep in older adults. A randomized controlled trial. JAMA. 1997; 277(1):32-7.

18. King AC et al. Effects of moderate-intensity exercise on polysomnographic and subjective sleep quality in older adults with mild to moderate sleep complaints. J Gerontol A Biol Sci Med Sci. 2008; 63(9):997-1004.

Effectiveness of Valerian on insomnia: a meta-analysis of randomized placebo-controlled trials. Fernández-San-Martín MI, Masa-Font R, Palacios-Soler L, Sancho-Gómez P, Calbó-Caldentey C, Flores-Mateo G. *Sleep Med. 2010 Jun;11(6):505-11.*

How effective is valerian for insomnia?

Subjects	Methods	Outcomes
18 published RCTs comparing valerian and placebo for treatment of insomnia	Search using Medline, Cochrane Library, Embase and Biosis Assessments: • SQ (qualitative and quantitative) • SOL	Mean differences in SOL between the valerian and placebo treatment: 0.70 min* Standardized mean difference in SOL VAS between valerian and placebo: -0.02** Compared with placebo, valerian was associated with a relative risk of SQ of 1.37***

RCT: randomized clinical trial; SOL: sleep onset latency; SQ: sleep quality; VAS: visual analogical scale; *95% CI, -3.44 to 4.83; **95% CI, -0.35 to 0.31; ***95% CI, 1.05-1.78

Conclusion
Metaanalysis of randomized controlled trials have not shown any objective improvement of sleep with valerian in persons with insomnia.

Commentary
Insomnia, which affects around 30% of the population[1], is the most frequent of sleep pathologies.[2] As family doctors, we find ourselves confronted with it in doctor-patient visits practically on a daily basis (some 50% of the primary care population refers to insomnia if asked[3]) and we have the feeling of not being able to offer a satisfactory response to our patients.

Given that they are the most effective treat, we think that there is a tendency to resort to the use of benzodiazepines[4] and not consider other medications with fewer secondary effects. Many patients prefer "natural remedies".[5] Thus, we decided to investigate the effectiveness of Valerian as popular culture has attributed sedative effects to it for a long time.

We came across few randomized clinical trials (RCT) in our search. Of those that we encountered, less than half fulfilled the inclusion criteria. In the majority of the instances, they were very heterogeneous studies[6-8] that evaluated distinct doses of Valerian in very different populations with a small sample size and disparate results. Therefore, we carried out this metaanalysis.

Three outcomes were evaluated. Two of them, *latency time until getting to sleep and improvement in the quality of sleep quantified with a visual analogical scale*, showed no statistically significant differences. On the other hand, *dichotomic sleep quality improvement (Yes/No)* did suggest that Valerian can be effective.

In conclusion, sufficient objective data on the effectiveness of Valerian in the treatment of insomnia was not found. However, given its safety profile and the subjective improvements that it produces in some cases, its use in determinant patients could be considered. Posterior publications have not provided greater evidence relative to the subject.[9] We believe that studies of higher quality are needed in order to evaluate the effectiveness of Valerian in front of insomnia. Furthermore, future investigations oriented towards evaluating other non-pharmacological interventions for insomnia are recommended.

Roser Masa-Font
Servicio de Atención Primaria Litoral
Institut Català de Salut, Barcelona

Laura Palacios-Soler
Consorci d'Atenció Primària de
Salut de l'Eixample, Barcelona

References
1. Hajak G. Insomnia in primary care. Sleep. 2000; 23(Suppl. 3):S54-63.
2. Sarrais F et al. El insomnio. An Sist Sanit Navar. 2007; 30(Suppl. 1):121-34.
3. Smith MT et al. Comparative meta-analysis of pharmacotherapy and behaviour therapy for persistent insomnia. Am J Psychiatry. 2002; 159(1):5-11.
4. Morin C et al. Behavioural and pharmacological therapies for late-life insomnia. JAMA. 1999; 281(11):991-9.
5. Borbély AA. Schlafgewohnheiten, Schlafqualität und Schlafmittelkonsum der Schweizer Bevölkerung. Ergebnisse einer Repräsentativumfrage. Ärztezeitung. 1984; 34:1606-13.
6. Stevinson C et al. Valerian for insomnia: a systematic review of randomized clinical trials. Sleep Med. 2000; 1(2):91-9.
7. Bent S et al. Valerian for sleep: a systematic review and meta-analysis. Am J Med. 2006; 119(12):1005-12.
8. Taibi DM et al. A systematic review of valerian as a sleep aid: safe but not effective. Sleep Med Rev. 2007; 11(3):209-30.
9. Salter S et al. Treating primary insomnia - the efficacy of valerian and hops. Aust Fam Physician. 2010; 39(6):433-7.

Habitual sleep duration and insomnia and the risk of cardiovascular events and all-cause death: report from a community-based cohort. Chien KL, Chen PC, Hsu HC, Su TC, Sung FC, Chen MF, Lee YT. *Sleep. 2010 Feb 1;33(2):177-84.*

Are risks of all-cause death and cardiovascular events related to sleep duration and severity of insomnia?

Subjects	Methods	Outcomes
3430 subjects • Age: $\geq$ 35 yrs	Community-based prospective cohort study	During the follow-up period (median 15.9 yrs): • 901 subjects died • 420 subjects developed CVD There was a U-shape association between sleep duration and all-cause death Adjusted relative risks (95% CI) with 7 hrs of daily sleep as reference) were: • Sleep < or = 5 hrs: 1.15*,## • Sleep = 6 hrs: 1.02**, ## • Sleep = 8 hrs: 1.05***,## • Sleep > or = 9 hrs: 1.43#,## There was a linear relationship between sleep duration and CVD risk. Compared to the reference 7-hr daily sleep duration, the age- and gender-adjusted RR (95% CI) of all-cause death for those with the following daily sleep durations were: • $\leq$ 5 h: 1.15*, ## • 6 h: 1.02**, ## • 8 h: 1.05***, ## • $\geq$ 9 h: 1.43#, ## Compared to subjects without insomnia, the RR (95% CI) for all-cause death were: • Occasional insomnia:

		$1.02^{\#\#\#,\wedge\wedge\wedge}$ • Frequent insomnia: $1.15^{\wedge,\wedge\wedge}$ • Nearly everyday insomnia: $1.70^{\wedge\wedge,\wedge\wedge\wedge}$ For subjects sleeping ≥ 9 hrs and for those with frequent insomnia, the RR (95% CI) were: • All-cause death: 2.53+ • CVD rate: 2.07++

CI: confidence interval; CVD: cardiovascular disease; RR: relative risk; *0.91-1.45; **0.85-1.25; ***0.88-1.27; #1.16-1.75; ##P for trend, 0.019; ###0.86-1.20; ^0.92-1.42; ^^1.16-2.49; ^^^P for trend, 0.028; +1.71-3.76; ++1.11-3.85

Conclusion
Among ethnic Chinese in Taiwan, both habitual sleep duration and insomnia severity were related to cardiovascular events and all-cause death, with the latter lesser with a 7 to 8-hour sleep duration.

Commentary
A number of cohort studies conducted in North American, European, and Asian countries and among different ethnicities have demonstrated that short or long sleep duration is associated with increased risk for cardiovascular disease (CVD) and/or mortality.[1-10] Similar studies assessing the relationship of insomnia to hypertension, CVD, and mortality have had more mixed results.[2,6,11-15] Varying methodologies and different operational definitions of insomnia, of course, may account for some discrepancies in the literature and leave room for ongoing inquiry to further clarify these relationships. In addition, the ability to control for multiple characteristics of epidemiologic samples enhances the strength and utility of any findings.

Just such an effort was undertaken by Chien et al. who capitalized on the community-based, prospective, Chin-Shan Community Cardiovascular Cohort study.[16] In 1990-1991, the parent study first assessed sleep (and a host of baseline demographic and health variables) via questionnaires and blood sample collections from 3,602 men and women of Chinese ethnicity aged 35 and above living in one township in Taiwan. The current study (n=3,430) includes as outcomes incident CVD events and stroke cases, verified by neurologists and internists, as well as deaths verified by official death certificates and home visits. These outcomes were assessed at a median of 15.9 years following initial assessment with an interquartile range of 13.1 to 16.9 years.

Importantly, sleep duration was a question with 5 answer categories (≤ 5, 6, 7, 8, and ≥ 9 hours of sleep and insomnia) and insomnia was defined for respondents as "difficulty falling asleep, staying asleep, or additional nonrefreshing sleep," and the insomnia frequency question had 4 response alternatives, (no insomnia, occasional insomnia [2-3 times each month], frequent insomnia [2-3 times each week], and insomnia nearly every day).

With respect to sleep duration, in models adjusting for demographic, lifestyle, and health risk factors, the authors report a U-shape association with all-cause death, wherein short ($\leq$ 5 h) and long ($\geq$ 9h) habitual sleep conferred heightened relative risk (RR) to 7 h habitual sleep duration. The relationship between sleep duration and CVD events was roughly linear with increased relative risk for CVD events associated with longer sleep duration. With respect to insomnia, the multivariate-adjusted RR (95% CI) for all-cause death was also linear and most pronounced (with no insomnia as the comparison group) for nearly daily insomnia 1.70 (1.16-2.49). A similar, though less robust and *ns* trend was observed for insomnia status and CVD events. Finally, and notably, similar adjusted models assessing together sleep duration (in these analyses categorized as $\leq$ 6 h, 7-8 h, or $\geq$ 9h) and insomnia (dichotomized as frequent or infrequent) found that individuals with frequent insomnia <u>and</u> sleeping $\geq$ 9 h had highest RR (95% CI) for all-cause death 2.53 (1.71-3.76) and for CVD occurrences 2.07 (1.11-3.85). RR for other groups did not, or barely reached, significance.

Taken together, the findings suggest that both sleep duration and insomnia frequency are indeed associated with all-cause death and CVD events in this study population. Given the extensive number and types of covariates used in the analytic models, these are important confirmatory data vis-à-vis the extant literature. The data are also unique in terms of the ethnic Chinese study population. The findings with respect to insomnia are especially striking as there have been inconsistent findings on this front.

Equally striking, however, is the observation in the joint analyses (insomnia and duration), that individuals with frequent insomnia and $\leq$ 6 h of habitual sleep duration were not at increased risk for all cause death (1.1 [0.8-1.5]) or CVD events (0.7 [0.4-1.1]). One would hypothesize that this group would represent the "worst" sleep group and, therefore, be associated with increased RR for both outcomes. Similarly, it is somewhat difficult to conceive of frequent insomnia in an individual sleeping more than 9 hours per night. Although models adjusted for BMI, alcohol use, tobacco use, exercise, hypertension, and clinical chemistry profiles, it is possible that such a group represents individuals who are more ill, sleep more, but have insomnia nonetheless. As the authors point out, it is also possible that the operationalization of insomnia which includes nonrefreshing sleep, a very nonspecific complaint, allows for forms of sleep disturbance that are not consistent with initiating and maintaining sleep more commonly associated with insomnia.

This, in turn, underscores the ongoing need for epidemiologic studies addressing sleep to include items which can distinguish both between individuals with insomnia complaints and those meeting diagnostic criteria for insomnia and between insomnia subtypes (including nonrefreshing sleep). Notwithstanding the ongoing need for such prospective investigations, the work of Chien et al. underscores the grave implications of sleeping less (or more) than the 7 to 8 hours that may be optimal. This work does also contribute to the small, but growing body of work implicating insomnia complaints as potential risk indicators for CVD and all cause mortality.

Wilfred R. Pigeon
Sleep & Neurophysiology Research Lab
University of Rochester Medical Center
Canandaigua VA Medical Center
Center for Integrated Healthcare
Syracuse VA Medical Center

References

1. Amagai Y et al. Sleep duration and mortality in Japan: the Jichi Medical School Cohort Study. J Epidemiol. 2004; 14:124-8.

2. Ayas NT et al. A prospective study of sleep duration and coronary heart disease in women. Arch Intern Med. 2003; 163:205-9.

3. Dew MA et al. Healthy older adults' sleep predicts all-cause mortality at 4 to 19 years of follow-up. Psychosom Med. 2003; 65(1):63-73.

4. Gangwisch JE et al. Sleep duration associated with mortality in elderly, but not middle-aged, adults in a large US sample. Sleep. 2008; 31:1087-96.

5. Ikehara S et al. Association of sleep duration with mortality from cardiovascular disease and other causes for Japanese men and women: the JACC study. Sleep. 2009; 32(3):295-301.

6. Kripke DF et al. Mortality associated with sleep duration and insomnia. Arch Gen Psychiatry. 2002; 59:131-6.

7. Patel SR et al. A prospective study of sleep duration and mortality risk in women. Sleep. 2004; 27:440-4.

8. Lan TY et al. Nighttime sleep, Chinese afternoon nap, and mortality in the elderly. Sleep. 2007; 30:1105-10.

9. Shankar A et al. Sleep duration and coronary heart disease mortality among Chinese adults in Singapore: a population-based cohort study. Am J Epidemiol. 2008; 168:1367-73.

10. Tamakoshi A et al. Self-reported sleep duration as a predictor of all-cause mortality: results from the JACCstudy, Japan. Sleep. 2004; 27:51-4.

11. Althuis MD et al. The relationship between insomnia and mortality among community-dwelling older women. JAGS. 1998; 46:1270-3.

12. Kripke DF et al. Short and Long Sleep and Sleeping Pills: Is Increased Mortality Associated? Archives of General Psychiatry. 1979; 36:103-16.

13. Phillips B et al. Do insomnia complaints cause hypertension or cardiovascular disease? J Clin Sleep Med. 2007; 3:489-94.

14. Phillips B et al. Insomnia did not predict incident hypertension in older adults in the cardiovascular health study. Sleep. 2009; 32(1):65-72.

15. Suka M et al. Persistent Insomnia Is a Predictor of Hypertension in Japanese Male Workers. J.Occup.Health. 2003; 45(6):344-50.

16. Lee YT et al. Chin-Shan Community Cardiovascular Cohort in Taiwan: baseline data and five-year follow-up morbidity and mortality. J Clin Epidemiol. 2000; 53:836-46.

Prospective associations of insomnia markers and symptoms with depression. Szklo-Coxe M, Young T, Peppard PE, Finn LA, Benca RM. *Am J Epidemiol. 2010 Mar 15;171(6):709-20.*

Are there specific insomnia markers that predict subsequent development of depression?

Subjects	Methods	Outcomes
555 subjects • Participants of the Wisconsin Sleep Cohort Study • Age: 33-71 yrs • Without depression or antidepressant use	Assessments: • Baseline and follow-up PSG • Questionnaire on insomnia and depression Definitions: • Depression: Zung scale score ≥ 50	At 4-year (average) follow-up, 4.7% of subjects (n = 26) developed depression Depression risk was predicted by the presence of 3-4 insomnia symptoms (vs. none): RR = 3.2* • Insomnia symptoms or markers were associated with a 2.2- to 5.3-fold increased risk of depression After multiple adjustments, the following factors predicted depression: • Frequent difficulty falling asleep: RR = 5.3** • PSG sleep latency, continuity and sleep duration: RRs = 2.2-4.7; P's ≤ 0.05** 1. Graded trends were noted for increasing number of symptoms, and difficulty falling asleep and returning to sleep***

PSG: polysomnography; RR : relative risk; SL : sleep latency; *95% CI: 1.1, 9.6; **95% CI: 1.1, 27.9; ***P's ≤ 0.05

Conclusion
Among persons with chronic insomnia, frequent difficulty falling asleep and polysomnographically-measured sleep latency, continuity and sleep duration increased risk of subsequent depression.

Commentary

Insomnia is a vastly under-treated and under-recognized disorder.[1,2] However, its adverse correlates and societal toll are wide-ranging and include increased functional impairment,[1,3] health care use[1], absenteeism[4], and mood disturbances.[5] Sleep disturbances are closely related to psychiatric disorders[5,6] more than to any other medical illnesses.[7] Insomnia and depression, in particular, are closely related, yet distinct,[8] disorders. Both are highly prevalent,[1,5,9,10] persistent,[8,10,11] and related to significant morbidity, even at mild or sub-threshold levels.[7,10,12] Thus, better understanding their association may have implications for preventing and treating both disorders.

Classically, insomnia symptoms have been considered diagnostic for, or constituting, criteria for depression/mood disturbances.[13] However, insomnia's role extends beyond that of accompanying clinical symptom for depression, or it's correlate. Increasingly, insomnia is considered comorbid with[8,14], rather than secondary to[8], depression. Clinical and epidemiologic studies suggest insomnia is a precursor[15] and prodrome[16] for new or recurrent depression before the latter's full clinical development. Notably, insomnia is the most prevalent residual symptom of depression[17], potentially increasing the risk for relapse.[18] Additionally, sleep abnormalities in depression relate to lower post-treatment remission.[19] Untangling insomnia's association to depression is important, albeit challenging, given their overlapping conceptualizations and criteria[20], high comorbidity[5,8], and chronic, intermittent courses.[8,10]

Epidemiologic studies have found insomnia to be related cross-sectionally[3,8] and prospectively[9,21,22,23] to depression across age groupss.[8,22] Prospective studies have contributed to our understanding of insomnia as a risk for depression. We aimed to extend epidemiologic research, heretofore based solely on self-reported insomnia, to an investigation of insomnia's polysomnographic biological markers (e.g., sleep latency and continuity) as predictors, including those corresponding to self-reported difficulty initiating and maintaining sleep. Sleep electroencephalographic (EEG) abnormalities had been correlated with depression in clinical samples[24], yet their predictive value for depression remained unknown, particularly in a population-based sample.

We investigated whether, in 555 Wisconsin Sleep Cohort participants aged 33-71 years, free of depression at baseline, insomnia--assessed both via self-reported and objective markers— would independently predict subsequent depression at 4-year follow-up. Other unique aspects of our work included examining individual insomnia symptoms representing early, middle, or late insomnia "subtypes"; previously correlated to psychiatric comorbidity[3] yet not examined as risk factors. We further hypothesized a new conceptualization, namely a graded ("dose-response") relationship between insomnia (frequency or number of symptoms) and depression. The Wisconsin Sleep Cohort Study's methods are described in detail elsewhere.[25]

In individuals free of depression at baseline, those with insomnia (self-reported) or its polysomnographic markers had 2.2 to 5.3-fold increased risk of developing subsequent depression at 4-year follow-up, after multiple adjustments. We had a longer follow-up than most other studies with rare exceptions.[21,23] A modified depression (Zung ≥ 50) scale excluded sleep-related items to preclude built-in associations. Moreover, individuals on antidepressants without depressive symptoms were excluded from follow-up analyses to prevent outcome misclassification

Polysomnographically-assessed sleep latency, continuity, and duration (Relative Risks=2.2–4.7; P's ≤ 0.05) predicted depression as did difficulty falling asleep (Relative Risk=5.3, 95% confidence interval: 1.1-27.9). Significant (P-trend ≤ 0.05) graded trends were found for number of insomnia symptoms, difficulty falling asleep, and difficulty returning to sleep. When we analyzed continuous depression scores, results were largely confirmatory, with graded trends observed for all insomnia symptoms, number of symptoms, and polysomnographic markers-- decreased sleep efficiency and increased waking after sleep onset.

Our findings strongly suggest insomnia symptoms and markers may be risk factors for subsequent depression in those free of depression (and anxiety) at baseline. Graded trends of incident depression with increased insomnia are suggestive of insomnia potentially having a causal role in depression onset. Given that the pathways and presentations of insomnia are important[8,26] yet poorly understood, findings regarding insomnia markers and subtypes may help identify those at risk for future depression and have implications for depression prevention. That difficulty initiating sleep was most predictive of depression may help guide intervention efforts, though there may be temporal variability in self-reported subtypes.[26,27] Additional insomnia subtypes, related to duration,[8] paradoxical insomnia, or other,[26] should be investigated.

Our study's key strengths include its prospective design; assessment and investigation of objective and self-reported measures; and conservative depression outcome measure. A limitation of our study is that it did not distinguish between first-onset or recurrent depression. However, as depression symptoms are characterized by dynamic, symptomatic flux,[10,12] this differentiation may less relevant. Sleep and depression are multidimensional.[28] Sleep continuity was assessed, yet other dimensions of sleep architecture[28] or depression (e.g., somatic, cognitive) were not.

The relationship of insomnia to depression is dynamic and considered bidirectional[6,8,18] though research on this, particularly within the context of insomnia's natural history, has been limited. Buysse et al.[8] recommend future studies on whether insomnia becomes increasingly severe or frequent with time. Benca and Petersen[6] recommend objective measures beyond polysomnography (e.g., topographic high-density EEG patterns). Future research is needed to elucidate mechanisms through which insomnia leads to future depression, including a common neurobiology.

Diverse explanations have been posited[2] for the link between insomnia and depression, including hypothalamo-pituitary-adrenal axis activation[29] or shared genetic bases (e.g., serotonin transporter length polymorphism[30], familial aggregations regarding vulnerability to stress-related sleep disturbances).[31] Studies on other areas of insomnia may have implications for insomnia-depression research. Chronic hyperarousal, described for insomnia[32], may relate to dysfunctional nocturnal blood pressure [33]and increased risk for psychiatric disorders, also recently predicted by sleep disturbance pre-trauma.[34] According to Bryant et al.[34] ,this increased risk might relate to increased cortisol (linked to sleep disturbance)[35] during trauma. An association has also been observed in insomnia between EEG activity in the β frequency, elevated in insomnia[36], and higher night-time systolic blood pressure.[33] This may have implications for depression which increases cardiovascular risk.[37]

Our study may help to provide some information on specific insomnia risk factors which might be targeted for depression prevention. Insomnia may be a modifiable risk factor.[9] Even sub-threshold or mild depression is associated with substantial morbidity and functional impairment (e.g., increased health care use, work loss).[10,12] The search for pathways[26] regarding how insomnia may lead to depression continues.

Insomnia and depression are highly interconnected disorders with a complex relationship on many levels including conceptually and temporally. Recent studies suggest that treating insomnia in depression may improve both insomnia and depression outcomes, relative to just depression.[38,39] Further intervention efforts and prevention program need to be developed and implemented to specifically examine whether recognizing or treating insomnia symptoms or markers could help prevent or mitigate depression (first-onset or recurrent), particularly as insomnia continues to be under-recognized and under-treated.[2]

Mariana Szklo-Coxe
School of Community and Environmental Health
College of Health Sciences
Old Dominion University
Division of Sleep Medicine
Department of Internal Medicine
Eastern Virginia Medical School

References

1. Simon GE et al. Prevalence, burden, and treatment of insomnia in primary care. Am J Psychiatry. 1997; 154(10):1417-1423.
2. Benca RM. Diagnosis and treatment of chronic insomnia: A review. Psychiatr Serv. 2005; 56(3): 332-343.
3. Roth T et al. Sleep problems, comorbid mental disorders, and role functioning in the national comorbidity survey replication.Biol Psychiatry. 2006; 60(12):1364-71.
4. Léger D et al. Professional correlates of insomnia. Sleep. 2006; 29(2):171-178.
5. Ohayon MM et al. Comorbidity of mental and insomnia disorders in the general population. Comprehensive Psychiatry. 1998; 39(4):185-197.
6. Benca RM et al. Insomnia and depression. Sleep Medicine. 2008; 9 Suppl. 1: S3–S9.
7. Katz DA et al. Clinical correlates of insomnia in patients with chronic insomnia. Arch Intern Med. 1998; 158(1):1099-1107.
8. Buysse DJ et al. Prevalence, course and comorbidity of insomnia and depression in young adults. Sleep. 2008; 31(4):473-480.9.
9. Ford DE et al. Epidemiologic study of sleep disturbances and psychiatric disorders. An opportunity for prevention? JAMA. 1989; 262(11):1479-1484..
10. Kessler RC et al. Prevalence, correlates, and course of minor depression and major depression in the national comorbidity survey. J Affect Disord. 1997; 45(1-2):19-30.
11. Morin CM et al. The natural history of insomnia: a population-based 3-year longitudinal study. Arch Intern Med. 2009; 169(5):447-453.
12. Judd LL et al. The role and clinical significance of subsyndromal depressive symptoms (SSD) in unipolar major depressive disorder. J Affect Disord. 1997; 45(1-2):5-17.
13. Diagnostic and Statistical Manual of Mental Disorders. 4th ed. Washington, DC: American Psychiatric Association Press, 1994.

14. Reynolds CF et al. The DSM-V sleep-wake disorders nosology: an update and an invitation to the sleep community. Sleep. 2010; 33(1):10-11.

15. Eaton WW et al. Prodromes and precursors: Epidemiologic data for primary prevention of disorders with slow onset. American J Psychiatry. 1995; 152(7):967-972.

16. Perlis ML et al. Self-reported sleep disturbance as a prodromal symptom in recurrent depression. J Affect Disord. 1997; 42(2-3):209-212.

17. Nierenberg AA et al. Trazodone for antidepressant-associated insomnia. Am J Psychiatry 1994; 151(7):1069-1072.

18. Ohayon MM et al. Place of chronic insomnia in the course of depressive and anxiety disorders. Journal of Psychiatric Research. 2003; 37(1):9-15.

19. Buysse DJ et al. Pretreatment REM sleep and subjective sleep quality distinguish depressed psychotherapy remitters and nonremitters. Biol Psychiatry 1999; 45(2):205-213.

20. The International Classification of Sleep Disorders: Diagnostic & Coding Manual, ICSD-2. 2nd ed. Westchester, IL: American Academy of Sleep Medicine; 2005.

21. Breslau N et al. Sleep disturbances and psychiatric disorders: A longitudinal epidemiologic study of young adults. Biol Psychiatry 1996; 39 (6):411-418.

22. Livingston G et al. Does sleep disturbance predict depression in elderly people? A study in inner London. British Journal of General Practice. 1993; 43(376):445-448.

23. Chang PP et al. Insomnia in young men and subsequent depression. Am J Epidemiology. 1997; 146 (2):105-114.

24. Thase ME et al. Identifying an abnormal electroencephalographic sleep profile to characterize major depressive disorder. Biol Psychiatry. 1997; 41(9):964-973.

25. Young T et al. The occurrence of sleep-disordered breathing among middle-aged adults. N Engl J Med. 1993; 328(17):1230-1235.

26. Pigeon WR. Insomnia as a predictor of depression: do insomnia subtypes matter? Commentary on Yokoyama et al. Association between depression and insomnia subtypes: a longitudinal study on the elderly in Japan. Sleep. 2010;33(12):1693-1702.

27. Hohagen F et al. Sleep onset insomnia, sleep maintaining insomnia and insomnia with early morning awakening--temporal stability of subtypes in a longitudinal study on general practice attenders. Sleep. 1994; 17(6):551-4.

28. Perlis ML et al. Which depressive symptoms are related to which sleep electroencephalographic variables? Biol Psychiatry. 1997; 42(10):904--913

29. Balbo M et al. Impact of sleep and its disturbances on hypothalamo-pituitary-adrenal axis activity. International Journal of Endocrinology. 2010; 759234.

30. Deuschle M et al. Association between a serotonin transporter length polymorphism and primary insomnia. Sleep. 2010; 33(3):343-347

31. Drake C et al. Vulnerability to insomnia: The role of familial aggregation. Sleep Medicine. 2008; 9(3):297-302.

32. Bonnet MH et al. Hyperarousal and insomnia: state of the science. Sleep Medicine Reviews. 2010; 14(1):9-15.

33. Lanfranchi PA et al. Nighttime blood pressure in normotensive subjects with chronic insomnia: implications for cardiovascular risk. Sleep. 2009; 32(6):760-766.

34. Bryant RA et al. Sleep disturbance immediately prior to trauma predicts subsequent psychiatric disorder. Sleep. 2010; 33(1):69-74.

35. Leproult R et al. Sleep loss results in an elevation of cortisol levels the next evening. Sleep. 1997; 20(10):865-70.

36. Perlis ML et al. Beta/gamma EEG activity in patients with primary and secondary insomnia and good sleeper controls. Sleep. 2001; 24(1):110-7.

37. Barefoot JC et al. Symptoms of depression, acute myocardial infarction, and total mortality in a community sample. Circulation. 1996; 93(11):1976-80.

38. Manber R et al. Cognitive behavioral therapy for insomnia enhances depression outcome in patients with comorbid major depressive disorder and insomnia. Sleep. 2008; 31(4):489-495.

39. Fava M et al. Eszopiclone co-administered with fluoxetine in patients with insomnia coexisting with major depressive disorder. Biol Psychiatry. 2006; 59(11):1052-60.

The efficacy of cognitive-behavioral therapy for insomnia in patients with chronic pain.
Jungquist CR, O'Brien C, Matteson-Rusby S, Smith MT, Pigeon WR, Xia Y, Lu N, Perlis ML. *Sleep Med. 2010 Mar;11(3):302-9.*

Is cognitive-behavioral therapy for insomnia also effective for sleep disturbance in patients with chronic pain?

Subjects	Methods	Outcomes
28 subjects non-malignant chronic neck and back pain	Parallel-groups, randomized, single blind trial Subjects were assigned to either: • CBT-I (8 weeks): n = 19 1. Sleep restriction 2. Stimulus control 3. Sleep hygiene 4. Cognitive therapy • Control condition: n = 9 Assessments: • Sleep diary (sleep continuity) • ISI • MPI • Mood • SF-36	Compared to controls, CBT-I was associated with: • Decrease in SL • Decrease in WASO • Decrease in number of awakenings • Increase in SE • Improvement in ISI * • Improvement in MPI Interference Scale** • No difference in TST and measures of mood or pain severity

CBT-I: cognitive-behavioral therapy for insomnia; ISI: Insomnia severity index; MPI: Multidimensional pain inventory; SE: sleep efficiency; SF-36: Short form 36; SL: sleep latency; TST: total sleep time; WASO: wake after sleep onset; *P = 0.05; **P = 0.03

Conclusion
Cognitive-behavioral therapy for insomnia improved several sleep parameters and daytime vigor in persons with chronic pain.

Commentary
Traditionally, clinicians have addressed sleep disturbance in the presence of pain by just treating the painful condition. In fact, often, the effectiveness of treatments for pain is often judged on a patients' improvement in sleep. This practice seems logical, as nocioceptive arousal is a precipitator and potentially a perpetuator of insomnia. But, currently, there is little evidence to base clinical practice guidelines on whether to treat sleep disturbance co-morbid with pain using pain treatments, or treat sleep disturbance directly.

To start to answer this clinical query, we recruited patients who had moderate to severe pain with insomnia that started after the painful condition. When this study was developed, the hope was that we would see improvements in sleep without aggravating pain. In addition, we hoped for improvements in pain intensity and function as insomnia symptoms dissipated. We were able to document the safe and effective delivery of CBT-I in patients with chronic pain. Additionally, the standardized form of 8-session CBT-I was successfully delivered by a nurse practitioner (her training includes a 24 hour CBT-I course and weekly supervision). Despite significant improvements in sleep, we did not find group differences in reports of pain intensity. The patients in the treatment group did exhibit clinically relevant improvement in pain intensity and function related to pain. This finding is encouraging as were concerned that sleep restriction would not be tolerated in patients with moderate to severe pain.

Since this study was published, we have looked at the follow up data, and are pleased to report that patients in the treatment group continued to improve. At the end of the study (6 months post treatment) they were experiencing on average 72 minutes more sleep than at baseline despite continuing with moderate pain.

In addition to a report of this study, this manuscript offers a summary of recent studies describing their types of therapy and therapists. This information will be helpful in the development of other studies testing cognitive and behavioral interventions for insomnia in patients with chronic pain. Future interventional studies comparing CBT-I and CBT for pain; briefer forms of therapy; therapy in the clinic setting by medical providers; and comparisons of behavioral and pharmaceutical therapies are needed. Additionally, studies seeking the neural basis of the relationship between pain and sleep as well as the development of biomarkers that can be used to determine individual differences in responses to treatment as well as to be used as objective outcome measures are needed.

Carla Jungquist
University of Rochester

Michael L. Perlis
University of Pennsylvania

Treatment effects of gabapentin for primary insomnia. Lo HS, Yang CM, Lo HG, Lee CY, Ting H, Tzang BS. *Clin Neuropharmacol. 2010 Mar-Apr;33(2):84-90.*

Should gabapentin be used in the treatment of primary insomnia?

Subjects	Methods	Outcomes
18 subjects with primary insomnia	Subjects received gabapentin for ≥ 4 weeks Assessments before and after treatment: • Biochemical blood testing • Heart rate • Neuropsychological testing • PSG	Compared to baseline, gabapentin treatment was associated with: • PSG features 1. Increase in SE 2. Increase in SWS 3. Decrease in WASO 4. Decrease in spontaneous AI 5. EEG power spectral analysis: increase in delta-2 and theta power in N1 and decreased sigma activity power in N2 and N3 • Biochemical blood testing 1. Decrease in prolactin levels in the morning after treatment • Heart rate variability analyses 1. Increase in normalized high frequency percentage in N2 and N3 2. Increase in low frequency-high frequency ratio in N2 • Neuropsychological testing 1. Increase in visual motor processing speed

AI: arousal index; EEG: electroencephalographic; HR: heart rate; N1: sleep stage 1; N2: sleep stage 2; N3: sleep stage 3; NPT: neuropsychological tests; PSG: polysomnography; SE: sleep efficiency; SWS: slow wave sleep; WASO: wake after sleep onset

Conclusion
Gabapentin increased slow wave sleep, improved sleep efficiency and decreased arousals in persons with primary insomnia.

Commentary

Insomnia is the most prevalent sleep disorder in the general adult population and is associated with medical and psychiatric morbidity, impaired daytime function, and reduced quality of life.[1] Additionally, in recent years, insomnia has achieved wide recognition as a comorbid condition requiring targeted intervention.[2] Although efficacious pharmacologic and behavioral treatments exist for the treatment of insomnia, many patients find these either intolerable or ineffective. Unique insomnia treatments are needed.

When compared to the sleep effects of other medications commonly prescribed for insomnia, the findings in this study represent a promising foundation for gabapentin as a unique treatment for insomnia. The physiologic findings of increased N3 sleep, increased Delta-2 and theta power, and increased parasympathetic activity strongly support gabapentin as having a unique effect profile. This particular constellation of effects is not documented for benzodiazepine and non-benzodiazepine hypnotics or frequently used antidepressant medications such as trazodone, amitriptyline and doxepin.

Gabapentin has been widely studied across a variety of psychiatric and medical conditions including restless leg syndrome, multiple pain conditions (i.e. fibromyalgia and neuropathic pain of various etiologies), menopausal symptoms, generalized anxiety disorder, posttraumatic stress disorder, panic disorder, and bipolar disorder.[3-7] Across studies and across disease states gabapentin has been associated with subjective and/or objective improvements in sleep.

Foldvary-Schaefer and colleagues published findings in 2002 that showed increased slow wave sleep and minor reductions in arousals, awakenings, and sleep stage shifts with administration of gabapentin in normal adults.[8] Despite these data indicating a primary effect of gabapentin on sleep architecture, there are no published reports of use of this drug explicitly for the treatment of insomnia. Accordingly, the findings of Lo and colleagues provide a much-needed examination of sleep specific effects of this drug on insomnia uncomplicated by medical or psychiatric comorbidity.

The authors suggest that the adverse event profile of gabapentin may be preferable to that of traditional sedative-hypnotic medications. However, no data exist to indicate that differences in adverse event profiles provide an advantage for gabapentin in terms of improved tolerance or reduced attrition in insomnia patients.

Although gabapentin has been shown to be relatively safe, caution is warranted before recommending this medication as a primary therapy for the treatment of insomnia.[9] There are a multitude of medications currently being prescribed off label for the treatment of insomnia with a paucity of data to support their use. Given some of the methodological questions in the current study, further evaluation – including double blinded studies – is warranted before recommending wide spread clinical use. Specifically, a double-blind placebo-controlled study would help to firmly establish this drug as an effective primary therapy for insomnia. Additionally, the majority of insomnia patients seen in clinical practice have comorbid rather than primary insomnia. Accordingly investigation of the effectiveness of gabapentin explicitly for treatment of chronic comorbid insomnia would have a high level of generalizeability and clinical relevance.

Robert N. Glidewell
Lynn Institute for Healthcare Research

Gregory A. Ruff
Pulmonary Associates, Colorado Springs

References

1. Partinen M et al. Epidemiology of Sleep Disorders. In Kryger MH, Roth T, and Dement WC (Eds) Principles and Practices of Sleep Medicine. Philadelphia: Elsevier-Saunders, 694-715.

2. NIH State of the Science Conference statement on Manifestations and Management of Chronic Insomnia in Adults statement. J Clin Sleep Med. 2005; 1(4):412-421.

3. Hamner MB et al. Gabapentin in PTSD: A retrospective clinical series of adjunctive therapy. Ann Clin Psych. 2001; 13:141-146.

4. Vieta E et al. A double-blind, placebo-controlled, prophylaxis study of adjunctive gabapentin for bipolar disorder. J Clin Psychiatry. 2006; 67(3):473-7.

5. Yurcheshen ME et al. Effects of gabapentin on sleep in menopausal women with hot flashes as measured by a Pittsburgh Sleep Quality Index factor scoring model. Journal of Women's Health. 2009; 18:1355-1360.

6. Gordh TE et al. Gabapentin in traumatic nerve injury pain: A randomized, double-blind, placebo-controlled, cross-over, multicenter study. Pain. 2008; 138:255-266.

7. Malcolm R et al. Self-reported sleep, sleepiness, and repeated alcohol withdrawals: A randomized, double blind, controlled comparison of lorazepam vs. gabapentin. J Clin Sleep Med. 2007; 3:24-32.

8. Foldvary-Schaefer I et al. Gabapentin increases slow-wave sleep in normal adults. Epilepsia. 2002; 43:1493-1497.

9. Wilton L et al. A postmarketing surveillance study of gabapentin as an add-on therapy for 3100 patients in England. Epilepsia. 2002; 43:983-99.

Sleep-Related Breathing Disorders

A multicenter, prospective study of a novel nasal EPAP device in the treatment of obstructive sleep apnea: efficacy and 30-day adherence. Rosenthal L, Massie CA, Dolan DC, Loomas B, Kram J, Hart RW. *J Clin Sleep Med. 2009 Dec 15;5(6):532-7.*

How effective is a nasal expiratory resistance device for the treatment of obstructive sleep apnea?

Subjects	Methods	Outcomes
34 subjects • Age: 27-67 yrs • AHI: ≥ 5	Protocol (30-day in-home trial): • 1 diagnostic PSG • 3 treatment PSGs • 1 PSG at end of trial	Compared to baselines, use of a nasal expiratory resistance device was associated with: • Decrease in AHI: 24.5 ± 23.6 to 13.5 ± 18.7* 1. AHI was 15.5 ± 18.9** at end of trial • Of 24 subjects with AHI > 10 at baseline, 13 and 10 had AHI < 10 on the initial and final treatment nights, respectively • Decrease in % of night snoring: 27.5 ± 23.2 to 11.6 ± 13.7*** on initial treatment nights and 14.6 ± 20.6# at end of trial • Decrease in ESS: 8.7 ± 4.0 to 6.9 ± 4.4## at end of trial • Improvement in PSQI: 7.4 ± 3.3 to 6.5 ± 3.6### • Increase in mean SaO_2: 94.8 ± 2.0 to 95.2 ± 1.9^ on initial treatment nights and 95.3 ± 1.9^^ at end of trial • No change in sleep architecture Subjects reported 94% all-night device use during the trial

AHI: apnea hypopnea index; ESS: Epworth sleepiness score; OSA: obstructive sleep apnea; PSG: polysomnography; PSQI: Pittsburgh sleep quality index; SaO_2: arterial oxygen saturation; *P < 0.001 ; **P = 0.001 ; ***P < 0.001 ; #P = 0.013 ; ##P < 0.001 ; ###P = 0.042 ; ^P = 0.023 ; ^^P = 0.003

Conclusion

A nasal expiratory resistance device improved snoring, apnea hypopnea indices, symptoms, oxygen saturation and subjective sleepiness in persons with obstructive sleep apnea.

Commentary

The study evaluated the efficacy of the Provent (Ventus Medical, Belmont CA) device in the treatment of OSA, which represents the newest available therapy for OSA. The device was approved by the FDA in 2008; it consists of two valves (one in each nostril) held in place by adhesive tape. The valves offer no resistance during inhalation but generate expiratory positive airway pressure, which were shown to offer therapeutic benefit in a pilot study of OSA patients.[1] Participants were recruited at 3-centers in metropolitan areas of the US. Subjects with an AHI of ≥ 5 (N = 34; age: 27 to 67) with no other co-morbid sleep conditions and in otherwise stable medical condition were included. Participants completed 4-nights of in-laboratory polysomnography (PSG) in random order (one control and 3-nights using expiratory resistances of 50, 80 and 110 cm H2O*sec/liter) followed by 30-days of in-home use of assigned device with an additional PSG at the end of the month. The assigned device was based on a pre-defined algorithm, which was based on maximal reduction of AHI with a bias toward using the lower possible resistance device. The AHI was reduced from 24.5 ± 24 to 15.5 ± 19 at 30 days. Only 10 of 24 subjects with control AHI >10 had a reduction in AHI to <10. While no improvement was noted in sleep architecture, sleep continuity, minimum SaO2 level or on the oxygen desaturation index (≥ 3%), the percent of time snoring was significantly decreased from 28 ± 23 to 15 ± 21%. Epworth scores showed a significant reduction from 8.7 ± 4.0 to 6.9 ± 4.4.

The availability of an additional therapeutic option for patients with OSA represents a welcome addition to the clinical armamentarium. However, the variable and inconsistent response documented in this cohort was greeted with caution in a commentary by Dr. David White.[2] He appropriately raises concerns about persistent sleep disruption and intermittent hypoxia in these subjects. In this context, it is surprising that subjects reported improved alertness on the Epworth scale. An additional critical issue relates to the mechanism by which nasal resistors improve ventilation during sleep. Efforts at characterizing the mechanism of action have yielded mixed results.[3] While it is clear that patients who benefit from the device need to be able to breathe through their nose in order to generate positive end expiratory pressure (PEEP), questions about the precise mechanism of action remain germane.

Additional data on the use of the device has been presented. Walsh et al reported on the outcome of 5-week use of the device in a cohort of OSA subjects who refused CPAP therapy. Therapeutic benefit was documented on the device.[4] In a critical 3-month, multi-center, sham-device study Berry et al confirmed therapeutic benefits in a large cohort.[5] Oximetry data, sleep continuity and sleep architecture were also significantly improved by the device. However, the unpredictable pattern of response has remained a critical issue. Data on the effectiveness of the device following alcohol consumption and/or CNS depressants remains unexplored.

The clinical experience with the device has been consistent with published data. There are no elements to enable the reliable identification of patients best suited for this therapy. Adaptation to the device is often difficult and many patients discontinue treatment. For those who find it tolerable, therapeutic response often falls short from desirable. On the other hand, those who tolerate it (and achieve adequate therapeutic response) become ardent proponents of this new treatment.

Leon Rosenthal
Sleep Medicine Associates of Texas
Dallas, TX

References
1. Colrain IM et al. A pilot evaluation of a nasal expiratory resistance device for the treatment of obstructive sleep apnea. J Clin Sleep Med. 2008; 4:426-33.
2. White DP. Auto-PEEP to Treat Obstructive Sleep Apnea. J Clin Sleep Med. 2009; 5(6):538-539.
3. Patel AV et al. Predictors of response to a nasal expiratory resistor device and its potential mechanisms of action for treatment of Obstructive Sleep Apnea (OSA). J Clin Sleep Med (in press).
4. Walsh JK et al. A convenient expiratory positive airway pressure nasal device for the treatment of sleep apnea in patients non-adherent with CPAP. Sleep Med. 2011; 12(2):147-52.
5. Berry RB et al. A Novel Nasal Expiratory Positive Airway Pressure (EPAP) Device for the Treatment of OSA: A Randomized Controlled Trial. Sleep (in press).

Adenotonsillectomy outcomes in treatment of obstructive sleep apnea in children: a multicenter retrospective study. Bhattacharjee R, Kheirandish-Gozal L, Spruyt K, Mitchell RB, Promchiarak J, Simakajornboon N, Kaditis AG, Splaingard D, Splaingard M, Brooks LJ, Marcus CL, Sin S, Arens R, Verhulst SL, Gozal D. *Am J Respir Crit Care Med. 2010 Sep 1;182(5):676-83.*

What factors predict successful outcomes following adenotonsillectomy for obstructive sleep apnea in children?

Subjects	Methods	Outcomes
578 children who underwent AT for OSA • Age: 6.9 ± 3.8 yrs • Weight: 50% were obese • BMI z-score: 1.35±1.74 • Mean AHI: 18.2±21.4 Exclusion criteria • Underlying medical condition • Inappropriate timing of repeat PSG	Multicenter retrospective review Assessments: • Preoperative and postoperative PSGs • Note: Repeat PSG performed > 40 days and < 720 days following AT	Results of AT • Decrease in AHI: 18.2 ± 21.4 vs. 4.1 ± 6.4* • 27.2% (n = 157) of subjects had complete resolution of OSA (AHI < 1) Factors that contributed to post-AT AHI • Age** • BMI z-score** • Presence of asthma • Pre-AT AHI (non-obese)***

AHI: apnea hypopnea index; AT: adenotonsillectomy; BMI: body mass index; OSA: obstructive sleep apnea; PSG: polysomnography; TST: total sleep time; US: United States; *P < 0.001; **P < 0.001; ***P < 0.05

Conclusion

Many children had incomplete resolution of obstructive sleep apnea following adenotonsillectomy, and risk factors associated with residual sleep disordered breathing were advanced age, obesity, presence of asthma and severity of underlying obstructive sleep apnea.

Commentary

Obstructive sleep apnea (OSA) is estimated to affect 2-3% of all children.[1,2] While this condition is associated with an increased burden to health care[3], it does lead to significant comorbidities in childhood including neurocognitive and behavioral disturbances[4], cardiovascular dysfunction[5], metabolic and inflammatory disease.[6]

Hypertrophy of adenotonsillar tissue constitutes the most significant risk factor to the development of OSA in children as impingement of the upper airway induced by these inflammatory tissues leads to profound increases in airway resistance and ultimately episodic airway collapse characteristic of OSA.[7] It is therefore not surprising that the guidelines established by the Task Force of the American Academy of Pediatrics recommend adenotonsillectomy (AT) as the first line of treatment in childhood OSA. Furthermore, OSA has become the current most common indication for AT in children, surpassing recurrent tonsillar infections as the primary indication.[8]

The purpose of this study was to examine not only the efficacy of AT in the treatment of OSA in children, but also to ascribe risk factors associated with residual sleep disordered breathing (SDB) in children undergoing AT. By selecting centers that routinely perform nocturnal polysomnography (NPSG) pre- and post- AT in children, the study coupled polysomnographic data from pre-AT NPSG to demographical data from retrospective chart review to create a multi-variate linear regression model in order to determine which factors were most strongly influential on the study primary outcome, post-AT AHI, as a marker of residual sleep disordered breathing following surgery.

Analysis of data available in 578 children revealed that while AT resulted in significant improvements in most parameters of SDB in children, AT only resulted in complete resolution, as defined by post-AT AHI<1 event/hr, in 27.2% of children, suggesting that the vast majority were left with some degree of residual SDB.

By order of influence, advancing age (particularly age > 7 years), advancing BMI z-score (a marker of obesity), presence of asthma, and severity of underlying OSA (as defined by pre-AT AHI) were all significantly associated with post-AT AHI, thereby emerging as the major risk factors determining the effectiveness of AT in the treatment of childhood OSA. Of note, the presence of asthma and the severity of underlying OSA were found to be particularly influential in non-obese children (BMI z-score < 1.65).

While debate remains on the utility of pre-AT AHI in the approach to pediatric OSA[9,10], this study does provide insights into the judicious implementation of post-AT NPSG in children with a higher risk for residual OSA.

Taken together, until prospective studies become available, the study supports the notion that older children, obese children, and non-obese children with asthma or severe OSA are at an elevated risk for residual SDB or overt OSA following AT, and may therefore benefit from polysomnography after surgery.

David Gozal
Department of Pediatrics
Comer Children's Hospital
The University of Chicago

Rakesh Bhattacharjee
Department of Pediatrics
Comer Children's Hospital
The University of Chicago

Leila Kheirandish-Gozal
Department of Pediatrics
Comer Children's Hospital
The University of Chicago

References

1. Lumeng JC et al. Epidemiology of pediatric obstructive sleep apnea. Proc Am Thorac Soc. 2008; 5(2):242-252.

2. Montgomery-Downs HE et al. Snoring and sleep-disordered breathing in young children: subjective and objective correlates. Sleep. 2004; 27(1):87-94.

3. Tarasiuk A et al. Elevated morbidity and health care use in children with obstructive sleep apnea syndrome. Am J Respir Crit Care Med. 2007; 175(1):55-61.

4. Gozal D. Sleep-disordered breathing and school performance in children. Pediatrics. 1998; 102(3 Pt 1):616-620.

5. Bhattacharjee R et al. Cardiovascular complications of obstructive sleep apnea syndrome: evidence from children. Prog Cardiovasc Dis. 2009; 51(5):416-433.

6. Gozal D et al. Metabolic alterations and systemic inflammation in obstructive sleep apnea among nonobese and obese prepubertal children. Am J Respir Crit Care Med. 2008; 177(10):1142-1149.

7. Marcus CL et al. Upper airway collapsibility in children with obstructive sleep apnea syndrome. J Appl Physiol. 1994; 77(2):918-924.

8. Erickson BK et al. Changes in incidence and indications of tonsillectomy and adenotonsillectomy, 1970-2005. Otolaryngol Head Neck Surg. 2009; 140(6):894-901.

9. Friedman NR. Polysomnography should not be required both before and after adenotonsillectomy for childhood sleep disordered breathing. J Clin Sleep Med. 2007; 3(7):678-680.

10. Hoban TF. Polysomnography should be required both before and after adenotonsillectomy for childhood sleep disordered breathing. J Clin Sleep Med. 2007; 3(7):675-677.

Automatic slow eye movement (SEM) detection of sleep onset in patients with obstructive sleep apnea syndrome (OSAS): comparison between multiple sleep latency test (MSLT) and maintenance of wakefulness test (MWT). Fabbri M, Pizza F, Magosso E, Ursino M, Contardi S, Cirignotta F, Provini F, Montagna P. *Sleep Med. 2010 Mar;11(3):253-7.*

How does automatic detection of slow eye movements compare with standard scoring criteria of sleep onset during multiple sleep latency test and maintenance of wakefulness test in persons with obstructive sleep apnea?

Subjects	Methods	Outcomes
20 subjects with severe OSA • 8 subjects had EDS (ESS)	Assessments: • MLST SOL • MWT SOL • Automatically detected SEM latency	Mean SEM latency was comparable to SOL in both MSLT* and MWT** Mean SEM latency correlated significantly with MSLT SOL*** and MWT SOL[#] ESS score correlated with MWT SEM latency[##] but not with MSLT

ESS: Epworth sleepiness scale; MSLT: Multiple sleep latency test; MWT: Maintenance of wakefulness test; OSA: obstructive sleep apnea; SEM: slow eye movement; SOL: sleep onset latency; *6.4+/-5.5 min vs. 7.4+/-5.1 min, P = 0.25; **25.2+/-14.5 min vs. 24.4+/-14.0 min, P = 0.45; ***R = 0.52, P < 0.05; [#]R = 0.74, P < 0.001; [##]R = -0.62, P < 0.01

Conclusion
Sleep onset based on automatically detected slow eye movement latency was comparable to, and correlated with, sleep onset latency identified during multiple sleep latency test and maintenance of wakefulness test in persons with obstructive sleep apnea.

Commentary
Daytime sleepiness is a problem reported by 10–25% of the population.[1] Excessive daytime sleepiness (EDS) is defined as sleepiness that occurs at a time when the individual is usually expected to be awake and alert.[2] EDS may adversely impact work, road safety and public health with relevant costs for the society.[3]

Psychomotor tests, subjective scales and neurophysiological measures are largely used to asses sleepiness, but the Multiple Sleep Latency Test (MSLT) and the Maintenance Wakefulness Test (MWT) are the only objective laboratory-based tools currently validated for the diagnosis and management of patients with EDS.[4] MSLT is used to measure "sleep propensity", whereas MWT explores the "ability to remain awake", and both use the standard visual scoring of sleep that requires sleep montage (EEG, EOG and chin EMG), dedicated technicians and a polysomnography laboratory.

Although the eyes are closed during sleep, oculomotor activity persists and is characterized by distinct eye movements. Slow eye movements (SEMs) are known to clinicians as a phenomenon typical of the wake–sleep transition.[5-7]

In the last 5 years of our studies on sleepiness, we developed and validated an automatic method for the detection of SEMs[8,9] based on a wavelet transform of the EOG tracings. This method allows an easy, reliable, off-line detection of SEMs and has already been applied to the detection of the sleep onset (SO) during the MSLT.[10]

In the present study, we compared the standard defined SO with the SEM-defined SO in order to confirm previous findings obtained on MSLT recordings[10] and to extend the applicability of this approach on MWT recordings, both performed in 20 patients with severe Obstructive Sleep Apnea Syndrome (OSAS).

The MSLT requires that patients lay with closed-eyes trying to fall asleep, whereas during the MWT patients are seated and instructed to remain awake keeping their eyes opened. Thus, the efficacious application of SEMs in both situations extends the reliability of this method in identifying drowsiness in two distinct physiological conditions.

On MSLT data, comparing our defined measure of "SEM latency" (elapsed time from lights-off to the first epoch with 50% of time occupied by SEMs) with the standard sleep latency (SL, elapsed time from lights-out to the occurrence of a single epoch of sleep stage 1 or any other sleep stage), we found that the "mean SEM latency" significantly correlated only with SL. Moreover, on MWT data, SL was significantly correlated with SEM latency, showing even closer relation than in the MSLT recordings. Finally, we found that subjective sleepiness evaluated with the Epworth Sleepiness Scale correlated with the MWT, but not with the MSLT results.

Our study, even if applied on a population of selected type of hypersomnia, proved that SEMs automatic detection could simplify the currently techniques for routine assessment of EDS opening the possibility to use a simpler and cheaper laboratory setting. Moreover, the strict correlation of SEMs with SL is in line with the occurrence of SEMs during the early phase of the wake-sleep transition, disclosing its potential in detecting the early process of falling asleep. Finally, we proved the reliability of SEMs analysis in both the MSLT and MWT recordings. The applicability of our method on open-eyes recordings discloses the possibility to apply the SEMs detection in a real-life setting. New and easy methods of real-time sleepiness detection could be largely useful in order to prevent sleepiness-related accident and to diminish its cost on the society.

Margherita Fabbri
Department of Neurological Sciences
University of Bologna

References

1. Roehr T et al. Daytime sleepiness and alertness. In: Kryger MH, Roth T, Dement WC, editors. Principles and practice of sleep medicine 4th ed. Elsevier Saunders, 2005.

2. American Academy of Sleep Medicine ICSD–2. International classification of sleep disorders, 2nd ed. Diagnostic and coding manual. Illinois: Westchester, American Academy of Sleep Medicine, 2005.

3. Akerstedt T et al. Sleep and sleepiness in relation to stress and displaced work hours. Physiol Behav. 2007; 92:250-5.

4. Littner MR et al. Standards of practice committee of the American Academy of Sleep Medicine. Practice parameters for clinical use of the multiple sleep latency test and the maintenance of wakefulness test. Sleep. 2005; 28:113-21

5. Liberson WT et al. EEG records, reaction times, eye movements, respiration, and mental content during drowsiness. Recent Adv Biol Psychiatry. 1965; 8:295-302.

6. Hori T. Electrodermal and electro-oculographic activity in hypnagogic state. Psychophysiology. 1982; 19:668-72.

7. De Gennaro L et al. Slow eye movements and EEG power spectra during wake–sleep transition. Clin Neuro-Physiol. 2000; 111:2107-15.

8. Magosso E et al. A wavelet method for automatic detection of slow eye movements: a pilot study. Med Eng Phys. 2006; 28:860-75.

9. Magosso E et al. Visual and computer-based detection of slow eye movements in overnight and 24-h EOG. Clin Neurophysiol. 2007; 118:1-11.

10. Fabbri M et al. Detection of sleep onset by analysis of slow eye movements: A preliminary study of MSLT recordings. Sleep Med. 2009; 10(6):637-40.

Auto-titrating continuous positive airway pressure for patients with acute transient ischemic attack: a randomized feasibility trial. Bravata DM, Concato J, Fried T, Ranjbar N, Sadarangani T, McClain V, Struve F, Zygmunt L, Knight HJ, Lo A, Richerson GB, Gorman M, Williams LS, Brass LM, Agostini J, Mohsenin V, Roux F, Yaggi HK. *Stroke. 2010 Jul;41(7):1464-70.*

What is the prevalence of sleep apnea in persons with acute transient ischemic attacks, and is recurrence rate of the former affected by automatic positive airway pressure therapy of sleep apnea?

Subjects	Methods	Outcomes
70 subjects with acute TIA	Subjects were assigned to one of 2 groups: • Intervention: n = 45 1. APAP for 2 nights 2. Subjects with OSA received APAP for 90 days • Control: n = 25 Assessments: • PSG at baseline and at 90 days after TIA Definitions: • Acceptable APAP adherence: ≥ 4 hours per night for ≥ 75% of nights • Vascular events: death, hospitalization for CHF, MI, recurrent TIA, stroke	Prevalence of SA • At baseline: 57% • At 90 days: 59% 30 subjects in the intervention group had airflow obstruction • 40% (n = 12) had acceptable APAP adherence • 60% (n = 18) had some use Recurrent events were noted in: • 12% (n = 3) of intervention group • 2% (n = 1) of control group* Vascular event rate among SA subjects: • No APAP use: 16% • Some APAP use: 5% • Acceptable APAP adherence: 0%**

APAP: auto-titrating continuous positive airway pressure; CHF: congestive heart failure; MI: myocardial infarction; PSG: polysomnography; SA: sleep apnea; TIA: transient ischemic attack; *P = 0.13; **P = 0.08

Conclusion
Sleep apnea was common during the post-acute transient ischemic attack period.

Commentary

Patients with transient ischemic attack (TIA) are at high risk of adverse events. An expected 25% of patients with TIA will have a cerebrovascular or cardiovascular event or death in the 90-days post-event.[1-3] Because patients with TIA have little neurological impairment, yet are at high risk of recurrent vascular events, they are ideal candidates for interventions to reduce their risk of adverse events. Given that half of the recurrent events occur in the first two days post-TIA,[3] new interventions are needed that can be applied in the acute TIA period.

The stroke community has long called for the development of new therapies for patients with acute cerebrovascular events. This article provides evidence to support a novel approach to improving outcomes for patients with acute TIA; namely, via treatment of sleep apnea. Sleep apnea occurs in at least 60% of patients with TIA. Auto-titrating continuous positive airway pressure (auto-CPAP) safely and effectively treats sleep apnea.

In this randomized controlled strategy trial, patients with acute TIA were randomly assigned to an intervention group and control group. All intervention patients received auto-CPAP for two nights. The auto-CPAP machine was interrogated after two nights. If there was no evidence of airflow limitation (apnea hypopnea index [AHI] < 5 or median pressure < 6 cmH$_2$0), then the auto-CPAP was discontinued. If there was evidence of airflow limitation, then the auto-CPAP was continued for the remainder of the 90-day period. Intervention patients received polysomnography at 90-days post-TIA. Control patients received polysomnography at baseline and at 90-days.

The results of our study demonstrated that it is feasible to diagnose and treat sleep apnea using auto-titrating continuous positive airway pressure (auto-CPAP) in the acute transient ischemic attack (TIA) period. Using auto-CPAP in the acute TIA setting appeared to be a therapeutic approach for which the majority of stroke patients were eligible, which could be delivered safely to patients, and which did not require any specialized infrastructure.

Two noteworthy aspects of this study merit additional commentary. First, the study was designed to use auto-CPAP on patients with TIA—as opposed to a focus on patients with known sleep apnea. Given that the prevalence of sleep apnea is very high in this population, the minority of patients were exposed to auto-CPAP without underlying sleep apnea. The diagnostic capability of the auto-CPAP units was used to identify the patients with some evidence of airflow obstruction; for these patients, the auto-CPAP was continued. Definitive sleep apnea diagnoses were made on the basis of unattended polysomnography 90-days after enrollment.

Second, the study was designed to enroll patients in the acute TIA period. Much of the prior research had focused on patients who were distant from a cerebrovascular event; however these results support the feasibility of using auto-CPAP early after a cerebrovascular event. This early application of treatment is key to reducing the post-TIA event rate, given the very high risk of events early in the post-TIA course. Protocols that require a polysomnography prior to initiation of CPAP therapy necessarily pose delays in providing therapy to patients. Although it is theoretically possible to perform an attended polysomnography at the TIA patient's bedside and then provide CPAP to patients with a preliminarily positive study, in reality, most centers require patients to be physically present within a sleep laboratory for the conduct of attended polysomnography and only patients with the most severe sleep apnea are provided CPAP in "split night" studies. The reading of the polysomnography usually confers additional delays in treatment. Therefore, our approach of using auto-CPAP without polysomnography in the acute TIA setting provided the earliest treatment to the greatest number of patients with minimal exposure of auto-CPAP to the minority without sleep apnea.

The current study was not designed to provide adequate sample size to evaluate the efficacy of this treatment strategy for the reduction of vascular events. A larger clinical trial is currently underway to examine the use auto-CPAP among patients with TIA that might provide additional information about the effectiveness of diagnosing and treating sleep apnea for the reduction of vascular events.

Dawn M. Bravata
VA Stroke Quality Enhancement Research Initiative (QUERI)
Indiana University School of Medicine
VA HSR&D Center of Excellence on Implementing Evidence-Based Practice
Richard L. Roudebush VA Medical Center

References

1. Johnston S et al Short-term prognosis after emergency department diagnosis of TIA. JAMA. 2000; 284:2901-2906.
2. Johnston S. Short-term prognosis after a TIA: a simple score predicts risk. Cleveland Clinic Journal of Medicine. 2007; 74(10):729-736.
3. Rothwell P et al. Transient ischemic attacks: stratifying risk. Stroke. 2006; 37(2):320-322.

Beneficial effects of adaptive servo ventilation in patients with chronic heart failure. Koyama T, Watanabe H, Kobukai Y, Makabe S, Munehisa Y, Iino K, Kosaka T, Ito H. *Circ J. 2010 Oct;74(10):2118-24.*

Can adaptive servo ventilation improve cardiac function and reduce the inflammatory response in persons with heart failure and sleep disordered breathing?

Subjects	Methods	Outcomes
17 subjects with CHF and SDB • NYHA II or III	Intervention: PSG with and without ASV • ASV – n = 10 • Non-ASV – n = 7 Assessments before and after ASV treatment: • BNP • EF • Hs-CRP	Correlation was noted between: • AHI and hs-CRP* • Increase in EF and decrease in hs-CRP## In the ASV group (but not in the ASV group), significant improvements were noted in: • BNP** • EF*** • hs-CRP# • NYHA class

AHI: apnea hypopnea index; ASV: adaptive servo ventilation; BNP: brain natriuretic peptide; CHF: congestive heart failure; EF: ejection fraction; hsCRP: high-sensitivity C-reactive protein; NYHA: New York Heart Association; PSG: polysomnography; SDB: sleep disordered breathing; *r=0.753, P=0.016; **212.1 ± 181.2 to 77.3 ± 54.0 pg/ml [P < 0.05]; ***43.5 ± 6.4 to 53.3 ± 6.1% [P = 0.002]; #0.85 ± 0.58 to 0.21 ± 0.19 mg/dl [P = 0.008]

Conclusion
In persons with heart failure and sleep disordered breathing, adaptive servo ventilation improved heart function and attenuated the inflammatory response.

Commentary
Heart failure is a highly prevalent disorder and a major public health burden in the United States. Among all cardiovascular diseases, heart failure is the second most common outpatient diagnosis, surpassed only by systemic hypertension. In 2007, the number of visits for heart failure was estimated at an astounding 3,434,000. In 2007, close to one million patients were discharged from hospitals with heart failure listed as the primary diagnosis.[1] Although the prevalence is 2% among general population, it is estimated to be 10% in individuals 65 years and older. Approximately 80% of heart failure patients are 65 or older, making heart failure the most common Medicare diagnosis-related group. The disease burden will increase considerably as the number of people over 65 years is estimated to increase to 77 million, 21% of the population, by 2040.

Due in part to its high prevalence, the economic impact of the heart failure was estimated at a staggering 39 billion US dollars in 2009.[2] In addition, heart failure is also associated with excess mortality estimated at 290000 in 2006 with more than 90% of mortality occurring in older people.

In summary, heart failure is a common disorder with increasing prevalence in an aging population, and is associated with excess morbidity and mortality in spite of recent triumphs in pharmacological and device therapy. Therefore the identification and treatment of heart failure co-morbidities which contribute to morbidity and mortality is one current challenge that needs to be pursued systematically and aggressively. The hope is that identification of these co-morbidities and appropriate therapy will further improve the survival of patients with heart failure. In this regard, there are multiple co-morbidities which have been identified including anemia, depression, renal dysfunction and sleep-related breathing disorders, with the last co-morbidity being the least recognized by cardiologists and primary care physicians who take care of patients with heart failure.

In the last several years worldwide studies have shown that in ambulatory patients with stable heart failure, sleep apnea is highly prevalent. Analysis of the studies from US[3-5], Great Britain[6], Canada[7], and Germany[8] indicates that out of 1,250 consecutive patients with systolic heart failure, 52% have an apnea hypopnea index of 15 or more per hour.[2] It is noted that a threshold of ≥ 15 per hour is considered moderate sleep apnea and individuals with an index of ≥ 30 per hour are considered to have severe sleep apnea. With respect to the two major phenotypes of sleep apnea, central sleep apnea accounts for about 31% and obstructive apnea for about 21% of the of sleep apnea in patients with heart failure and low left ventricular ejection fraction.

Data in patients with heart failure and preserved left ventricular ejection fraction has been scarce; in the largest study[9] of 244 consecutive patients, 48% had an apnea hypopnea index of 15 or more per hour, of whom 23 had CSA and 25% OSA. However, there is considerable variability in the reported proportions of central versus obstructive sleep apnea in heart failure. This difference is multifactorial and in part due to the inherent difficulty in differentiating the two kinds of hypopneas.

Nonetheless, the aforementioned studies make heart failure one of the most common risk factors for sleep apnea. Yet, sleep apnea remains under diagnosed in heart failure patients. A retrospective cohort study[10], which used the 2004-2005 Medicare Standard Analytical Files (these files contain a 5 % sample of randomly selected Medicare beneficiaries) found that among a population of 30,719 newly diagnosed HF patients, only 1,263 (4%) were clinically suspected to have sleep apnea.[10] Of these, 553 (only 2% of the total cohort) were tested for sleep apnea. The reasons for under-diagnosis are multiple and one major factor is that CSA is an occult disorder.[10] Such patients are commonly thin, do not snore much and do not have excessive day time sleepiness.[11]

Meanwhile, multiple studies[12-19] have shown that co-morbid sleep apnea independent of other confounders decreases survival of patients with systolic heart failure. In regards to CSA, we followed 88 consecutive male heart failure patients in Veterans Affairs Medical Center in Cincinnati, 56 with and 32 without CSA. The median follow-up was 51 months.[12] In multiple regression analysis controlling for 24 confounding variables, CSA was independently associated with excess mortality (hazard ratio=2.14, P = 0.02). The average survival of heart failure patients without CSA was 90 months compared to 45 months of those with CSA. That CSA contributes to excess mortality in systolic heart failure is supported by the observation that effective treatment of CSA improves survival.[14]

Treatment of CSA in heart failure with positive airway pressure (PAP) devices. Several PAP devices, including continuous positive airway pressure (CPAP), bilevel pressure, and adaptive pressure support servoventilation (ASV) have been used to treat central sleep apnea in patients with heart failure.[20-22] However, only CPAP has been subjected to a long-term randomized clinical trial and unfortunately with unfavorable results.[23] In this study 258 patients were randomized into 2 arms, a control group and the CPAP arm. Patients were followed for an average of 2 years. At 3 months, when the first CPAP polysomnography was performed, only 57% of heart failure patients with CSA were CPAP-responsive. In these patients AHI decreased below 15/hour. In the remaining 47% of patients in whom CSA persisted (consistent with a prior report[24], a post-hoc analysis[14] demonstrated higher mortality. It has been suggested that the adverse hemodynamic effects of CPAP contributed to the excess mortality in the CPAP non-responders.[25] CPAP increases intrathoracic pressure which could impede venous return and decrease cardiac output and cause hypotension. The effect of CPAP on hemodynamics depends on multiple factors including ventricular preload and intravascular volume. In any case the treatment of CPAP resistant CSA in heart failure (almost 50% of the patients) remains a challenge. Currently we treat such patients with adaptive servo ventilation devices.

ASV devices to treat CPAP resistant CSA. There are 2 such devices available in US: BiPAP auto SV Advanced and VPAP Adapt ASV Enhanced (Autoset CS in Japan). These devices have been used to effectively treat CSA in idiopathic CSA[26], sleep apnea associated with opioids[27] and central sleep apnea in congestive heart failure[28-36], generally with favorable results. They have different algorithms, however. In general, these devices provide varying amounts of inspiratory support during different phases of periodic breathing. The support is proportional, being minimal during the hyperpneic phase of periodic breathing and maximal during periods of diminished breathing. This is in contrast to bilevel devices which provide fix preset inspiratory support independent of the patient ventilation. Meanwhile, the expiratory pressure is to titrated either manually (in ASV) or automatically (In BiPap auto SV Advanced) to eliminate obstructive disordered breathing events. In addition, both ASV devices can initiate mandatory breaths on a timely basis preventing development of a central apnea.

Koyama and associates[37] used an ASV device (Autoset CS) to treat central sleep apnea in patients with heart failure and low left ventricular systolic function. This was a nonrandomized study of 17 patients, 10 of whom used ASV for 4 weeks. The other 7 patients did not agree to use the device or were intolerant. Patients had a mildly reduced left ventricular ejection fraction of about 44%. About 30% to 40% of these patients were on beta blockers. They had severe sleep apnea with an average AHI of 35 per hour. The central apnea index was about 17 per hour. There was mild arterial oxyhemoglobin desaturation with a minimum SaO_2 of about 84%. ASV settings included an expiratory pressure which ranged from 4 cm H_2O to 6 cm H_2O and the inspiratory support was set on a default status. This means that there was a minimum support of 3 cm H_2O and a maximum support of 8 cm H_2O which was variable across the night based on the algorithm of the device. After 4 weeks of use of ASV (the compliance hours were not reported), the AHI decreased from about 37 per hour to 5 per hour in the ASV-treated group and remained unchanged at about 33 per hour in the non-ASV group. As a result, the arousal index decreased from about 28 per hour to 10 per hour in the ASV treated and remained essentially unchanged in the non-ASV group at about 30 per hour. The important cardiac findings were: 1) ejection fraction increased by a striking 10% in the ASV-treated group from 43.5% to 53.3% and remained essentially unchanged at about 46% in the non-ASV treated group; 2) that the proportion of patients moving from higher class to lower functional class of the New York Heart Association increased significantly in the ASV group; 3) BNP decreased, and 4) CRP decreased significantly in the ASV group. The change in CRP correlated with the rise in LVEF. These parameters remained unchanged in the non-ASV group.

The aforementioned findings of Koyoma and associates[37] are extremely important. Once myocardial damage, e.g., ischemic injury, has lead to heart failure, progression of left ventricular dysfunction becomes dependent on an interplay of complex processes including neurohormonal stimulation, inflammation, and oxidative stress. Chronic heart failure is an inflammatory disorder and CRP and other biomarkers of inflammation including TNFα, IL 1,6,and 18 play an important role in the progression of heart failure and CRP is an independent predictor of adverse outcomes in heart failure.[38] Similarly, BNP, a peptide hormone released primarily from ventricular myocytes in response to cellular stretch, is an independent predictor of poor outcomes in heart failure.[39] Finally, a clinically important increase in ejection fraction occurred in the ASV group, which if confirmed should have important prognostic value of improved survival in patients with heart failure.

Therefore, in the absence of long-term trials, it is based on these findings and other similar reports in the literature that I recommend a trial with an ASV device in *first night CPAP nonresponders*. As noted above, 43% to 57% of heart failure patients with CSA are CPAP non-responsive and continuation therapy with CPAP could be associated with excess mortality.

Do we need more ASV trials? Yes, we need randomized clinical trials. Observational studies should open the gate for randomize clinical trials. It is quite common that the results of observational studies are different from randomize clinical trials. Currently there is only one randomized clinical trial with ASV[29]; Pepperell et al performed an excellent study which involved using sham ASV in the control group. After 1 month, there was no significant change in left ventricular ejection fraction, in contrast to Koyoma's observation, but BNP decreased consistent with koyoma's observation.

What is needed are both short- term and long-term randomized clinical trials to determine whether in the short –term trials, surrogates of mortality such as left ventricular ejection fraction, New York Heart association functional class, signatures of neurohormonal activation, inflammation and oxidative stress , and in the long-term trials, quality of life, number of hospitalizations and mortality are affected. We anxiously wait for the results two long-term studies which currently are ongoing. Stay tuned.

Shahrokh Javaheri
University of Cincinnati
Sleepcare Diagnostics

References

1. Heart Disease and Stroke Statistics 2011 Update: A Report from the American Heart Association. Circulation. 2011; 123:e1-e192.

2. Heart Disease and Stroke Statistics 2010 Update: A Report from the American Heart Association. Circulation. 2010; 121:e46-e215.

3. Javaheri S et al. Sleep apnea in 81 ambulatory male patients with stable heart failure: Types and their prevalences, consequences, and presentations. Circulation. 1998; 97:2154-2159.

4. Javaheri S. Sleep disorders in systolic heart failure: A prospective study of 100 male patients. The Final Report. Int J Cardiol. 2006; 106:21-28.

5. MacDonald M et al. The current prevalence of sleep disordered breathing in congestive heart failure patients treated with beta-blockers. J Clin Sleep Med. 2008; 4:38-42.

6. Vazir A et al. A high prevalence of sleep disorder breathing in men with mild symptomatic chronic heart failure due to left ventricular systolic dysfunction. Eur J Heart Failure. 2007; 9: 243-250.

7. Wang H et al. Influence of obstructive sleep apnea on mortality in patients with heart failure. J Am Coll Cardiol. 2007; 49:1625-1631.

8. Oldenburg O et al. Sleep disordered breathing in patients with symptomatic heart failure: a contemporary study of prevalence in and characteristics of 700 patients. Eur J Heart Fail. 2007; 9:251-257.

9. Bitter T et al. Sleep-disordered breathing in heart failure with normal left ventricular ejection fraction. European Journal of Heart Failure. 2009; 11:602-608.

10. Javaheri S et al. Sleep apnea testing and outcomes in a large cohort of Medicare beneficiaries with newly diagnosed heart failure . Am J Respir Crit Care Med. 2011; 183(4):539-46.

11. Javaheri S et al. Occult sleep-disordered breathing in stable congestive heart failure. Ann Intern Med. 1995; 122:487-492.

12. Javaheri S et al. Central sleep apnea, right ventricular dysfunction and low diastolic blood pressure are predictors of mortality in systolic heart failure. J Am Coll Cardiol. 2007; 49:2028-2034.

13. Lanfranchi PA et al. Prognostic value of nocturnal Cheyne-Stokes respiration in chronic heart failure. Circulation. 1999; 99:1435-1440.

14. Arzt M et al. Suppression of central sleep apnea by continuous positive airway pressure and transplant-free survival in heart failure. A post-hoc analysis of the Canadian Continuous Positive Airway Pressure for patients with central sleep apnea and heart failure trial (CANPAP). Circulation. 2007; 115:3173-3180.

15. Hanly PJ et al. Increased mortality associated with Cheyne-Stokes respiration in patients with congestive heart failure. Am J Respir Crit Care Med. 1996; 153:272-276.

16. Sin DD et al. Effects of continuous positive airway pressure on cardiovascular outcomes in heart failure patients with and without Cheyne-Stokes respiration. Circulation. 2000; 102:61-66.

17. Leite JJ et al. Periodic breathing during incremental exercise predicts mortality in patients with chronic heart failure evaluated for cardiac transplantation. J Am Coll Cardiol. 2003; 41:2175-2181.

18. Brack T et al. Daytime Cheyne-Stokes respiration in ambulatory patients with severe congestive heart failure is associated with increased mortality. Chest. 2007; 132:1463-1471.

19. Corra U et al. Sleep and exertional periodic breathing. Circulation. 2006; 113:44-50.

20. Javaheri S. Treatment of obstructive and central sleep apnoea in heart failure: practical options. Eur Respir Rev. 2007; 16:183-188.

21. Javaheri S. Heart failure. In: Kryger MH et al (eds). Principles and Practices of Sleep Medicine. WB Saunders, Philadelphia. 2010; pp 1400-1414.

22. Javaheri S. Positive airway pressure treatment of central sleep apnea with emphasis on heart failure, opioids, and complex sleep apnea. Sleep Medicine Clinics. 2010; 407-417.

23. Bradley T et al. Continuous positive airway pressure for central sleep apnea and heart failure. N Engl J Med. 2006; 353:2025-2033.

24. Javaheri S. Effects of continuous positive airway pressure on sleep apnea and ventricular irritability in patients with heart failure. Circulation. 2000; 101:392-397.

25. Javaheri S. CPAP should not be used for central sleep apnea in congestive heart failure patients. J Clin Sleep Med. 2006; 2:399-402.

26. Banno K et al. Adaptive servo-ventilation in patients with idiopathic Cheyne-Stokes breathing. J Clin Sleep Med. 2006; 2:181-186.

27. Javaheri S et al. Adaptive pressure support servoventilation: a novel treatment for sleep apnea associated with use of opioids. J Clin Sleep Med. 2008; 4:305-310.

28. Teschler H et al. Adaptive pressure support servo-ventilation. Am J Respir Crit Care Med. 2001; 64:614-619.

29. Pepperell J et al. A randomized controlled trial of adaptive ventilation for Cheyne-Stokes breathing in heart failure. Am J Respir Crit Care Med. 2003; 168:1109-1114.

30. Szollosi I et al. Adaptive servo-ventilation and deadspace: effects on central sleep apnoea. J Sleep Res. 2006; 15:199-205.

31. Kasai T et al. First experience of using new adaptive servo-ventilation device for Cheyne-Stokes respiration with central sleep apnea among Japanese patients with congestive heart failure. Circ J. 2006; 70:1148-1154.

32. Fietze I et al. Bi-level positive pressure ventilation and adaptive servo ventilation in patients with heart failure and Cheyne-Stokes respiration. Sleep Med. 2008; 9:652-659.

33. Oldenburg O et al. Adaptive servoventilation improved cardiac function in patients with chronic heart failure and Cheyne-Stokes respiration. Eur J Heart Fail. 2008; 10:581-586.

34. Arzt M et al. Effects of dynamic bilevel positive airway pressure support on central sleep apnea in men with heart failure. Chest. 2008; 134:61-66.

35. Randerath W et al. Adaptive servo-ventilation in patients with coexisting obstructive sleep apnoea/hypopnoea and Cheyne-Stokes respiration. Sleep Med. 2008; 9:823-830.

36. Philippe C et al. Compliance with and effectiveness of adaptive servoventilation versus continuous positive airway pressure in the treatment of Cheyne-Stokes respiration in heart failure over a six month period. Heart. 2006; 92:337-342.

37. Koyama T et al. Beneficial effects of adaptive servoventilation in patients with chronic heart failure. Circ J. 2010; 74:2118-2124.

38. Tsutamoto T et al. Attenuation of compensation of endogenous cardiac naturetic peptide system in chronic heart failue: prognostic role of plasma brain naturetic peptide concentration in patients with chronic symptomatic left ventricular dysfunction. Circulation. 1997; 96:509-516.

39. Anand IS et al. C-reactive protean in heart failure;prognostic value and the effect of valsartan. Circulation. 2005; 112:1428-1434.

Cheyne-Stokes respiration and obstructive sleep apnoea are independent risk factors for malignant ventricular arrhythmias requiring appropriate cardioverter-defibrillator therapies in patients with congestive heart failure. Bitter T, Westerheide N, Prinz C, Hossain MS, Vogt J, Langer C, Horstkotte D, Oldenburg O. *Eur Heart J. 2010 Sep 16.*

Does sleep disordered breathing increase the risk of malignant ventricular arrhythmias in persons with congestive heart failure?

Subjects	Methods	Outcomes
472 subjects with CHF 6 months after implantation of CD • 283 with untreated SDB • 170 with mild or no SDB • 113 declined ventilation therapy	Assessments during 48 months of follow-up: • Number of ventricular arrhythmias • Number of CD therapies	Of 255 subjects, subjects with OSA or CSA had significantly shorter time to 1st monitored ventricular arrhythmias and 1st CD therapy CSA and OSA were independently correlated with: • Monitored ventricular arrhythmias 1. AHI ≥ 5: CSA HR 2.15* and OSA HR 1.69** 2. AHI ≥ 15: CSA HR 2.06*** and OSA HR 1.69[#] • Appropriate CD therapies 1. AHI ≥ 5: CSA HR 3.24[##] and OSA HR 2.07[###] 2. AHI ≥ 15: CSA HR 3.41[^] and OSA HR 2.10[^^]

AHI: apnea-hypopnea index; CD: cardioverter-defibrillator; CHF: congestive heart failure; CSA: central sleep apnea; OSA: obstructive sleep apnea; SDB: sleep disordered breathing; *95% CI 1.40-3.30, P < 0.001; **95% CI 1.64-1.75, P = 0.001; ***95% CI 1.40-3.05, P < 0.001; [#]95% CI 1.14-2.51, P = 0.02; [##]95% CI 1.86-5.64, P < 0.001; [###]95% CI 1.14-3.77, P = 0.02; [^]95% CI 2.10-5.54, P < 0.001; [^^]95% CI 1.17-3.78, P = 0.01

Conclusion
Both obstructive and central sleep apnea increased the risk for ventricular arrhythmias in persons with congestive heart failure.

Commentary
Heart failure is one of the fastest growing cardiac disorders with a prevalence of approximately 2% and is associated with a high public cost burden upwards of 30 billion dollars annually related in large part to hospitalizations and high re-hospitalization rates of up to 50%. It is also

associated with an overall 5-year mortality rate of 50%. Several mainly clinic-based studies have demonstrated a high prevalence of both obstructive sleep apnea and central sleep apnea in heart failure which appears to portend a poor prognosis. The specific pathophysiologic underpinnings remain unclear, however, are likely due to direct sleep apnea effects of intermittent hypoxia, recurrent intrathoracic swings resulting in alterations in intrathoracic pressures thereby disadvantaging myocardial performance and/or sympatho-excitation. A plausible indirect mechanism leading to poorer prognosis of those individuals with heart failure and sleep apnea is a state of enhanced arrhythmogenicity, particularly ventricular irritability leading to malignant ventricular arrhythmias and increased mortality.

The aim of the current investigation was to assess the event-free survival time period to the first cardioverter-defibrillator therapy and also the event-free survival time period to the first appropriately monitored ventricular arrhythmia over a 4-year follow-up period in 255 participants (n=82 with obstructive sleep apnea, n = 87 with central sleep apnea and n=86 without sleep apnea based upon unattended sleep study data) with heart failure and implantation of a cardioverter-defibrillator device six months prior to the sleep study. This is after exclusion of 189 individuals with moderate to severe sleep apnea electing to be treated with positive airway pressure therapy. The authors concluded that obstructive sleep apnea and central sleep apnea are independently (after consideration of age, ischemic cardiac etiology, body mass index, NYHA classification class, blood pressure, heart rate, atrial fibrillation, medications, left ventricular ejection fraction, left ventricular end diastolic diameter, creatinine, NT-pro BNP, C-reactive protein, etc) associated with both a shorter event-free survival time period to the first cardioverter-defibrillator therapy and also first monitored ventricular arrhythmia.

This is a well-done prospective study examining important relationships of sleep apnea and ventricular arrhythmias in a heart failure group. An interesting finding is the lack of a statistically significant difference in the obstructive sleep apnea versus central sleep apnea in the ventricular arrhythmia outcomes after consideration of a vast range of potential confounders including objective measures of cardiac function based upon echocardiography. This is in contrast to our findings in the large epidemiologic cohort, the MrOS Sleep Study, which demonstrated differential relationships such that obstructive sleep apnea and hypoxia were more closely associated with ventricular arrhythmias and central sleep apnea with atrial fibrillation after consideration of confounders including self-reported heart failure and cardiac disease. These differences may be attributed to the differences in populations (all male cohorts versus men and women with heart failure), investigation of cross-sectional versus longitudinal sleep apnea- arrhythmia relationships and differences in scoring methodology and definitions used to characterize obstructive versus central sleep apnea.

Study limitations should be taken into consideration when interpreting these findings some of which were recognized by the authors. These include the use of portable sleep monitoring, use of a hypopnea definition that is inconsistent with American Academy of Sleep Medicine recommendations, differentiation of central versus obstructive hypopneas without use of gold standard methods (such as esophageal balloon monitoring) and selection bias given inclusion of a sample that chose not to pursue treatment for sleep apnea. The validity and reliability of methods used to obtain sleep data and score respiratory events are very important, particularly with respect to distinctions of obstructive versus central sleep apnea, as if this is compromised then this can contribute to measurement error and misclassification of these categories. The generalizeability of the reported findings should also be considered as 189 of 472 (40%) of the sample elected to consider sleep apnea treatment and only those who did not pursue treatment were included in the study. The differences in subject characteristics between those that chose treatment versus not are unclear. As the authors acknowledge, those that elected not to pursue sleep apnea treatment may also be less likely to engage in other healthy behaviors such as taking medications, diet and exercise which may have influenced the study findings. The ethical issues and implications of implementing a randomized controlled trial in sleep apneics in the setting of heart failure are duly noted. Investigating responses to sleep apnea therapy of intermediate cardiac and arrhythmia outcomes over a shorter time period may, however, be a reasonable paradigm with which to design a randomized study. Furthermore, comparative effectiveness research studies could potentially provide important mechanistic insights, e.g. comparing various sleep apnea treatment modalities such as continuous positive airway pressure versus supplemental oxygen therapy which could help identify the benefits of addressing sleep apnea-related upper airway obstruction versus solely addressing the intermittent hypoxia/hyperoxia on arrhythmic outcomes in sleep apnea.

Reena Mehra
Division of Pulmonary, Critical Care and Sleep Medicine
University Hospitals Case Medical Center
Case School of Medicine

Cognitive function and sleep related breathing disorders in a healthy elderly population: the SYNAPSE study. Sforza E, Roche F, Thomas-Anterion C, Kerleroux J, Beauchet O, Celle S, Maudoux D, Pichot V, Laurent B, Barthélémy JC. *Sleep. 2010 Apr 1;33(4):515-21.*

What is the impact of sleep-related breathing disorders on cognitive function in the elderly adult?

Subjects	Methods	Outcomes
827 subjects • Age (mean): 68 yrs at study entry • Gender: 41% men • No history of SRBD, CHD and neurological disorders (stroke and dementia)	Cross sectional study Assessments: • Clinical interview • Cognitive tests • Neurological assessment • PSG Definitions: • SRBD: AHI > 15	SRBD was present in 53% (n = 445) of subjects • 37% had AHI > 30 • Most had no significant EDS: only 9.2% had ESS score > 10 • There was no significant association between AHI, nocturnal hypoxemia and cognitive scores • Compared to mild OSA, those with AHI > 30 had lower cognitive scores

AHI: apnea hypopnea index; CHD: coronary heart disease; EDS: excessive daytime sleepiness; ESS: Epworth sleepiness scale; NPT: neuropsychological battery testing; SRBD: sleep related breathing disorders

Conclusion
Except for severe cases, obstructive sleep apnea was not associated with significant impairments in cognition among healthy older adults.

Commentary
Sleep-related breathing disorder (SRBD) is becoming increasingly recognized as a health condition because it affects a considerable proportion of the population, in particular older subjects. The prevalence of SRBD itself increases with age to a degree of approximately 20% in older patients, relative to 5-10% in younger populations. SRBD has also been linked to cardiovascular morbidity and mortality as well as to cognitive dysfunction. Research studies on cognitive SRBD consequences have been more equivocal, some authors reporting a relationship between cognitive impairment and SRBD severity, others suggesting an age-related physiological decline in cognition. Differences in results may be explained by the differences in cognitive testing, the limited number of patients examined and the worsening of sleep quality in the oldest patients recorded in the laboratory. Moreover, since previous studies on SRBD and cognition have been done in predominantly middle-aged clinical populations with co-morbid conditions, the association of a specific effect of SRBD on cognitive function may have been over-estimated.

It is, therefore, not known if cognitive alterations related to SRBD in older populations are a specific entity or whether the presence of SRBD exaggerates the aging-related physiological changes in cognitive abilities. Understanding the cognitive consequences of SRBD in the elderly is crucial for identifying at-risk patients needing prompt therapy.

To understand better the relationship between SRBD and cognition, we conducted a cross sectional study on 827 community-dwelling healthy subjects free of clinically diagnosed SRBD and dementia. The homogeneity of age (68 yr) at the inclusion time, the large sample, and the extended cognitive assessment were chosen to identify whether a cognitive decline in elderly SRBD subjects occurs and if this decline is related to SRBD severity.

The results of the present study are the following: First, despite minimal symptoms (Epworth = 6/24), SRBD is prevalent in our community-dwelling elderly, 54% percent of the subjects having an AHI ≥ 15/hr, suggesting that SRBD may still be largely undiagnosed in the community. Second, comparison of subjects with and without SRBD showed no differences between groups in daytime sleepiness, anxiety and depression. Moreover, any statistically significant differences were found in all measures of attention, memory, and executive function, except a light impairment in episodic memory in severe SRBD subjects. Third, within this healthy elderly cohort, neither AHI nor nocturnal hypoxemia was related to cognitive scores and impaired episodic memory, suggesting more an age-related change in cognition than a hypoxemic effect on brain function.

There are many possible explanations that could explain why older SRBD subjects had better-preserved cognitive and alertness scores compared to middle-aged SRBD cases. First, the age-related changes in the circadian and homeostatic processes of sleep control resulted in older adults being less vulnerable to sleepiness and performance impairment. Second, SRBD in older subjects may exist as both an *age-dependent* process that is relatively benign and an *age-related* process that is associated with significant sequelae. Our finding of a light cognitive impairment only in severe cases, and previous studies showing a decline in mortality risk in older SRBD patients, support this theory.

In conclusion, our population-based study confirmed that SRBD is very common among subjects over 68 years. Compared to previous longitudinal and cross-sectional surveys, our study did not demonstrate any significant association between SRBD and cognitive decline in a healthy older population. The lack of a strong link between SRBD and cognition in contrast to the reported link in younger populations raised questions regarding the appropriate management strategy for sleep-related breathing disorders in the elderly. Presence of clinical symptoms, i.e., memory and attention deficit, sleepiness and alertness impairment, must be the only substantial factors attributing a clinical significance of an elevated apnea hypopnea index in older adults, and the treatment must not be simply decreasing the AHI, but improving the daytime consequences.

Emilia Sforza
Department of Clinical Physiology
Department of Neurology
University of Lyon

Frédéric Roche
Department of Clinical Physiology

Department of Neurology
University of Lyon

Catherine Thomas-Anterion
Department of Clinical Physiology
Department of Neurology
University of Lyon

Judith Kerleroux
Department of Clinical Physiology
Department of Neurology
University of Lyon

Olivier Beauchet
Department of Clinical Physiology
Department of Neurology
University of Lyon

Sébastien Celle
Department of Clinical Physiology
Department of Neurology
University of Lyon

Delphine Maudoux
Department of Clinical Physiology
Department of Neurology
University of Lyon

Vincent Pichot
Department of Clinical Physiology
Department of Neurology
University of Lyon

Bernard Laurent
Department of Clinical Physiology
Department of Neurology
University of Lyon

Jean Claude Barthélémy
Department of Clinical Physiology
Department of Neurology
University of Lyon

Comparison of positional therapy to CPAP in patients with positional obstructive sleep apnea.
Permut I, Diaz-Abad M, Chatila W, Crocetti J, Gaughan JP, D'Alonzo GE, Krachman SL. *J Clin Sleep Med. 2010 Jun 15;6(3):238-43.*

Is positional therapy as effective as continuous positive airway pressure therapy in the treatment of patients with positional obstructive sleep apnea?

Subjects	Methods	Outcomes
38 subjects with positional OSA • Age: 49 ± 12 yrs • Gender: 66% male • BMI: 31 ± 5 • Nonsupine AHI < 5 and 50% decrease in AHI compared to nonsupine position • AHI (mean) : 13 ± 5 • Supine AHI: 31 ± 19 • Nonsupine AHI: 2 ±1	Subjects were randomized to either (1 night each): • PD • CPAP (10 ± 3 cm H_2O)	Compared to CPAP, PD was equivalent at decreasing AHI to < 5 • PD: 92% • CPAP: 97%* Decrease in AHI (from median of 11* at baseline) • PD: to 2*** • CPAP: to 0[#] • Note: significant difference between treatments[##] Percent of TST in supine position (from 40% at baseline[###]) • PD: to 0%[^,^^] • CPAP: to 51%[^^^] (unchanged) Lowest SaO_2 (from 85% at baseline[@]) • PD: to 89%[@@] • CPAP: to 89%[@@,%] Change in TST (from 338 min[%%] at baseline) • PD: to 334 min[%%%] • CPAP: 319 min[$,$$] No changes in SE, spontaneous AI and sleep architecture were seen with both groups 50% of patients preferred

		the positional device compared to 34% who preferred CPAP therapy

AHI: apnea hypopnea index; AI: arousal index; BMI: body mass index; CPAP: continuous positive airway pressure; OSA: obstructive sleep apnea; PD: positional device; PSG: polysomnography; SaO_2: arterial oxygen saturation; SE: sleep efficiency; TST: total sleep time; *P = 0.16; **interquartile range 9-15, range 6-26 ; ***1-4, 0-8 ; #0-2, 0-7 ; ##P < 0.001 ; ###23%-67%, 7%-82% ; ^0%-0%, 0%-27% ; ^^P < 0.001 ; ^^^36%-69%, 0%-100% ; @83%-89%, 76%-93% ; @@86%-9%1, 78%-95% ; @@@87%-91%, 81%-95% ; %P < 0.001 ; %%303-374, 159-449 ; %%%287-366, 194-397 ; $266-343, 170-386 ; $$P= 0.02

Conclusion

Positional therapy was equivalent to continuous positive airway pressure therapy at normalizing apnea hypopnea indices and in improving sleep quality and nocturnal oxygenation in patients with positional obstructive sleep apnea.

Commentary

While obstructive sleep apnea (OSA) is highly prevalent in the general population, the number of treatment options is relatively limited. Continuous positive airway pressure (CPAP) remains the most widely used form of therapy; however, compliance is relatively poor.[1] Positional therapy has been evaluated in the treatment of OSA, but mostly in studies that have defined positional OSA as merely a decrease in the AHI by 50% in the non-supine compared to the supine position.[2,3] The use of such a definition, along with the lack of an effective positional device, has contributed to the relatively infrequent use of positional therapy as a primary treatment for OSA.

The rationale for our study is based on a rather unappreciated prevalence of positional OSA using a definition of normalizing the AHI to < 5 events/hr in addition to decreasing the AHI by more than 50%.[4] Using this definition, 27% of patients overall, with 50% of patients with mild, and 19% of patients with moderate OSA have positional OSA.[4] Therefore, these patients could benefit from the use of positional therapy as a primary treatment modality. We therefore developed a positional device, the Zzoma Positional Sleeper, which is made of lightweight semi-rigid synthetic foam contained in a backpack-type material with an associated Velcro elastic belt. The positional device is worn on the back with elastic belts brought around each side and secured anteriorly. The advantage of this new device relates to its particular size and wedge-shaped design on both sides, which keeps the patient comfortably positioned on their side and prevents them from going on their back.

We decided to do an equivalence (noninferiority) trial comparing the positional device to CPAP in regards to normalization of the AHI, since CPAP is the most commonly used treatment modality, and an AHI to < 5 events/hr would be a primary goal for effective therapy. We found that the positional device was equivalent to CPAP at normalizing the AHI to < 5 events/hr (92% and 97%, respectively (p=0.16). In addition, similar effects were seen with the 2 treatments in regard to measurements of sleep quality and nocturnal oxygenation.

An interesting finding in our study was the minimal night-to-night variability in the non-supine AHI between the baseline and positional therapy night studies (2 ± 1 and 2 ± 2 events/hr, respectively). These findings reflect the ability of our device to maintain the non-supine position during the night, with only 1 of 38 patients moving through the device for a short period during their device night study ($1 \pm 4\%$ of total sleep time supine for all 38 patients).

We do stress the limitations with our study, the most important of which is that it is a single night study. Whether effectiveness would be maintained over more prolonged use, as well as the issue of compliance with the device and assessment on daytime function will need to be determined.

Our study suggests that the use of positional therapy, with a device that is effective at maintaining the patient in the non-supine position, can be considered an appropriate primary treatment in patients with positional OSA.

Samuel Krachman
Division of Pulmonary and Critical Care
Temple University School of Medicine

References
1. Kribbs NB et al. Objective measurement of patterns of nasal CPAP use by patients with obstructive sleep apnea. Am Rev Respir Dis. 1993; 147: 887-895.
2. Jokic R et al. Positional treatment vs continuous positive airway pressure in patients with positional obstructive sleep apnea. Chest. 1999; 115: 771-781.
3. Skinner MA et al. Efficacy of the 'tennis ball technique' versus NCPAP in the management of position-dependent obstructive sleep apnoea syndrome. Respirology. 2008; 13:708-715.
4. Mador MJ et al. Prevalence of positional sleep apnea in patients undergoing polysomnography. Chest. 2005; 128:2130-2137.

Consequences of comorbid sleep apnea in the metabolic syndrome--implications for cardiovascular risk. Trombetta IC, Somers VK, Maki-Nunes C, Drager LF, Toschi-Dias E, Alves MJ, Fraga RF, Rondon MU, Bechara MG, Lorenzi-Filho G, Negrão CE. *Sleep. 2010 Sep 1;33(9):1193-9.*

Does obstructive sleep apnea increase cardiovascular risk in persons with metabolic syndrome?

Subjects	Methods	Outcomes
36 subjects with MetSyn • Female: 47% • Age (mean): 47 ± 2 yrs • BMI (mean): 33 ± 0.8 • 18 MetSyn and OSA 1. PSG: AHI > 15 • 18 MetSyn without OSA Exclusion criteria : • Chronic medication use • Smoking • Excessive alcohol consumption • Cardiovascular disease	Prospective clinical study Assessments: • BP • BRS • HR • MSNA • PSG	Compared to MetSyn without OSA, MetSyn + OSA was associated with: • Higher MSNA* • Higher mean BP** • Lower spontaneous BRS for increases*** and decreases[#] in BP There were correlations between MSNA and: • AHI[##] • Minimum nocturnal SaO2[###]

AHI: apnea hypopnea index; BP: blood pressure (Finapres); BRS: baroreflex sensitivity; HR: heart rate; MetS: metabolic syndrome; MSNA: muscle sympathetic nerve activity (microneurography); OSA: obstructive sleep apnea; PSG: polysomnography; SaO_2: arterial oxygen saturation; *34 ± 2 vs. 28 ± 1 bursts/min, P = 0.02; **111 ± 3 vs. 99 ± 2 mm Hg, P = 0.003; ***7.6 ± 0.6 vs. 12.2 ± 1.2 msec/mm Hg, P = 0.003; [#]7.2 ± 0.6 vs. 11.9 ± 1.6 msec/mm Hg, P = 0.01; [##]R= 0.48; P = 0.009; [###]R= -0.38, P = 0.04

Conclusion
The presence of obstructive sleep apnea in persons with metabolic syndrome gave rise to several factors, including higher blood pressure and sympathetic activity and reduced baroreflex sensitivity, which can potentially increase cardiovascular risk.

Commentary
Obstructive sleep apnea (OSA) and metabolic syndrome (MetSyn) are each increasingly common. There is a striking comorbidity of these conditions, perhaps more than would be expected by chance. Both of these conditions have been linked to increased cardiovascular risk.[1] Whether comorbid OSA increases the cardiovascular risk profile in patients with the MetSyn has not previously been investigated.

We therefore examined how the presence of OSA in patients with the MetSyn affected hemodynamic and autonomic variables associated with elevated cardiovascular risk. We compared those patients with and without polysomnographically proven OSA. Both groups were of similar age, sex, and body mass index and had comparable severity of the MetSyn.

We found that patients with the MetSyn with comorbid OSA had higher blood pressure (BP), higher sympathetic drive, and diminished baroreflex sensitivity (BRS), as compared with MetSyn patients without OSA.

Despite the high prevalence of OSA in patients with MetSyn[2,3,4], previous studies did not take into consideration the presence of occult sleep disorders. In the present study, we investigated whether OSA would have any additional excitatory effect on sympathetic drive in patients with MetSyn and found that patients with MetSyn and OSA have greater sympathetic activity than do patients with MetSyn without OSA, suggesting that sympathetic excitation is likely elicited through different mechanisms in these 2 conditions. Although hypertension[5], obesity[6], and hyperinsulinemia[7] may be accompanied by increased sympathetic activity in humans, it seems unlikely that these conditions explain the difference in sympathetic activity in patients with MetSyn+OSA versus patients with MetSyn-OSA. Multivariate analysis showed that none of the abnormalities that constitute the MetSyn correlated with sympathetic activity. OSA was, in fact, the only differentiating characteristic. Increased sympathetic nervous activity in patients with MetSyn+OSA could be secondary to hypoxemia during sleep. MSNA was positively correlated with AHI (apnea hypopnea index), and apnea and hypoxemia increase sympathetic nervous activity.[8] Thus, sympathetic excitatory effects of recurrent hypoxemic apneas may carry over into daytime wakefulness. Therefore, it is likely that the higher MSNA in patients with MetSyn+OSA was not due to the metabolic disturbances but, rather, to the coexisting sleep disorder.

We cannot rule out the alternative possibility that the augmented sympathetic activation in patients with MetSyn and OSA was due to baroreflex impairment. Although the inverse association between BRS and MSNA does not confirm a cause-and-effect relationship, it suggests that impaired baroreflex control may be involved, at least in part, in the augmented sympathetic activity in patients with MetSyn and OSA. Arterial baroreceptors exert a beat-to-beat inhibitory modulation of efferent sympathetic nervous activity. Thus, a consequence of impaired baroreflex control may include an exacerbation in sympathetic outflow. Impaired baroreflex gain is itself an important risk predictor for cardiovascular disease[9], including hypertension[10] and coronary artery disease.[11] Thus, the diminished baroreflex gain may represent an additional risk factor in patients with MetSyn and OSA.

The present study suggests that the treatment of patients with MetSyn+OSA should also aim for reduction in sympathetic nervous activity and improvement in BRS. Clearly, continuous positive airway pressure, the standard treatment for OSA, would be an important therapeutic approach. An adjunct may be non-pharmacologic therapy based on diet and exercise, since previous observations have shown that this combined strategy reduces MSNA in obese individuals.[12] In addition, exercise has been shown to improve BRS and attenuate sleep disorders in patients with established cardiovascular disease.[10,13] However, whether this approach is effective in patients with MetSyn and OSA awaits further studies.

Ivani C. Trombetta
Heart Institute (InCor)
University of São Paulo Medical School

Virend K. Somers
Division of Cardiovascular Diseases
Department of Internal Medicine
Mayo Clinic and Foundation

Carlos E. Negrão
Heart Institute (InCor)
University of São Paulo Medical School
School of Physical Education and Sports
University of São Paulo

References

1. Grundy SM et al. American Heart Association; National Heart, Lung, and Blood Institute. Diagnosis and management of the metabolic syndrome: an American Heart Association/National Heart, Lung, and Blood Institute Scientific Statement. Circulation. 2005; 112:2735-52.
2. Drager LF et al. Obstructive sleep apnea is highly prevalent and correlates with poor glycemic control in consecutive patients with metabolic syndrome. J Cardiometab Syndr. 2009; 4:89-95.
3. Venkateswaran S et al. The prevalence of syndrome Z (the interaction of obstructive sleep apnoea with the metabolic syndrome) in a teaching hospital in Singapore. Postgrad Med J. 2007; 83:329-31.
4. Vgontzas AN et al. Sleep apnea is a manifestation of the metabolic syndrome. Sleep Med Rev. 2005; 9:211-24.
5. Rondon MU et al. Abnormal muscle metaboreflex control of sympathetic activity in never-treated hypertensive subjects. Am J Hypertens. 2006; 19:951-7.
6. Ribeiro MM et al. Muscle sympathetic nerve activity and hemodynamic alterations in middle-aged obese women. Braz J Med Biol Res. 2001; 34:475-8.
7. Scherrer U et al. Insulin as a vascular and sympathoexcitatory hormone: implications for blood pressure regulation, insulin sensitivity, and cardiovascular morbidity. Circulation. 1997; 96:4104-13.
8. Narkiewicz K et al. Baroreflex control of sympathetic nerve activity and heart rate in obstructive sleep apnea. Hypertension. 1998; 32:1039-43.
9. Grassi G et al. Sympathetic activation and loss of reflex sympathetic control in mild congestive heart failure. Circulation. 1995; 92:3206-11.
10. Laterza MC et al. Exercise training restores baroreflex sensitivity in never-treated hypertensive patients. Hypertension. 2007; 49:1298-306.
11. Katsube Y et al. The decreased baroreflex sensitivity in patients with stable coronary artery disease is correlated with the severity of coronary narrowing. Am J Cardiol. 1996; 78:1007-10.
12. Trombetta IC et al. Weight loss improves neurovascular and muscle metaboreflex control in obesity. Am J Physiol Heart Circ Physiol. 2003; 285:H974-82.
13. Ueno LM et al. Effects of exercise training in patients with chronic heart failure and sleep apnea. Sleep. 2009; 32:637-47.

Continuous positive airway pressure deepens sleep in patients with Alzheimer's disease and obstructive sleep apnea. Cooke JR, Ancoli-Israel S, Liu L, Loredo JS, Natarajan L, Palmer BS, He F, Corey-Bloom J. *Sleep Med. 2009 Dec;10(10):1101-6.*

Does continuous positive airway pressure therapy of obstructive sleep apnea affect sleep architecture of persons with Alzheimer's disease?

Subjects	Methods	Outcomes
52 subjects with AD and OSA • Age: 77.8 ± 7.3 yrs	Randomized placebo-controlled trial Subjects were randomized to: • 3 weeks of therapeutic CPAP • 3 weeks placebo CPAP followed by 3 weeks of therapeutic CPAP Assessments: • PSG	After 1 treatment night, compared to placebo, therapeutic CPAP was associated with: • Less % N1* • More % N2** 3 weeks of therapeutic CPAP was associated with: • Decrease in WASO*** • Decrease in % N1[#] • Decrease in arousals[##] • Increase in % N3[###]

AD: Alzheimer's disease; CPAP: continuous positive airway pressure; N1: sleep stage 1; N2: sleep stage 2; N3: sleep stage 3; OSA: obstructive sleep apnea; PSG: polysomnography; SE: sleep efficiency; SOL: sleep onset; SP: sleep period; TIB: time in bed; TST: total sleep time; WASO: wake time after sleep onset; *P = 0.04 ; **P = 0.02 ; ***P = 0.005 ; [#]P = 0.001 ; [##]P = 0.005 ; [###]P = 0.006

Conclusion

Continuous positive airway pressure therapy of obstructive sleep apnea improved a number of sleep parameters, including greater deeper stages of sleep and decrease in arousals, in persons with Alzheimer's disease.

Commentary

Alzheimer's disease (AD) patients have disrupted sleep. In particular, they have less slow wave sleep (SWS), more frequent awakenings and spend more time awake during the night than non-demented older adults. Some have hypothesized that there is a positive association between the severity of these sleep disruptions and worsening cognitive function in AD.[1]

Patients with AD also have an increased incidence of obstructive sleep apnea (OSA).[2] Our laboratory has been studying sleep in patients with AD and OSA. One of the findings was that sleep of AD patients with OSA is characterized by less rapid eye movement (REM) sleep compared to AD patients without OSA.[3]

As part of a larger study exploring the effect of CPAP on cognitive functioning in patients with mild to moderate AD and OSA[4], this study examined the effect of CPAP on sleep parameters in this population of patients. Since it is known that continuous positive airway pressure (CPAP) is the most effective treatment for OSA and its effect on restoring consolidated sleep in patients without dementia is characterized by an increase in SWS and REM[5], the hypothesis of this study was that treatment with CPAP would result in deeper, less disrupted sleep (manifested by increases in SWS and REM sleep and decreases in Stage 1 sleep, WASO, and arousals). Patients with AD and OSA were randomized to either 3 weeks placebo CPAP (pCPAP) followed by 3 weeks therapeutic CPAP or to 6-weeks of therapeutic CPAP. Polysomnography data from a screening night, after one night of CPAP and after three weeks of CPAP were analyzed and a randomized design comparing one night of placebo CPAP to one night of therapeutic CPAP was performed along with a paired analysis combining 3 weeks of therapeutic CPAP in both groups. The results showed that after one CPAP treatment night, the therapeutic CPAP group had significantly less % Stage 1 (p=0.04) and more % Stage 2 sleep (p=0.02) when compared to the placebo group. In the paired analysis, 3-weeks of CPAP resulted in significant decreases in wake time (p=0.005), % Stage 1 (p=0.001), and arousals (p=0.005), and in an increase in % Stage 3 (p=0.006) sleep. In other words, there was an increase in SWS with CPAP treatment.

There are several exciting points that arise from this study. First, the study demonstrated that in mild to moderate AD patients with OSA, a single night of treatment with therapeutic CPAP, when compared to placebo CPAP, will result in an immediate deepening of sleep. Second, these improvements in sleep were maintained following three weeks of therapeutic CPAP. Third, three weeks of therapeutic CPAP resulted not only in deeper sleep, but in more consolidated sleep. While other studies have found similar results in OSA patients, this has not previously been tested in elderly or in patients with dementia. Other reports from this study have shown that AD patients are compliant with CPAP, and that CPAP treatment also improved daytime sleepiness and cognition.[4,6,7] This was the first study to confirm that treating OSA in Alzheimer's disease can be effective and have many benefits.

The main impact of this series of studies is to reinforce that no group of patients, no matter their age or physical or mental condition, should be denied treatment of their sleep disorder. This is an important lesson especially for geriatricians or other health care professionals who treat older patients. No matter the age or the cognitive level, the older adult with sleep apnea should be treated. This may result in better quality of life, postponement of institutionalization, and savings of thousands, if not millions, of health care dollars.

Sonia Ancoli-Israel
Gillin Sleep and Chronomedicine Research Center
Department of Psychiatry
University of California, San Diego

References
1. Prinz PN et al. Sleep, EEG and mental function changes in senile dementia of the Alzheimer's type. Neurobiol Aging. 1982; 3:361-70.
2. Ancoli-Israel S et al. Dementia in institutionalized elderly: Relation to sleep apnea. J Am Geriatr Soc. 1991; 39(3):258-263.
3. Cooke JR et al. The effect of sleep disordered breathing on sleep stages in patients with Alzheimer's disease. Behavioral Sleep Medicine. 2006; 4:219-227.
4. Ancoli-Israel S et al. Effect of Treating Sleep Disordered Breathing on Cognitive Functioning

in Patients with Alzheimer's Disease: A Randomized Controlled Trial. J Am Geriatr Soc. 2008; 56(11):2076-2081.

5. Verma A et al. Slow wave sleep rebound and REM rebound following the first night of treatment with CPAP for sleep apnea: correlation with subjective improvement in sleep quality. Sleep Med. 2001; 2:215-223.

6. Ayalon L et al. Adherence to continuous positive airway pressure treatment in patients with Alzheimer's disease and obstructive sleep apnea. American Journal of Geriatric Psychiatry. 2006; 14:176-180.

7. Chong MS et al. Continuous positive airway pressure reduces subjective daytime sleepiness in patients with mild to moderate Alzheimer's disease with sleep disordered breathing. J Am Geriatr Soc. 2006; 54:777-781.

Craniofacial Changes After 2 Years of Nasal Continuous Positive Airway Pressure Use in Patients With Obstructive Sleep Apnea. Tsuda H, Almeida FR, Tsuda T, Moritsuchi Y, Lowe AA. *Chest. 2010; 138;870-874.*

Does chronic use of continuous positive airway pressure for adult persons with obstructive sleep apnea lead to changes in craniofacial characteristics?

Subjects	Methods	Outcomes
46 subjects with OSA who used CPAP via nasal mask for ≥ 2 yrs (> 4 hrs per day and >5 days a week) • Gender: 89.1% males • Age (mean): 56.3 ± 13.4 yrs • BMI (mean): 26.8 ± 5.6 • AHI (mean): 42.0 ± 18.6 • Average duration of CPAP use: 35.0 ± 6.7 months	Prospective study Assessments: • Baseline and follow-up lateral cephalometric radiographs • Demographic characteristics	Compared to baseline, at follow-up, CPAP use was associated with: • Decrease in maxillary-mandibular discrepancy • Decrease of convexity • Retroclination of maxillary incisors • Retrusion of the anterior maxilla • Setback of the supramentale and chin positions No significant correlations were noted between these craniofacial changes and duration of CPAP use There were no self-reported permanent changes in occlusion or facial profile

OSA: obstructive sleep apnea; CPAP: continuous positive airway pressure; BMI: body mass index; AHI: apnea hypopnea index

Conclusion
Chronic use of continuous positive airway pressure produced significant changes in certain craniofacial measurements in adults with obstructive sleep apnea.

Commentary
Nasal continuous positive airway pressure (nCPAP) has been shown to produce midfacial hypoplasia in children.[1] The first line therapy for patients with obstructive sleep apnea is nCPAP. The common noted side effects of nCPAP include air leakage, skin abrasions, mouth dryness, rhinitis, pressure intolerance and aerophagia. This is the first study to date that looked into the craniofacial changes caused by long term nCPAP use.

This was a prospective study that looked into the craniofacial changes following long term use of nCPAP. Their hypothesis was that the pressure of the mask could affect the anterior maxillary and mandibular incisors and the position of the mandible resulting in decrease tongue space and worsening of OSA symptoms. They used cephalometric analysis to study the skeletal and pharyngeal dimensions in patients before and after two years of using nCPAP. Correlations between cephalometric changes and demographic variables, such as age, sex, BMI, baseline AHI, nCPAP pressure, duration of nCPAP use, and pretreatment cephalometric variables were evaluated. Out of 46 patients, mask types used in the study include: Mirage Activa (n = 21), comfort gel (n = 21), comfort select (n = 1) and comfort fusion (n=3). In this study auto CPAP and average nCPAP pressure was used in the analysis. During data analysis they did not look into the craniofacial changes caused by different mask types.

Few limitations were noted in the study. To better understand the dental arch changes a three dimensional analysis was required, but in this study they used 2 dimensional analysis with which it is impossible to know the lateral direction changes. Average pressure from the Auto PAP was used to know this effect and did not look into the band pressure from the mask directly on the face. Other limitations of the study include absence of control, short duration and small sample size. This study was done in Japanese patients only, so we need studies across different ethnic groups to apply in clinical practice.

One of the confounding factors of this study is the dental and skeletal changes that occurred with aging. As per the authors, based on their references no significant changes occurred in 10 years of observation or an opposite direction change occurred in > 25 years of observation[2-4], so they concluded that the 3 year period of the study is not causing any age related changes.

Since the craniofacial changes are not fully investigated with the limitations mentioned above we need a detailed study looking into the limitation of this study to apply this in practice. Since the benefit of using CPAP is more, like reducing the cardiovascular consequences and excessive daytime sleepiness which in turn improve the quality of life of these patients we think it's appropriate to continue the treatment now.

It will be interesting to look into the craniofacial changes produced by different masks, the effect of mask pressure and the changes caused by different dental conditions in different ethnic groups.

Manju Pillai
National Jewish Health
University of Colorado Denver School of Medicine

References

1. Li KK et al. An unreported risk in the use of home nasal continuous positive airway pressure and home nasal ventilation in children: mid-face hypoplasia. Chest. 2000; 117 (3):916 - 918.
2. Bondevik O. Growth changes in the cranial base and the face: a longitudinal cephalometric study of linear and angular changes in adult Norwegians. Eur J Orthod. 1995; 17(6):525-532.

3. Kollias I et al. Adult craniocervical and pharyngeal changes—a longitudinal cephalometric study between 22 and 42 years of age. Part I: Morphological craniocervical and hyoid bone changes. Eur J Orthod . 1999; 21 (4):333-344.
4. Formby WA et al. Longitudinal changes in the adult facial profile. Am J Orthod Dentofacial Orthop.1994; 105(5):464-476.

Effect of a very low energy diet on moderate and severe obstructive sleep apnoea in obese men: a randomised controlled trial. Johansson K, Neovius M, Lagerros YT, Harlid R, Rössner S, Granath F, Hemmingsson E. *BMJ. 2009 Dec 3;339:b4609.*

How does weight loss secondary to a very low energy diet affect obese persons with moderate to severe obstructive sleep apnea?

Subjects	Methods	Outcomes
63 obese male subjects with moderate to severe OSA treated with CPAP • Age: 30-65 yrs • BMI: 30-40 • AHI: 37 ± 15	Parallel, randomized, controlled, open label trial Subjects were randomized to either (for 9 weeks): • Intervention (n = 30): very low energy liquid diet (2.3 MJ daily) for 7 weeks followed by 2 weeks of gradually normal food (reaching 6.3 MJ daily at week 9) • Control (n = 33): usual diet o 2 subjects discontinued with the study Assessment: • AHI • Weight	At week 9, compared to controls, intervention group had: • 20 kg lower mean body weight * • 23 events per hour lower mean AHI AHI at week 9 • Intervention group 1. 17% (n = 5) had AHI <5 2. 50% (n = 15) had AHI 5-14.9 3. 33% (n = 10) had AHI 15-30 • Control group 1. All except one had AHI ≥ 15 In the intervention group, greater improvements in AHI with similar weight loss ** were seen in those with AHI > 30 at baseline than in those with AHI 15-30 at baseline***

AHI: apnea hypopnea index; BMI: body mass index; CPAP: continuous positive airway pressure; OSA: obstructive sleep apnea; VLED: very low energy diet; *95% confidence interval 18 to 21; **-19.2 vs. -18.2 kg, P = 0.55; ***-38 vs. -12, P < 0.001

Conclusion

Weight loss from a low energy diet improved obstructive sleep apnea among obese persons, with greater reductions in the apnea hypopnea indices in those with severe disease compared to mild-moderate disease.

Commentary

Sixty to seventy percent of patients with obstructive sleep apnea have been reported to be either overweight or obese.[1][2] During the last 20 years uncontrolled studies have shown that weight loss is associated with improvements obstructive sleep apnea.[3] Randomized controlled trials supporting this effect has been lacking until 2009, when three trials[4 5 6] on the effects of weight loss in obstructive sleep apnea were published in different subgroups. A Finnish study by Tuomilehto et al[4] investigated the effect of very low energy diet (VLED) followed by supervised lifestyle counselling for one year in overweight or obese patients with mild obstructive sleep apnea. Thereafter, a US study by Foster et al[5] investigated the effects of intensive lifestyle change in overweight or obese patients with type 2 diabetes and mild to severe obstructive sleep apnea for one year. Finally, we investigated the effects of VLED during 9 weeks in obese Swedish men with moderate to severe obstructive sleep apnea,[6] the conditions associated with increased mortality.[7,8]

The aim of our randomized controlled study was to investigate if weight loss induced by VLED (2,3MJ/d = 554kcal/d) during nine weeks could be used in the treatment for moderate and severe obstructive sleep apnea.

We included 63 obese men (body mass index 30-40 kg/m^2; age 30-65 years) with moderate to severe obstructive sleep apnea (apnea hypopnea index, AHI, ≥15) treated with continuous positive airway pressure. Thirty were randomized to the very low energy diet and 33 to control. Two patients in the control group were dissatisfied with allocation and immediately discontinued. All other patients completed the trial. Data from all randomized patients were included in an intention to treat analysis (baseline carried forward for missing data). AHI, the primary outcome, was derived from two consecutive nocturnal sleep studies in the home at baseline and after nine weeks. After nine weeks, there was a 67% reduction in AHI after 19 kg weight loss in the group allocated to VLED, with the greatest effect seen in patients with severe disease, whereas no change occurred in the weight stable control group. In the intervention group, five patients (17%) were disease free after the intervention (AHI <5) and 15 (50%) had mild disease (AHI 5-14.9), whereas AHI remained at 15 or greater in all controls.

In conclusion, the findings of this randomized trial showed that VLED-induced weight loss resulted in a significant reduction of moderate to severe obstructive sleep apnea in obese men. Patients with severe obstructive sleep apnea benefitted most from the intervention. Long term treatment studies are needed to validate weight loss as a primary treatment strategy for obstructive sleep apnea. However, all obese patients with obstructive sleep apnea should be informed about the beneficial effect of weight loss.

Kari Johansson
Department of Medicine
Karolinska Institutet, Stockholm

Erik Hemmingsson
Department of Medicine
Karolinska Institutet, Stockholm

Martin Neovius
Department of Medicine
Karolinska Institutet, Stockholm

References

1. Pillar G et al. Abdominal fat and sleep apnea: the chicken or the egg? Diabetes Care. 2008; 31 Suppl 2:S303-9.
2. Lindberg E et al. Epidemiology of sleep-related obstructive breathing. Sleep Med Rev. 2000; 4(5):411-33.
3. Veasey SC et al. Medical therapy for obstructive sleep apnea: a review by the Medical Therapy for Obstructive Sleep Apnea Task Force of the Standards of Practice Committee of the American Academy of Sleep Medicine. Sleep. 2006; 29(8):1036-44.
4. Tuomilehto HP et al. Lifestyle intervention with weight reduction: first-line treatment in mild obstructive sleep apnea. Am J Respir Crit Care Med. 2009;.179(4):320-7.
5. Foster GD et al. A randomized study on the effect of weight loss on obstructive sleep apnea among obese patients with type 2 diabetes: the Sleep AHEAD study. Arch Intern Med. 2009; 169(17):1619-26.
6. Johansson K et al. Effect of a very low energy diet on moderate and severe obstructive sleep apnoea in obese men: a randomised controlled trial. BMJ. 2009; 339:b4609.
7. Young T et al. Sleep disordered breathing and mortality: eighteen-year follow-up of the Wisconsin sleep cohort. Sleep. 2008; 31(8):1071-8.
8. Marshall NS et al. Sleep apnea as an independent risk factor for all-cause mortality: the Busselton Health Study. Sleep. 2008; 31(8):1079-85.

Effect of episodic hypoxia on the susceptibility to hypocapnic central apnea during NREM sleep. Chowdhuri S, Shanidze I, Pierchala L, Belen D, Mateika JH, Badr MS. *J Appl Physiol. 2010 Feb;108(2):369-77.*

Does episodic hypoxia produce ventilatory long-term facilitation as well as change apneic threshold, carbon dioxide reserve, and hypocapnic/hypoxic ventilatory responses that contribute to breathing instability during non-rapid eye movement sleep?

Subjects	Methods	Outcomes
11 healthy subjects • Gender: 37% males • Age (mean): 26.1 ± 4.2 yrs • BMI: 22.1 ± 2.0 • AHI: 0.7 ± 1.4	NIPPV was adjusted to induce hypocapnia and CA during stable NREM sleep before and after exposure to EH (15 1-min episodes of isocapnic hypoxia [mean SaO_2: $87.0 \pm 0.5\%$]) Assessments: • Eupneic $PetCO_2$, AT, $PetCO_2$, CO_2 reserve, and hypocapnic ventilatory response before and after EH • Hypoxic ventilatory response during EH Definitions: • AT: $PetCO_2$ demarcating CA • CO_2 reserve: difference between AT and baseline $PetCO_2$ immediately before onset of MV • Eupneic $P_{ET}CO_2$: average of breaths during the control room air period immediately before onset of NIPPV • Hypocapnic ventilatory response: change in MV for every change in $PetCO_2$ ($\Delta MV/\Delta PetCO_2$) • Hypoxic ventilatory response: change in MV for each change in SaO_2	MV values increased during EH and remained elevated during post-EH: • Pre-EH control: 6.2 ± 0.4 l/min • During EH: 7.9 ± 0.5 l/min • Post-EH: $6.7 +/- 0.4$ l/min* Changes associated after EH: • No change in AT • Significant decline in CO_2 reserve 1. Pre-EH: -3.1 ± 0.5 mmHg 2. Post-EH: -2.3 ± 0.4 mmHg** • Increased hypocapnic ventilatory response*** No significant change in hypoxic ventilatory response during EH

	(ΔMV)/ΔSaO$_2$) Sham studies on room air were completed in 8 individuals	

AHI: apnea-hypopnea index; AT: apneic threshold; BMI: body mass index; CA: central apnea; CO_2: carbon dioxide; EH: episodic hypoxia; MV: minute ventilation; NIPPV: noninvasive positive pressure mechanical ventilation; NREM: non-rapid eye movement sleep; PetCO$_2$: end-tidal partial pressure of carbon dioxide; SaO$_2$: arterial oxygen saturation; *P < 0.05; **P < 0.001; ***3.3 +/- 0.6 vs. 1.8 +/- 0.3 l x min(-1) x mmHg(-1), P < 0.001

Conclusion
Episodic hypoxia led to an increase in hypocapnic ventilatory response and decrease in carbon dioxide reserve, both of which might destabilize breathing and promote central apneas during non-rapid eye movement sleep.

Commentary
Long-term facilitation is a form of respiratory plasticity that is characterized by a sustained increase in ventilatory motor output following exposure to repetitive acute exposures to episodic hypoxia and can last up to 90 min after the termination of hypoxia.[1,2] This model of hypoxia mimics sleep apnea and has been used to study the effects of episodic hypoxia on ventilatory stability and/or upper airway collapsibility in animals as well as in humans.[2-5]

The experimental findings from our study have important physiological implications. Specifically, the increased hypocapnic ventilatory response and narrowed CO_2 reserve in the aftermath of EH renders the ventilatory control system more susceptible to recurrent central apnea and may perpetuate instability, even after the initial perturbation produced by hypoxia is removed. An increased hypocapnic ventilatory response promotes the development of central apnea because the decrease in ventilation for a given reduction in P$_{ET}$CO$_2$ is enhanced.[6,7] Similar changes were absent after sham intervention in the study participants. Thus, susceptibility to apnea may be evident in the presence of ventilatory LTF, indicating that LTF may be a marker for ventilatory instability after EH. It is possible that enhanced susceptibility to central apnea after EH may contribute to increased apnea severity across the night in patients with sleep apnea. It is important to clarify that our study investigated effects of acute EH and did not address the effects of chronic intermittent hypoxia.[8]

Potential mechanism for the observed changes may be related to a reduced cerebral reactivity to CO_2,[9] enhanced production of ROS[10] or increased activity via oxygen sensing neurons in the central nervous system.[11] In animal models, LTF is mediated via serotonergic receptors[8,12], N-methyl-D-aspartate receptors[13] or ROS.[10] These mechanisms may provide potential targets for pharmacological manipulations of LTF. While our protocol does not permit us to definitively identify a specific mechanism to explain the increased chemoreflex sensitivity after EH in healthy humans during sleep, it does allow us to clarify the role of LTF on breathing stability in humans during sleep.[1] Elucidation of the components and mechanisms of LTF in humans during sleep potentially provides an understanding toward the development of pharmacological therapies for sleep apnea.

Susmita Chowdhuri
John D Dingell VA Medical Center
Wayne State University

M.Safwan Badr
John D Dingell VA Medical Center
Wayne State University

References

1. Chowdhuri S et al. Effect of episodic hypoxia on the susceptibility to develop central apnea during NREM sleep. J Appl Physiol. 2010; 108:369-77.
2. Cao KY et al. Increased normoxic ventilation induced by repetitive hypoxia in conscious dog. J Appl Physiol. 1992; 73:2083–2088.
3. Fuller D et al. Long term facilitation of phrenic motor output. Respir Physiol. 2000; 121:135–146.
4. Babcock MA et al. Long-term facilitation of ventilation in humans during NREM sleep. Sleep. 1998; 21:709–716.
5. Chowdhuri S et al. Long-term facilitation of genioglossus activity is present in normal humans during NREM sleep. Respir Physiol Neurobiol. 2008; 160:65–75.
6. Dempsey JA. Crossing the apnoeic threshold: causes and consequences. Exp Physiol. 2005; 90:13–24.
7. Khoo MCK et al. Sleep-induced breathing and apnoea: a theoretical study. J Appl Physiol. 1991; 70:2014–2024.
8. Ling L et al. Chronic intermittent hypoxia elicits serotonin-dependent plasticity in the central neural control of breathing. J Neurosci. 2001; 21:5381–5388.
9. Ainslie PN et al. Integration of cerebrovascular CO2 reactivity and chemoreflex. Control of breathing: mechanisms of regulation, measurement, and interpretation. Am J Physiol Regul Integr Comp Physiol. 2009; 296:R1473–R1495.
10. MacFarlane PM et al. Reactive oxygen species and respiratory plasticity following intermittent hypoxia. Respir Physiol Neurobiol. 2008; 164: 263–271.
11. Neubauer JA et al. Oxygen-sensing neurons in the central nervous system. J Appl Physiol. 2004; 96: 367–374.
12. Bach KB et al. Hypoxia-induced long-term facilitation of respiratory activity is serotonin dependent. Respir Physiol. 1996; 104:251–260.
13. McGuire M et al. Phrenic long-term facilitation requires NMDA receptors in the phrenic motonucleus in rats. J Physiol. 2005; 567:599–611.

Effect of flow-triggered adaptive servo-ventilation compared with continuous positive airway pressure in patients with chronic heart failure with coexisting obstructive sleep apnea and Cheyne-Stokes respiration. Kasai T, Usui Y, Yoshioka T, Yanagisawa N, Takata Y, Narui K, Yamaguchi T, Yamashina A, Momomura SI; JASV Investigators. *Circ Heart Fail. 2010 Jan;3(1):140-8.*

Does adaptive servo ventilation affect heart function in persons with heart failure and sleep disordered breathing?

Subjects	Methods	Outcomes
31 subjects with CHF • LVEF < 50% • NYHA class ≥ II • Coexisting OSA and CSR-CSA	Subjects were randomized to (a) CPAP or (b) ASV during a 3-month period Assessments: • Respiratory events • Cardiac function • Compliance	Compared to CPAP, ASV was associated with: • Greater effectiveness in decreasing respiratory events* • Better compliance** • Greater improvements in QOL and LVEF***

AHI: apnea hypopnea index; ASV: flow-triggered adaptive servo ventilation; CHF: chronic heart failure; CPAP: continuous positive airway pressure; CSR-CSA: Cheyne-Stokes respiration-central sleep apnea; LVEF: left ventricular ejection fraction; NYHA: New York Heart Association; OSA: obstructive sleep apnea; QOL: quality of life; SBD: sleep disordered breathing; *-35.4 ± 19.5 vs. -23.2 ± 12.0, P < 0.05; **5.2 ± 0.9 vs. 4.4 ± 1.1 h/night, P < 0.05; ***+9.1 ± 4.7% vs. +1.9 ± 10.9%

Conclusion
Adaptive servo ventilation was more effective than continuous positive airway pressure in improving respiratory events, quality of life and left ventricular function in persons with congestive heart failure and coexisting obstructive sleep apnea or Cheyne-Stokes respiration-central sleep apnea.

Commentary
It has been reported that approximately 50% of chronic heart failure (CHF) patients have sleep-disordered breathing (SDB)[1-4], which consists of obstructive sleep apnea (OSA) and Cheyne-Stokes respiration (CSR)-central sleep apnea (CSA). The presence of SDB, including both OSA and CSR-CSA, is known to be associated with increased mortality in CHF patients.[5-8]

Treating SDB by continuous positive airway pressure (CPAP) has been shown to attenuate sympathetic overactivity, and improve left ventricular systolic function in CHF patients with either OSA or CSR-CSA.[9-12] However, it is still unknown whether CPAP should be recommended for all CHF patients with SDB, because randomized clinical trials assessing the long-term outcomes of CPAP therapy in CHF patients with OSA are lacking, and because a large-scale randomized clinical trial in which the long-term efficacy of CPAP therapy in CHF patients with CSR-CSA was investigated, failed to show the efficacy of CPAP therapy on the transplant-free survival probably in association with its insufficient alleviation of SDB.[13] On the other hand, it is well recognized that compliance with CPAP is one of the important issue in CHF patients because they usually do not have excessive daytime sleepiness. Therefore, studies assessing the efficacy of other therapies that can suppress SDB more effectively and can produce better compliance than CPAP are of interest.

From this perspective, adaptive servo-ventilation (ASV) may be an effective alternative for suppression of SDB.[14] Other groups have reported the efficacy of ASV for suppressing SDB using two different types of ASV: volume-triggered ASV, and flow-triggered ASV, which has been developed based on the concept of normalizing breathing in patients with both OSA and CSR-CSA.[15-17] Although several reports have demonstrated the efficacy of volume-triggered ASV for improving compliance with the device and cardiac function in patients with predominant CSR-CSA[18-20], there are no data showing such efficacies using flow-triggered ASV . Moreover, no data about the efficacy of ASV for CHF patients with coexisting OSA and CSR-CSA are available.

Therefore, we compared the efficacy of flow-triggered ASV to CPAP for cardiac function in CHF patients with coexisting OSA and CSR-CSA in this parallel randomized multi-center trial.

In addition to the greater alleviation of SDB, we found better compliance with the devices during the 3-month study period in patients who were allocated to the flow-triggered ASV (flow-triggered ASV group) than those who were allocated to the CPAP (CPAP group). Flow-triggered ASV group also showed greater increase in left ventricular ejection fraction, greater reduction in plasma level of brain natriuretic peptide and greater gain in the distance walked in 6 minutes as compared with CPAP group. Furthermore, improvements of scales for quality of life were also greater in the flow-triggered ASV group than in CPAP group.

Differences in the alleviation of SDB and compliance with the device between two groups may have contributed to the improvements in cardiac function and QOL in the flow-triggered ASV group. These results also suggest that CHF patients with coexisting OSA and CSR-CSA may receive greater benefit from treatment with flow-triggered ASV than with CPAP.

Takatoshi Kasai
Sleep Center
Toranomon Hospital, Tokyo
Department of Cardiology
Juntendo University
School of Medicine, Tokyo

Endothelial repair capacity and apoptosis are inversely related in obstructive sleep apnea.
Jelic S, Lederer DJ, Adams T, Padeletti M, Colombo PC, Factor P, Le Jemtel TH. *Vasc Health Risk Manag. 2009;5:909-20.*

Does obstructive sleep apnea affect endothelial repair capacity and apoptosis?

Subjects	Methods	Outcomes
16 subjects with newly diagnosed OSA • BMI: < 30 16 controls subjects	Assessments (before and after 4 weeks of CPAP therapy): • Endothelial repair capacity: circulating levels of endothelial progenitor cells • Endothelial apoptosis: endothelial microparticles • Endothelial cell apoptotic rate in freshly harvested venous endothelial cells • Vascular reactivity: flow-mediated dilation	At baseline, compared to controls, OSA was associated with: • Greater endothelial microparticle levels* • Lower endothelial progenitor cell levels* • Note: There was an inverse correlation between levels of endothelial microparticles and progenitors cells** CPAP therapy results in increased levels of endothelial progenitor cells***

BMI: body mass index; CPAP: continuous positive airway pressure; OSA: obstructive sleep apnea; *P < 0.001; **R = -0.67, P < 0.001; ***P = 0.036

Conclusion
Obstructive sleep apnea was associated with abnormal endothelial repair capacity and apoptosis.

Commentary
Increased rates of endothelial apoptosis and reduced endothelial repair capacity may mediate well-documented accelerated atherosclerosis and cardiovascular morbidity in patients with obstructive sleep apnea (OSA). Whether OSA affects endothelial apoptosis and repair capacity independently from obesity is controversial. Elevated levels of circulating endothelial apoptotic microparticles (EMPs), a marker of endothelial apoptosis, have been reported in obese individuals who were not systematically evaluated for OSA. Considering a high prevalence of OSA in obesity, unrecognized OSA may have contributed to increased rate of endothelial apoptosis. We aimed to determine the effects of OSA on endothelial apoptosis and repair capacity in the absence of any conditions known to affect the vascular endothelium, including obesity.

Circulating levels of endothelial progenitor cells (EPCs), a marker of endothelial repair capacity, and EMPs were quantified before and after four-week therapy with continuous positive airway pressure in otherwise healthy non-obese patients with OSA and healthy controls matched for age, gender and adiposity. Before treatment, levels of EMPs were greater and levels of EPCs were lower in patients with OSA than in controls. Levels of EMPs and EPCs were inversely related, suggesting that enhanced endothelial apoptosis may exhaust the repair capacity of the vascular endothelium in OSA thereby resulting in continuous endothelial damage. Furthermore, the significant correlation between levels of EMPs and endothelium-dependent vasodilation suggests that enhanced endothelial apoptosis impairs endothelial vasomotor function. Levels of EPCs increased significantly after effective treatment of OSA, suggesting that treatment of OSA restores endothelial repair capacity.

These findings indicate that OSA independently promotes vascular endothelial apoptosis and impairs endothelial repair capacity and that short-term treatment of OSA in part alleviates these changes. By restoring endothelial repair capacity, treatment of OSA may prevent or at least delay the development and progression of cardiovascular complications of OSA.

Sanja Jelic
Division of Pulmonary, Allergy, and Critical Care Medicine
Columbia University College of P&S

Evaluation of sham-CPAP as a placebo in CPAP intervention studies. Rodway GW, Weaver TE, Mancini C, Cater J, Maislin G, Staley B, Ferguson KA, George CF, Schulman DA, Greenberg H, Rapoport DM, Walsleben JA, Lee-Chiong T, Kuna ST. *Sleep. 2010 Feb 1;33(2):260-6.*

Is sham-continuous positive airway pressure an acceptable placebo intervention in studies of persons with obstructive sleep apnea?

Subjects	Methods	Outcomes
First 104 subjects with OSA in the CATNAP trial randomized to sham CPAP • AHI: 5-30	Assessments: • Analysis of PSGs with and without sham CPAP	Compared to PSG without sham-CPAP, first night with sham-CPAP was associated with: • Decrease in SE • Increase in arousal index • Increase in N1 sleep • Prolonged latency to REM sleep • Increase in hypopneas • Decrease in apneas

AHI: apnea hypopnea index; AI: arousal index; CATNAP: CPAP Apnea Trial North American Program; CPAP: continuous positive airway pressure; N1: sleep stage 1; OSA: obstructive sleep apnea; PSG: polysomnography; REM SL: latency to REM sleep; SE: sleep efficiency

Conclusion
The use of sham-continuous positive airway pressure in intervention trials of persons with obstructive sleep apnea was associated with differences in sleep architecture and respiratory events that were statistically significant but most likely of minimal clinical significance.

Commentary
Sham-CPAP is currently the placebo intervention of choice in randomized controlled trials (RCTs) evaluating the effectiveness of CPAP treatment.[1-4] Although these studies uniformly report no difference in apnea hypopnea index (AHI) on polysomnograms (PSGs) with and without sham-CPAP in patients randomized to the placebo intervention arm, no systematic evaluation in a large number of subjects has assessed the effect of sham-CPAP on multiple other PSG measures that might influence clinical outcomes. Thus, the primary purpose of this study was to perform a comprehensive evaluation of sham-CPAP effects on PSG outcomes in subjects with obstructive sleep apnea (OSA). To make this comparison, we used data obtained from participants in the CPAP Apnea Trial North American Program (CATNAP), a multi-center, randomized, triple-blind study utilizing sham-CPAP as the placebo intervention.

After our study data had been analyzed, it became apparent that the most interesting study finding may have concerned the respiratory parameters – specifically, the decrease in the number of obstructive apneas (39.3 [SD 51.0] vs. 67.7 [SD 63.7], P < 0.001) and the increase in the number of hypopneas (158.7 [SD 92.0] vs. 140.7 [SD 68.5], P = 0.029) on the sham-CPAP PSG compared to the PSG without sham-CPAP. Despite the changes in the type of respiratory event, the AHI determinations on the sham-CPAP PSG were, nevertheless, either similar or minimally increased compared to those on the study without sham-CPAP (Total AHI: 34.0 [SD 20.1] vs. 33.8 [SD 13.8], P = 0.921).

The shift from apneas to hypopneas was not explained by differences in sleep staging or time spent in the supine position, but one can speculate that the change in the type of respiratory event may have been due to other factors. For instance, the swing from apneas to hypopneas may have been due to increased inhaled carbon dioxide on the sham-CPAP study because of mask dead space, the application of the small positive airway pressure delivered by the sham-CPAP device (< 1 cm H_2O), the increase in arousal index and wakefulness after sleep onset episodes on the sham-CPAP PSG, or the different methods used to record airflow with sham-CPAP (within the mask) and without sham-CPAP (via nasal cannula). In addition, we must consider the possible influence of night-to-night variability in PSG outcome measures in subjects and patients with OSA.[5-8] In studies comparing multiple PSG study nights in the same subjects without *any* intervention, there is evidence of broad inter-PSG variation in AHI between nights.[7,9]

Furthermore, the changes in sleep staging variables suggested decreased sleep quality during the subjects' first night using sham-CPAP compared to the preceding PSG without sham-CPAP. For instance, sleep efficiency and minutes in slow wave sleep decreased, while arousal index, latency to REM sleep, episodes of wakefulness, and minutes in stage 1 NREM sleep increased during the sham-CPAP PSG. We suggest that the probable explanation for these findings is a "mask effect" of wearing the CPAP apparatus for the first time. The novel experience of wearing this device may have accounted for the participants' decrease in sleep quality on the sham-CPAP study. It is likely that similar effects of the initial mask intervention on sleep would be present on a PSG with "active" CPAP. Such a possible device-driven alteration in sleep may in some respects be analogous to the so-called "first night effect" on diagnostic PSG results.[10-12] It is therefore conceivable that the sleep stage differences seen on the first night using sham-CPAP *compared* to the diagnostic PSG would not have been present if the sham-CPAP PSG had been performed following several nights of use.

Using a fixed order study design similar to that in the current study, Henke and colleagues[13] compared the outcome measures from PSGs without and with sham-CPAP in 18 subjects with OSA (mean AHI on the PSG without sham-CPAP 68.1 ± 25.2 events/hr) and found that the placebo intervention in this relatively small sample did not significantly affect any of the measured sleep parameters. No studies, however, have previously examined the effect of sham-CPAP on other potentially important PSG measures such as arousal index, AHI during REM, and AHI events associated with oxygen desaturation > 3%. In addition to our larger sample size than the study of Henke et al.[13], the subjects studied by Henke and coworkers had more severe OSA than the subjects in this investigation. It is conceivable that limiting our comparison to patients with mild to moderate OSA may have contributed to the more notable PSG changes in our study.

In summary, in order to account for the placebo and possible therapeutic effects on sham-CPAP, determination of clinically-related outcomes on CPAP treatment in RCTs should be based on comparison of the change in the selected outcome measures between participants randomized to the active and sham-CPAP intervention arms. While the results of this study support the use

132

of sham-CPAP as a placebo in RCTs evaluating the effects of CPAP treatment in patients with OSA, future RCTs using sham-CPAP might consider assessing the effect of this intervention on PSG measures following a week or more of participant use in order to rule out influences such as the "first night (or mask) effect."

This work was supported by NIH grant R01 HL076101 and the Respironics Sleep and Respiratory Foundation.

George W. Rodway
University of Utah College of Nursing

Terri E. Weaver
University of Illinois at Chicago College of Nursing

Samuel T. Kuna
Philadelphia Veterans Affairs Medical Center and
University of Pennsylvania

References

1. Campos-Rodriguez F et al. Effect of continuous positive airway pressure on ambulatory BP in patients with sleep apnea and hypertension: a placebo-controlled trial. Chest. 2006; 129:1459-67.
2. Loredo JS et al. Effect of continuous positive airway pressure vs placebo continuous positive airway pressure on sleep quality in obstructive sleep apnea. Chest. 1999; 116:1545-9.
3. Profant J et al. A randomized, controlled trial of 1 week of continuous positive airway pressure treatment on quality of life. Heart Lung. 2003; 32:52-8.
4. Ziegler MG et al. Effect of continuous positive airway pressure and placebo treatment on sympathetic nervous activity in patients with obstructive sleep apnea. Chest. 2001; 120:887-93.
5. Bliwise DL et al. Factors associated with nightly variability in sleep-disordered breathing in the elderly. Chest. 1991; 100:973-6.
6. Le Bon O et al. Mild to moderate sleep respiratory events: one negative night may not be enough. Chest. 2000; 118:353-9.
7. Mendelson WB. Use of the sleep laboratory in suspected sleep apnea syndrome: is one night enough? Cleve Clin J Med. 1994; 61:299-303.
8. Meyer TJ et al. One negative polysomnogram does not exclude obstructive sleep apnea. Chest. 1993; 103:756-60.
9. Mosko SS et al. Night-to-night variability in sleep apnea and sleep-related periodic leg movements in the elderly. Sleep. 1988; 11:340-8.
10. Agnew HWJ et al. The first night effect: an EEG study of sleep. Psychophysiology. 1966; 2:263-6.
11. Le Bon O et al. The first-night effect may last more than one night. J Psychiatr Res. 2001; 35:165-72.
12. Lorenzo JL et al. Variability of sleep parameters across multiple laboratory sessions in healthy young subjects: the "very first night effect". Psychophysiology. 2002; 39:409-13.

13. Henke KG et al. Effect of nasal continuous positive airway pressure on neuropsychological function in sleep apnea-hypopnea syndrome. A randomized, placebo-controlled trial. Am J Respir Crit Care Med. 2001; 163:911-7.

Gender differences in obstructive sleep apnea and treatment response to continuous positive airway pressure. Ye L, Pien GW, Ratcliffe SJ, Weaver TE. *J Clin Sleep Med. 2009 Dec 15;5(6):512-8.*

Are there gender differences in clinical features of obstructive sleep apnea and response to treatment with continuous positive airway pressure?

Subjects	Methods	Outcomes
176 subjects with severe OSA • Gender: 86% males	Assessments (at baseline and at 3 months after treatment): • FOSQ • SIP • ESS • MSLT • POMS • Multivariable apnea prediction index • PVT	Despite comparable age, BMI and AHI, compared to men, female subjects had at baseline: • Lower functional status • Greater subjective daytime sleepiness • More apnea symptoms • Greater mood disturbance • Worse neurobehavioral performance For both genders, CPAP treatment was associated with similar improvements in: • Functional status • Symptoms

AHI: apnea hypopnea index; BMI: body mass index; CPAP: continuous positive airway pressure; ESS: Epworth sleepiness scale; FOSQ: Functional outcomes of sleep questionnaire; MSLT: Multiple sleep latency test; OSA: obstructive sleep apnea; POMS: Profile of mood states; PVT: psychomotor vigilance task; SDB: sleep disordered breathing; SIP: Sickness impact profile

Conclusion
Although women with obstructive sleep apnea had lower functional status and more severe apnea symptoms compared to men, response to continuous positive airway pressure therapy was similar in both genders.

Commentary
In 2009 we conducted an analysis of data on a sample of 152 men and 24 women who participated in a multicenter continuous positive airway pressure (CPAP) effectiveness study. We questioned whether gender differences might exist in clinical manifestations of obstructive sleep apnea (OSA) and whether women's responses to CPAP are similar to those of men. We will primarily discuss three aspects of our findings from this analysis here: clinical manifestations, treatment response, and treatment adherence. Hopefully this will bring insights to future investigations on this topic and help to decrease gender-based bias in clinical practice.

OSA Clinical Manifestations Gender differences in the clinical manifestation of OSA may contribute to the clinical under-diagnosis of OSA in women, and thus have important implications for education, clinical practice, and research.[1] We found that despite similarities in age, degree of obesity, and OSA severity, women had significantly lower functional status, more subjective daytime sleepiness, higher frequency of apnea symptoms, more mood disturbance, and poorer neurobehavioral performance when compared to men. Our finding of more impaired functional status in women was similar to findings reported in a Swedish population.[2] Further studies are needed to examine how functional status is impaired in each gender with OSA, in order to design gender-specific supports to improve patient quality of life. If women do report more daytime sleepiness, as is suggested by our analysis and other studies[3,4], it is critical to examine why current clinical practice, which emphasizes sleepiness as a feature of OSA, does not facilitate the diagnosis of women with this disorder. It is possible that women may report their sleepiness differently and have a tendency to emphasize fatigue or lack of energy more than sleepiness.[5] Additional studies should examine how men and women report sleepiness, which will contribute to rectifying the problem of clinical under recognition of OSA in women. A gender-based referral bias may contribute to our finding, as well as the high male-to-female ratio (6.3:1) in this study. Referral bias needs to be considered when examining gender differences in OSA manifestations when using clinical samples. This referral bias may be caused by the lack of understanding of gender differences in clinical presentation, and a low awareness of OSA in women due to the stereotype held by health care providers that OSA is a male disease. A larger sample size, ideally from a community sample, could clarify further analyses by controlling for other important covariates such as menopausal status and comorbidities.

CPAP Treatment Response Remarkably few studies have examined gender differences in therapeutic management for OSA. We found that CPAP treatment significantly improved impaired functional status, daytime sleepiness, mood state, apnea symptoms, and neurobehavioral performance in both men and women. A tendency toward greater improvement in each outcome was observed in women compared to men, but none of the comparisons were statistically significant. Our examination of gender differences in treatment response was an exploratory analysis due to the small number of women in the sample. Ideally, to evaluate gender differences in treatment response, it would have been better to consider the placebo effect, which may be different between genders. Additional studies are needed to extend these findings by including more female patients in a large sample with different OSA severity levels, and with special consideration of potential gender differences in placebo effects on subjective outcomes.

CPAP adherence We did not find any gender difference in CPAP adherence in this study. A limited body of research suggests that there are gender-based differences in CPAP adherence, but the results are conflicting.[6,7] Different sample characteristics and methodological differences among studies have likely contributed to the lack of consistency in findings. Although most studies exclusively examine the average hours of CPAP used, CPAP adherence patterns may differ between genders. For example, continued CPAP use has been found to be associated with male gender, and women are more likely to initially refuse CPAP.[8] In addition, men and women may present with different levels of motivation and dissimilar psychological responses to CPAP treatment.[9] Future studies examining gender differences in CPAP adherence should consider the patterns of use and the motivation underlying its use (self-efficacy).

Findings of our study add to the growing evidence of gender differences in clinical manifestations. Understanding these differences will not only contribute to greater recognition in women with OSA by clinicians, but also help to develop gender-sensitive interventions and consultations aimed to improve quality of life in this population. Adequately powered studies considering possible referral and response bias are necessary to examine gender differences in OSA clinical manifestations and response to CPAP treatment. Additional studies are needed to examine the effect of gender on CPAP adherence behavior, especially in adherence patterns and motivations.

Lichuan Ye
Boston College
William F. Connell School of Nursing

References

1. Ye L et al. Gender differences in the clinical manifestation of obstructive sleep apnea. Sleep Med. 2009; 10:1075-84.
2. Grunstein RR et al. Impact of self-reported sleep-breathing disturbances on psychosocial performance in the Swedish Obese Subjects (SOS) Study. Sleep. 1995; 18:635-43.
3. Young T et al. The occurrence of sleep-disordered breathing among middle-aged adults. N Engl J Med. 1993; 328:1230-5.
4. Larsson LG et al. Gender differences in symptoms related to sleep apnea in a general population and in relation to referral to sleep clinic. Chest. 2003; 124:204-11.
5. Chervin RD. Sleepiness, fatigue, tiredness, and lack of energy in obstructive sleep apnea. Chest. 2000; 118:372-9.
6. Pelletier-Fleury N et al. The age and other factors in the evaluation of compliance with nasal continuous positive airway pressure for obstructive sleep apnea syndrome. A Cox's proportional hazard analysis. Sleep Med. 2001; 2:225-32.
7. Sin DD et al. Long-term compliance rates to continuous positive airway pressure in obstructive sleep apnea: a population-based study. Chest. 2002; 121:430-5.
8. McArdle N et al. Long-term use of CPAP therapy for sleep apnea/hypopnea syndrome. Am J Respir Crit Care Med. 1999; 159:1108-14.
9. Ye L et al. Gender differences in adherence to positive airway pressure treatment in obstructive sleep apnea. Sleep. 2011; 34:A903.

Impact of sleeping position on central sleep apnea/Cheyne-Stokes respiration in patients with heart failure. Joho S, Oda Y, Hirai T, Inoue H. *Sleep Med. 2010 Feb;11(2):143-8.*

Do different sleeping positions affect central sleep apnea in persons with heart failure?

Subjects	Methods	Outcomes
71 subjects with HF • EF: < 45% • Positional OSA: n = 12 • Non-positional: n = 13	Assessments: • AHI during different body positions during sleep using cardiorespiratory polygraphy 25 subjects with predominantly CSA were classified as having positional or non-positional CSA: • CAI: 10 per hr • OAI: < 5 per hour Definitions: • Positional CSA: lateral to supine AHI ratio < 50% • Non-positional: ratio ≥ 50%	Compared to the positional group, subjects with non-positional CSA had: • Higher BNP level • Lower EF • Higher trans-tricuspid pressure gradient Factors that predicted the degree of positional CSA were: • Advanced age* • BNP** • Lung-to-finger circulation time*** In 8 subjects, therapy of HF converted non-positional CSA to positional CSA In 7 positional CSA subjects, one night of positional therapy resulted in: • Reduced CSA[#] • Lower BNP level[##]

AHI: apnea hypopnea index; BNP: brain natriuretic peptide; CAI: central apnea index; CRP: cardiorespiratory polygraphy; CSA: central sleep apnea; EF: ejection fraction; HF: heart failure; OAI: obstructive apnea index; TTPG: trans-tricuspid pressure gradient; *$P = 0.006$; **$P = 0.017$; ***$P = 0.020$; [#]$P < 0.05$; [##]$P = 0.07$

Conclusion
Sleep-position dependency of central sleep apnea correlated with severity of heart failure, and therapy of the latter converted non-positional to positional central sleep apnea.

Commentary
Up to 50% of patients with heart failure (HF) have sleep-related breathing disorders; 40% exhibit central sleep apnea (CSA) or Cheyne-Stokes respiration, and 10% have obstructive sleep apnea (OSA).[1,2] The level of respiratory distress during sleep among patients with OSA varies

according to position. Cartwright defined "positional sleep apnea" as a 50% decrease in apnea hypopnea index (AHI) in the lateral position compared with the supine position.[3] In contrast, patients in whom AHI in the lateral position does not decrease by ≥50% relative to the supine position are defined as having "non-positional sleep apnea".[4] Those with non-positional OSA have lower mean oxygen saturation, higher AHI and worse sleep quality than those with positional OSA.[4]

Similarly to OSA, the effect of body position on Cheyne-Stokes respiration was firstly described in patients with stroke.[5] Several reports also indicate that CSA is improved in patients with various diseases when sleeping in the lateral position compared with the supine position.[6,7] Interestingly, the AHI does not decrease in some patients when sleeping in the lateral position. Additionally, sleeping position could affect the severity of CSA in patients with HF. The present study therefore examined the influence of sleeping position on CSA with Cheyne-Stokes respiration in patients with HF.

Sahlin et al.[6] reported that sleep in the supine position increased the frequency of CSA in 20 patients with cardiovascular disease. Szollosi et al. also showed similar findings in 20 patients with HF.[7] Although the severity of HF was similar between the present findings and that of Sahlin's study (6), the prevalence of non-positional CSA was greater in Sahlin's study (80%) than in ours (52%). In addition, the severity of positional CSA seemed to be higher in Sahlin's study (0.63) than in our (0.53) and in Szollosi's studies (0.36). The difference might be explained by a high prevalence of stroke in Sahlin's study (40%). In fact, because stroke is another cause of CSA[8], such patients were excluded from the present study.

Optimal treatment for HF might improve or abolish CSA.[9,10] Animal studies suggest that elevated left atrial pressure could directly stimulate hyperventilation and hypocapnia leading to a decrease in the $PaCO_2$ level to below the apneic threshold, thus triggering periodic breathing.[11] These findings indicated a highly significant relationship between pulmonary capillary wedge pressure and degree of CSA. Increased left ventricular end-diastolic or left atrial pressure might contribute to hyperventilation and subsequent hypocapnia via direct stimulation of the J-receptors in the lungs.[12] Congestion also interferes with gas exchange and with the ability to store gases, particularly carbon dioxide, in the functional residual capacity of the lungs. The net effect of such impairment is that the ability of the lungs to manage variations of partial pressures of oxygen and carbon dioxide is reduced.

Why AHI in the supine and lateral positions responds differently to medical treatment remains unknown. The close correlation between log_{10} BNP levels and the severity of positional central apnea in the present study suggested that the level of end-diastolic pressure alters the degree of positional central apnea. Both right and left lateral positions decreased pulmonary capillary wedge pressure compared with the supine position in patients with normal cardiac output and a normal range of pulmonary capillary wedge pressure.[13] In contrast, pulmonary capillary wedge pressure did not change in patients with severe HF after moving from the supine, to the lateral position.[14] Thus, the abolished positional change of left atrial pressure might result in non-positional CSA in patients with severe HF. On the other hand, intensive medical therapy might result in a switch to positional CSA through recovery of positional change of left atrial pressure.

Although continuous positive airway pressure is the main treatment modality for patients with

HF and central apnea[15], positional therapy presents another option for patients with positional CSA. However, additional treatment for HF might be needed for patients with non-positional CSA. This could represent an important therapy for both positional and non-positional patients that become positional after intensive therapy.

These findings suggest that as cardiac dysfunction progresses, severity of CSA also increases and positional CSA becomes position-independent. Positional therapy could decrease CSA, thereby having a valuable effect on HF.

Shuji Joho
Second Department of Internal Medicine
Toyama University Hospital

References

1. Javaheri S et al. Sleep apnea in 81 ambulatory male patients with stable heart failure. Types and their prevalences, consequences, and presentations. Circulation. 1998; 97:2154-9.
2. Sin DD et al. Risk factors for central and obstructive sleep apnea in 450 men and women with congestive heart failure. Am J Respir Crit Care Med. 1999;160: 1101-6.
3. Cartwright R et al. A comparative study of treatments for positional sleep apnea. Sleep. 1991; 14:546-52.
4. Oksenberg A et al. Association of body position with severity of apneic events in patients with severe nonpositional obstructive sleep apnea. Chest. 2000; 118:1018-24.
5. Oksenberg A et al. Cheyne-Stokes respiration during sleep: a possible effect of body position. Med Sci Monit. 2002; 8:CS61-65.
6. Sahlin C et al. Cheyne-Stokes respiration and supine dependency. Eur Respir J. 2005; 25:829-33.
7. Szollosi I et al. Lateral sleeping position reduces severity of central sleep apnea / Cheyne-Stokes respiration. Sleep. 2006; 29:1045-51.
8. Parra O et al. Time course of sleep-related breathing disorders in first-ever stroke or transient ischemic attack. Am J Respir Crit Care Med. 2000; 161:375-80.
9. Solin P et al. Influence of pulmonary capillary wedge pressure on central apnea in heart failure. Circulation 1999; 99:1574-9.
10. Olson TP et al. Effects of acute changes in pulmonary wedge pressure on periodic breathing at rest in heart failure patients. Am Heart J. 2007; 153:104.e1-7.
11. Chenneul B et al. Increased propensity for apnea in response to acute elevations in left atrial pressure during sleep in the dog. J Appl Physiol. 2006; 101:76-83.
12. Yu J et al. Stimulation of breathing by activation of pulmonary peripheral afferents in rabbits. J Appl Physiol. 1998; 85:1485-92.
13. Nakao S et al. Effects of supine and lateral positions on cardiac output and intracardiac pressures: an experimental study. Circulation. 1986; 73:579-85.
14. Gawlinski A et al. Effect of positioning on SvO_2 in the critically ill patient with a low ejection fraction. Nurs Res. 1998; 47:293-9.
15. Sin DD et al. Effects of continuous positive airway pressure on cardiovascular outcomes in heart failure patients with and without Cheyne-Stokes respiration. Circulation. 2000; 102:61-66.

Long-term effect of continuous positive airway pressure in hypertensive patients with sleep apnea. Barbé F, Durán-Cantolla J, Capote F, de la Peña M, Chiner E, Masa JF, Gonzalez M, Marín JM, Garcia-Rio F, de Atauri JD, Terán J, Mayos M, Monasterio C, del Campo F, Gomez S, de la Torre MS, Martinez M, Montserrat JM; Spanish Sleep and Breathing Group. *Am J Respir Crit Care Med. 2010 Apr 1;181(7):718-26.*

Does continuous positive airway pressure therapy improve blood pressure in non-sleepy persons with hypertension and obstructive sleep apnea?

Subjects	Methods	Outcomes
359 subjects with nonsymptomatic OSA and hypertension • Age: 56 ± 10 yrs • BMI: 32 ± 5 • AHI: 45 ± 20 • ESS: 7 ± 3 • One of the following 1. On antihypertensive treatment 2. SBP > 140 or DBP > 90 mm Hg	Controlled trial Subjects were randomized to: • CPAP: n = 178 • Conservative treatment: n = 181 Assessments: • BP at baseline and at 3, 6, and 12 months	At 1 yr, CPAP treatment was associated with: • Decrease in SBP: by 1.89 mm Hg* • Decrease in DBP: by 2.19 mmHg** Good CPAP compliance (> 5.6 hrs per night) was associated with the greatest reduction in BP

AHI: apnea hypopnea index
BMI: body mass index; BP: blood pressure; CPAP: continuous positive airway pressure; DBP: diastolic blood pressure; ESS: Epworth sleepiness scale; OSA: obstructive sleep apnea; SaO_2: arterial oxygen saturation; SBP: systolic blood pressure; *95% CI: -3.90, 0.11 mm Hg; P = 0.0654; **95% CI: -3.46, -0.93 mm Hg; P = 0.0008

Conclusion
One year of continuous positive airway pressure therapy for nonsymptomatic severe obstructive sleep apnea produced a small decrease in blood pressure in hypertensive persons.

Commentary
Continuous positive airway pressure (CPAP) is the current treatment for patients with symptomatic obstructive sleep apnea (OSA). Its use for all subjects with sleep-disordered breathing, regardless of daytime symptoms, is unclear. The effects of CPAP on blood pressure are moderate and variable. Short-term studies performed in subjects with severe OSA but without daytime sleepiness failed to show any effect of CPAP on 24-hour ambulatory blood pressure. These studies infer that CPAP in not useful in nonsleepy patients.

This multicenter controlled trial assesses the effects of 1 year of CPAP treatment on blood pressure (BP) in nonsymptomatic, hypertensive patients with OSA. The goal of this study was to assess whether CPAP treatment produces a clinically significant reduction in blood pressure in nonsleepy hypertensive patients with OSA. To this end, we have analyzed the long-term effects of CPAP treatment on a large group of hypertensive patients with OSA included in the Spanish cohort of nonsleepy patients with OSA. This would establish whether there is likely to be a cardiovascular benefit to treating hypertensive patients with OSA, even when they do not report significant daytime hypersomnolence.

We evaluated 359 patients with OSA. Inclusion criteria consisted of an apnea hypopnea index (AHI) greater than 19 hour^{-1}, an Epworth Sleepiness Scale score less than 11, and one of the following: under antihypertensive treatment or systolic blood pressure greater than 140 or diastolic blood pressure greater than 90 mm Hg. Patients were randomized to CPAP (n=178) or to conservative treatment (n=181). BP was evaluated at baseline and at 3, 6, and 12 months of follow-up.

Mean (SD) values were as follows: age, 56 $\pm$ 10 years; body mass index (BMI), 32 $\pm$ 5 Kg.m^{-2}; apnea hypopnea index (AHI), 45 $\pm$ 20 h^{-1}; and Epworth Sleepiness Scale score, 7 $\pm$ 3. After adjusting for follow-up time, baseline blood pressure values, AHI, time with arterial oxygen saturation less than 90%, and BMI, together with the change in BMI at follow-up, CPAP treatment decreased systolic blood pressure by 1.89 mm Hg (95% confidence interval: -3.90, 0.11 mm Hg; P = 0.0654), and diastolic blood pressure by 2.19 mm Hg (95% confidence interval: -3.46, -0.93 mm Hg; P = 0.0008). The most significant reduction in BP was in patients who used CPAP for more than 5.6 hours per night. CPAP compliance was related to AHI and the decrease in Epworth Sleepiness Scale score.

This study shows that CPAP treatment is associated with a decrease in systolic and diastolic blood pressure in nonsleepy hypertensive patients with OSA. This effect is evident only in patients who use CPAP more than 5.6 hours per night.

Ferran Barbé
IRB Lleida, Lleida and CIBERes, Madrid

Manuel Sánchez de la Torre
IRB Lleida, Lleida and CIBERes, Madrid

References
1. Young T et al. The occurrence of sleep-disordered breathing among middle- aged adults. N Engl J Med. 1993; 328:1230-1235.
2. Duran J et al. Obstructive sleep apnea-hypopnea and related clinical features in a population-based sample of subjects aged 30 to 70 yr. Am J Respir Crit Care Med. 2001; 163:685-689.
3. Nieto FJ et al. Association of sleep-disordered breathing, sleep apnea, and hypertension in a large community-based study. JAMA. 2000; 283:1829-1836.
4. Lavie P et al. Obstructive sleep apnoea syndrome as a risk factor for hypertension: population study. British Med J. 2000; 320:479-482.
5. Peppard PE et al. Prospective study of the association between sleep-disordered breathing and hypertension. N Engl J Med. 2000; 342:1378-1384.
6. Hedner J et al. The link between sleep apnea and cardiovascular disease - Time to target the nonsleepy sleep apneics? Am J Respir Crit Care Med. 2001; 163:5-6.
7. Marin JM et al. Long-term cardiovascular outcomes in men with obstructive sleep apnoea-hypopnoea with or without treatment with continuous positive airway pressure: an

observational study. Lancet. 2005; 365:1046-1053.

8. Monasterio C et al. Effectiveness of Continuous Positive Airway Pressure in Mild Sleep Apnea-Hypopnea Syndrome. Am J Respir Crit Care Med. 2001; 164:939-943.

9. Hui DS et al. Nasal CPAP reduces systemic blood pressure in patients with obstructive sleep apnoea and mild sleepiness. Thorax. 2006; 61:1083-1090.

10. Barbe F et al. Treatment with continuous positive airway pressure is not effective in patients with sleep apnea but no daytime sleepiness. A randomized, controlled trial. Ann Intern Med. 2001; 134:1015-1023.

11. Robinson GV et al. Continuous positive airway pressure does not reduce blood pressure in nonsleepy hypertensive OSA patients. Eur Respir J. 2006; 27:1229-1235.

Nasopharyngoscopic evaluation of oral appliance therapy for obstructive sleep apnoea. Chan AS, Lee RW, Srinivasan VK, Darendeliler MA, Grunstein RR, Cistulli PA. *Eur Respir J. 2010 Apr;35(4):836-42.*

What are the effects of mandibular advancement splints (MAS) on upper airway structure during wakefulness in persons with obstructive sleep apnea?

Subjects	Methods	Outcomes
35 subjects with OSA (AHI ≥ 10) using MAS • Responders: n = 18 • Nonresponders: n = 17 Definition: • Responder: ≥ 50% reduction in AHI	Assessment: • Nasopharyngoscopy in a supine position during wakefulness	Use of MAS was associated with: • Increase in velopharyngeal caliber (+40 ± 10%) • Greater increase in velopharyngeal cross-sectional area in responders than nonresponders: +56 ± 16% vs. +22 ± 13%* • Minor changes occurring in oropharynx and hypopharynx • Greater upper airway collapse compared to baseline cross-sectional area during Müller maneuver in nonresponders than responders in the: 1. Velopharynx (-94 ± 4% vs. -69 ± 9%**) 2. Oropharynx (-37 ± 6% vs. -16 ± 3%***) • Greater upper airway collapse during the Müller man oeuvre with MAS in nonresponders than responders in the: 1. Velopharynx (-80 ± 11% vs. +9 ± 37%[#]), 2. Oropharynx (-36 ± 6% vs. -20 ± 5%[##]) 3. Hypopharynx (-64 ± 6% vs. -42 ± 6%[###])

AHI: apnea hypopnea index; MAS: mandibular advancement splints; OSA: obstructive sleep apnea; UA: upper airway; *P < 0.05; **P < 0.01; ***P < 0.01; #P < 0.001; ##P < 0.05; ###P < 0.05

Conclusion
Mandibular advancement splints increased the caliber of the velopharynx in persons with obstructive sleep apnea.

Commentary
While continuous positive airway pressure (CPAP) is a highly efficacious treatment for obstructive sleep apnea (OSA), there is a need for other treatment options because the clinical effectiveness of CPAP is often limited by poor patient acceptance and tolerance, and sub-optimal compliance.[1-3] Mandibular advancement splints (MAS) are an alternative to CPAP for the treatment of OSA.[4] With increasing recognition of the role of craniofacial factors in the pathogenesis of OSA, there has been an expansion of the research evidence to support the use of MAS in clinical practice.[5] On the basis of this evidence, clinical practice parameters of the American Academy of Sleep Medicine currently recommend the use of MAS for the treatment of mild to moderate OSA; or for patients with severe OSA who are unable to tolerate or refuse treatment with CPAP.[6]

A consistent finding across all studies is that success with MAS is not achievable in all patients.[5,7] Previous studies have identified a range of anthropomorphic, physiologic and polysomnographic parameters associated with a better treatment outcome. Such predictors of successful oral appliance treatment outcome include female gender, lower age, lower body mass index, smaller neck circumference, lower baseline apnea hypopnea index, supine-dependent OSA and primary oropharyngeal collapse of the upper airway during sleep.[8-11] However, there have been no published prospective studies demonstrating the ability to predict the outcome of oral appliance treatment using any parameter, either singly or in combination. Hence, while the findings of these studies provide general guidance for clinicians, it is not possible to reliably apply them in clinical decision-making for individual patients. This represents a major deficiency in clinical practice in this area, and there is a critical need for research to resolve this. A better understanding of the biomechanical mechanisms that mediate the efficacy of MAS may have important clinical implications, including the development of more efficacious appliances, and may improve the selection of patients for this treatment modality.

We have previously used upper airway magnetic resonance imaging (MRI) to study the effect of mandibular advancement on upper airway anatomy. We found that the mechanism of action of mandibular advancement was to increase the caliber of the upper airway, predominantly as a result of an increase in the volume of the velopharynx and was mediated by an increase its lateral dimensions.[12]

In the present study, nasopharyngoscopy was used to assess the upper airway during wakefulness. This imaging modality was chosen as, although upper airway MRI is a powerful research tool, it is expensive and not widely available, and, as such, is not likely to be a method that can be readily translated to clinical practice. In contrast, an evaluation of the upper airway with nasopharyngoscopy can be easily performed in the clinical setting. Nasopharyngoscopy also provides real-time imaging, allowing the effect of dynamic maneuvers to be assessed. The results confirm the findings of our previous study, namely that mandibular advancement causes an increase in the caliber of the velopharynx, with relatively minor changes occurring in the oropharynx and hypopharynx. In addition, nasopharyngoscopy performed during wakefulness was able to discern structural differences in the upper airway between those who respond to treatment with MAS and those who do not.

The findings from these studies challenge the traditional understanding of the mechanism of action of mandibular advancement. The precise reason for this effect on velopharyngeal patency is unclear. However, soft tissue connections exist between the mandible, tongue, lateral pharyngeal walls and soft palate within the palatoglossal and palatopharyngeal arches. It has been proposed that such soft tissue connections may be stretched by mandibular advancement[13], resulting in enlargement of the velopharynx, particularly in the lateral dimension. Variations in these structures may account for the observed differences between responders and non-responders.

Given the anatomical basis of OSA[14], and the differences between responders and non-responders observed in this study, upper airway imaging has the potential to be useful for predicting treatment outcome. However, before the prediction model derived in this study can be recommended for clinical use, it needs to be validated in a prospective cohort. This is important as, in this study, mandibular advancement was provided using the custom-made MAS. In a prospective study, nasopharyngoscopic prediction would need to be made prior to construction of the MAS.

Andrew S. L. Chan
Centre for Sleep Health and Research
Department of Respiratory Medicine
Royal North Shore Hospital

Peter A. Cistulli
Woolcock Institute of Medical Research
University of Sydney

References
1. McArdle N et al. Long-term use of CPAP therapy for sleep apnea/hypopnea syndrome. Am J Respir Crit Care Med. 1999; 159(4 Pt 1):1108-1114.
2. Weaver TE et al. Night-to-night variability in CPAP use over the first three months of treatment. Sleep. 1997; 20(4):278-283.
3. Kribbs NB et al. Objective measurement of patterns of nasal CPAP use by patients with obstructive sleep apnea. American Review of Respiratory Disease. 1993; 147(4):887-895.
4. Cistulli PA et al. Treatment of snoring and obstructive sleep apnea with mandibular repositioning appliances. Sleep Medicine Reviews. 2004; 8(6):443-457.
5. Ferguson KA et al. Oral appliances for snoring and obstructive sleep apnea: a review. Sleep. 2006; 29(2):244-262.
6. Kushida CA et al. Practice parameters for the treatment of snoring and Obstructive Sleep Apnea with oral appliances: an update for 2005. Sleep. 2006; 29(2):240-243.

7. Cistulli PA et al. Treatment of snoring and obstructive sleep apnea with mandibular repositioning appliances. Sleep Med Rev. 2004; 8(6):443-457.
8. Mehta A et al. A randomized, controlled study of a mandibular advancement splint for obstructive sleep apnea. Am J Respir Crit Care Med. 2001; 163(6):1457-1461.
9. Marklund M et al. Mandibular advancement devices in 630 men and women with obstructive sleep apnea and snoring: tolerability and predictors of treatment success. Chest. 2004; 125(4):1270-1278.
10. Liu Y et al. Cephalometric and physiologic predictors of the efficacy of an adjustable oral appliance for treating obstructive sleep apnea. Am J Orthod Dentofacial Orthop. 2001; 120(6):639-647.
11. Ng AT et al. Oropharyngeal collapse predicts treatment response with oral appliance therapy in obstructive sleep apnea. Sleep. 2006; 29(5):666-671.
12. Chan ASL et al. The effect of mandibular advancement on upper airway structure in obstructive sleep apnoea. Thorax. 65(8); 726-732.
13. Isono S et al. Pharyngeal patency in response to advancement of the mandible in obese anesthetized persons. Anesthesiology. 1997; 87(5):1055-1062.
14. Schwab RJ. Pro: sleep apnea is an anatomic disorder. Am J Respir Crit Care Med. 2003; 168(3): 270-271.

Natural history and predictors for progression of mild childhood obstructive sleep apnoea. Li AM, Au CT, Ng SK, Abdullah VJ, Ho C, Fok TF, Ng PC, Wing YK. *Thorax. 2010 Jan;65(1):27-31.*

What is the clinical course of mild childhood obstructive sleep apnea?

Subjects	Methods	Outcomes
56 children with mild OSA • Age: 6-13 yrs • AHI: 1-5 45 children were included in the follow-up study	Assessment: • Repeat evaluation 2 years after initial diagnosis	At follow-up, OSA was noted to be worse in 29% (13 of 45) of subjects Compared with subjects with stable OSA, those with worse OSA had: • Greater increase in waist circumference • Greater prevalence of large tonsils [occupying ≥ 50% of the airway] (at both baseline and follow-up) • Greater prevalence of habitual snoring (at both baseline and follow-up) For worsening OSA at 2-yr follow-up, the presence of large tonsils was associated with: • PPV: 53% • NPV: 83% With multivariate linear regression analysis, change in AHI was associated with the following factors: • Age at baseline* • Gender** • Presence of large tonsils at baseline*** • Change in waist circumference[#] • Persistently large tonsils[##]

AHI: apnea hypopnea index; NPV: negative predictive value; OSA: obstructive sleep apnea; PPV: positive predictive value; *beta (SE) = -0.92 (0.34), P = 0.009; **male = 1; female = 0) (beta (SE) = 4.69 (1.29), P < 0.001; ***beta (SE) = 4.36 (1.24), P = 0.001; [#]beta (SE) = 0.30 (0.09), P = 0.002; [##]beta (SE) = 5.69 (1.36), P < 0.001

Conclusion

Mild obstructive sleep apnea in children tended to persist, and the presence of large tonsils predicted worsening of the disease.

Commentary

The amount of research in the field of childhood obstructive sleep apnea (OSA) has increased substantially over the past 10 years. It has become apparent that the condition is prevalent with important sequelae if left untreated.[1-2] The 'gold standard' for diagnosing childhood OSA remains overnight polysomnography (PSG), but it has not been properly standardized with regard to its performance and interpretation. In children, normative standards for PSG cut-offs have been selected on the basis of the statistical distribution of data. However, validity of these standards as predictors for long-term outcome / presence of complications had not been established.

One of the most commonly used diagnostic criteria for childhood OSA is obstructive apnea hypopnea index (OAHI) more than or equal to 1/h of total sleep time.[3] Children with OAHI between 1 and 5/h are arbitrary classified as having mild OSA, while OAHI > 5/h represents moderate-to-severe disease. There is accumulating evidence to suggest children with OAHI > 5/h are at increased risk for cardiovascular abnormalities including hypertension and ventricular dysfunction and remodeling.[4-5] Moreover, some recent studies reported that these abnormalities are reversible following appropriate intervention[6-7], supporting prompt diagnosis and treatment for these cases. On the other hand, for children with mild OSA existing evidence on its complications is less robust. Certain studies suggested that children with mild OSA exhibited behavioral problems that improved after surgical intervention.[8-9] However, similar positive findings were not documented by other research groups.[10-11] Furthermore, natural history of mild childhood OSA is poorly defined, and the continual argument relates to whether it needs to be treated or not. Understanding the natural progression of OSA and ascertainment of factors that are associated with disease worsening would allow a more scientific approach for future patient care.

This study published in the January 2010 issue of Thorax examined the natural history of mild OSA over a 2-year period, and to investigate important risk factors that influenced disease progression.[12] Subjects were recruited from participants of an epidemiologic study that set out to evaluate the prevalence of OSA in Chinese children aged 6-13 years. The first 56 consecutive children identified to have mild OSA were invited for a repeat assessment 2 years after the diagnosis. Forty-five subjects agreed to participate, in 13 of whom (29%) their OSA worsened, defined as an increase in OAHI of > 2.38/h, which was the estimated measurement error of OAHI in children with mild OSA. The estimated error was derived from an earlier study involving children undergoing 2 consecutive nights of PSG.[13]

Male gender, younger age, large tonsils (soft tissue occupying > 50% of the oropharyngeal airway) and weight gain were found to be predictors of worsened OSA in a 2-year period.[12] The presence of large tonsils had a positive predictive value of 53% and a negative predictive value of 83% for worsening of OSA. These findings may help physicians to decide which mild cases should have earlier intervention and which could be managed under watchful monitoring.

Although this study was the first to examine natural progression of mild OSA in children, it was limited to a period of 2 years. Furthermore the sample size might not have allowed detection of other potential important risk factors for disease progression. Further studies should explore OSA progression over a longer time period, and assess different possible associated outcomes / complications for example behavioral or cognitive dysfunction. It may also be important to bring into the study protocol a treatment arm in order to answer the very relevant clinical question of whether mild OSA needs to be treated or not.

Chun T Au
Department of Pediatrics
Prince of Wales Hospital
The Chinese University of Hong Kong

Albert M. Li
Department of Pediatrics
Prince of Wales Hospital
The Chinese University of Hong Kong

References

1. Bhattacharjee R et al. Cardiovascular complications of obstructive sleep apnea syndrome: evidence from children. Prog Cardiovasc Dis. 2009; 51(5):416-433.
2. Owens JA. Neurocognitive and behavioral impact of sleep disordered breathing in children. Pediatr Pulmonol. 2009; 44(5):417-422.
3. American Academy of Sleep Medicine. International Classification of Sleep Disorders, diagnostic and coding manual. 2nd ed. Westchester, Illinois: American Academy of Sleep Medicine, 2005, pp.56-59.
4. Li AM et al. Ambulatory blood pressure in children with obstructive sleep apnoea: a community based study. Thorax. 2008; 63(9):803-809.
5. Amin R et al. Activity-adjusted 24-hour ambulatory blood pressure and cardiac remodeling in children with sleep disordered breathing. Hypertension. 2008; 51(1):84-91.
6. Chan JY et al. Cardiac remodelling and dysfunction in children with obstructive sleep apnoea: a community based study. Thorax. 2009; 64(3):233-239.
7. Ng DK et al. Ambulatory blood pressure before and after adenotonsillectomy in children with obstructive sleep apnea. Sleep Med. 2010; 11(7):721-725.
8. Hogan AM et al. Cerebral blood flow velocity and cognition in children before and after adenotonsillectomy. Pediatrics. 2008; 122(1):75-82.
9. Huang YS et al. Attention-deficit/hyperactivity disorder with obstructive sleep apnea: a treatment outcome study. Sleep Med. 2007; 8(1):18-30.
10. Calhoun SL et al. No relationship between neurocognitive functioning and mild sleep disordered breathing in a community sample of children. J Clin Sleep Med. 2009; 15;5(3):228-234.
11. Kohler MJ et al. Adenotonsillectomy and neurocognitive deficits in children with Sleep Disordered Breathing. PLoS One. 2009; 4(10):e7343.

12. Li AM et al. Natural history and predictors for progression of mild childhood obstructive sleep apnoea. Thorax. 2010; 65(1):27-31.
13. Li AM et al. Is a 2-night polysomnographic study necessary in childhood sleep-related disordered breathing? Chest. 2004; 126(5):1467-1472.

Nocturnal rostral fluid shift: a unifying concept for the pathogenesis of obstructive and central sleep apnea in men with heart failure. Yumino D, Redolfi S, Ruttanaumpawan P, Su MC, Smith S, Newton GE, Mak S, Bradley TD. *Circulation. 2010 Apr 13;121(14):1598-605.*

Does overnight rostral fluid displacement and subsequent increase in neck circumference affect the severity of obstructive and central sleep apnea in persons with heart failure?

Subjects	Methods	Outcomes
57 subjects with HF • Gender: 100% males • Age: ≥ 18 yrs • EF ≤ 45% • NYHA class: 1-3 • Stable on medical therapy Exclusion criteria: • Treated OSA • MI, coronary angioplasty or cardiac surgery within prior 3 months	Prospective observational study Subjects were divided into 2 groups: • Obstructive-dominant (≥ 50% of events are obstructive) • Central-dominant (>50% of events are central) Subjects with OSA received CPAP Assessments: • Before and after PSG 1. Leg fluid volume (bio-electrical impedance) 2. Neck circumference • During PSG 1. $TcCO_2$	Among subjects in the obstructive-dominant group, overnight change in leg fluid volume was inversely related to: • Overnight change in neck circumference* • AHI** • But not $TcCO_2$ Among subjects in the central-dominant group, overnight change in leg fluid volume was inversely related to: • Overnight change in neck circumference*** • AHI[#] • But directly related to $TcCO_2$[##] Overnight reduction in LFV was twice as high in the central as in the obstructive-dominant group[###] In both groups, change in leg fluid volume was the only significant independent correlate of AHI CPAP prevented the overnight increase in neck circumference[^]

AHI: apnea-hypopnea index; CPAP: continuous positive airway pressure; CSA: central sleep apnea; EF: ejection fraction; HF: heart failure; MI: myocardial infarction; NYHA: New York Heart Association; OSA: obstructive sleep apnea; PCO_2: partial pressure of carbon dioxide; PSG: polysomnography; $TcCO_2$: transcutaneous partial pressure of carbon dioxide; *r=-0.780, P <

0.001; **r=-0.881, P < 0.001; *** r=-0.568, P = 0.013; [#] r=-0.919, P < 0.001; [##]r=0.569, P = 0.009; [###]P < 0.001; [^]P < 0.001

Conclusion

In persons with heart failure, the development of obstructive and central sleep apnea were related to nocturnal rostral fluid shift and the accompanying increase in neck circumference.

Commentary

OSA and CSA occur commonly in patients with HF and are associated with increased mortality.[1-3] However, causes of these breathing disorders are not well established in the setting of HF but are thought to arise through different mechanisms: OSA through obesity and anatomic narrowing of the pharynx, and CSA through pulmonary congestion, hypocapnia and increased chemoreceptor sensitivity.[1,4,5] However, the observation that OSA and CSA can occur simultaneously in HF patients suggested a common pathophysiological mechanism linking these 2 disorders.[6]

Because HF is a fluid-retaining state, we hypothesized that overnight displacement of fluid from the legs into the neck might lead to OSA by narrowing the pharynx [7,8] and to CSA if fluid shifted into the lungs and caused stimulation of vagal receptors that stimulate hyperventilation and lower PCO_2.[1,5] In 57 patients with HF (ejection fraction $\leq$ 45%) we measured change in LFV and neck circumference before and after polysomnography, and $PtcCO_2$ during polysomnography. Patients were divided into an obstructive-dominant group ($\geq$ 50% of apneas and hypopneas obstructive) and a central-dominant group (> 50% of events central). Patients with OSA received continuous positive airway pressure (CPAP). In obstructive-dominant patients, the AHI was related inversely with both overnight changes in LFV (r = -0.881, P < 0.001), and in neck circumference (r = -0.623, P < 0.001), but not with $PtcCO_2$. In central-dominant patients, the AHI was inversely related to overnight change in LFV (r = -0.919, P < 0.001) and directly with $PtcCO_2$ (r = 0.569, P = 0.009), but not with overnight change in neck circumference. CPAP alleviated OSA in association with prevention of the overnight increase in neck circumference (P < 0.001).

In conclusion, these findings suggest the novel concept that nocturnal rostral fluid shift contributes to the pathogenesis of both OSA and CSA in patients with HF. In the case of OSA, this was through a concomitant increase in neck circumference. In the case of CSA, this was through an inverse relationship with $PtcCO_2$, presumably because of fluid movement into the lungs. The degree of fluid movement out of the legs at night was in turn related to inactivity and leg edema. In patients with OSA, CPAP alleviates OSA partly through preventing fluid accumulation in the neck. These findings suggest that manipulation of fluid status may be a novel means by which to treat OSA and CSA in HF patients.

Dai Yumino
Department of Cardiology
Tokyo Women's Medical University

T. Douglas Bradley
Sleep Research Laboratory of Toronto Rehab Institute
Centre for Sleep Health and Research
Toronto General Hospital of the University Health Network

References

1. Yumino D et al. Central sleep apnea and Cheyne-Stokes respiration. Proc Am Thorac Soc. 2008; 5:226-236.
2. Wang H et al. Influence of obstructive sleep apnea on mortality in patients with heart failure. J Am Coll Cardiol. 2007; 49:1625-1631.
3. Lanfranchi PA et al. Prognostic value of nocturnal Cheyne-Stokes respiration in chronic heart failure. Circulation. 1999; 99:1435-1440.
4. Yumino D et al. Prevalence and physiological predictors of sleep apnea in patients with heart failure and systolic dysfunction. J Card Fail. 2009; 15:279-285.
5. Solin P et al. Influence of pulmonary capillary wedge pressure on central apnea in heart failure. Circulation. 1999; 99:1574-1579.
6. Tkacova R et al. Overnight shift from obstructive to central apneas in patients with heart failure: role of PCO_2 and circulatory delay. Circulation. 2001; 103:238-243.
7. Shiota S et al. Alterations in upper airway crosssectional area in response to lower body positive pressure in healthy subjects. Thorax. 2007; 62:868-872.
8. Redolfi S et al. Relationship between overnight rostral fluid shift and obstructive sleep apnea in nonobese men. Am J Respir Crit Care Med. 2009; 179:241-246.

Obstructive sleep apnea and risk of motor vehicle crash: systematic review and meta-analysis.
Tregear S, Reston J, Schoelles K, Phillips B. *J Clin Sleep Med. 2009 Dec 15;5(6):573-81.*

Does obstructive sleep apnea increase the risk of motor vehicular crashes in commercial drivers?

Subjects	*Methods*	*Outcomes*
Publications that evaluated crash risk in CMV drivers with OSA	Systematic review of controlled studies Publications through 5-27-09 were searched using MEDLINE, PubMed, EMBASE, PsycINFO, CINAHL, TRIS and Cochrane by 2 independent analysts	Risk for crash was increased in persons with OSA • Mean crash-rate ratio associated with OSA is 1.21 to 4.89 Predictors of crash risk in persons with OSA include: • AHI • BMI • Daytime sleepiness (possible) • SaO_2

AHI: apnea hypopnea index; BMI: body mass index; CMV: commercial motor vehicle; MVA: motor vehicle accident; OSA: obstructive sleep apnea; SaO_2: arterial oxygen saturation

Conclusion
Untreated obstructive sleep apnea was associated with an increased risk of motor vehicle crashes.

Commentary
This report is result of an effort to get some of the excellent research that is conducted by the Federal Motor Carrier Safety Administration (FMCSA) of the Department of Transportation (DOT) into the peer-reviewed literature. A systematic review about obstructive sleep apnea and driving risk was commissioned by the FMCSA as part of the process by which the medical guidelines and standards for commercial motor vehicle drivers are developed. The results of this report were used to inform recommendations that were made to the FMCSA by a medical expert panel and by the medical review board.[1] This paper is certainly not the first one to show an increased risk for crash in individuals with obstructive sleep apnea[2], but it is the first to demonstrate the body mass index (BMI), self-reported sleepiness, degree of hypoxemia, and the apnea plus hypopnea index are correlated with crash risk. Indeed, BMI alone predicts crash, independent of its association with sleep-disordered breathing. A companion paper[3] was subsequently published from this systematic review; that report demonstrated that continuous positive airway pressure (CPAP) markedly reduces crash risk in individuals with obstructive sleep apnea. On the other hand, evidence for the efficacy of other treatments in reducing crash risk is not compelling. The FMCSA has taken this information and recommendations under advisement, and hopefully will issue regulations related to sleep apnea screening and management in commercial drivers in the near future. For the curious reader, many other

excellent, meticulous reports about the relationship between various medical conditions and moving vehicle crash languish on the FMCSA website.[4]

Barbara Phillips
Division of Pulmonary, Critical Care and Sleep Medicine
Department of Internal Medicine
University of Kentucky College of Medicine

References
1. http://www.fmcsa.dot.gov/rules-regulations/TOPICS/mep/report/Sleep-MEP-Panel-Recommendations-508.pdf.
2. Ellen RB et al. Systematic review of motor vehicle crash risk in persons with sleep apnea. J Clin Sleep Med. 2006; 2:193-200.
3. Tregear S et al. Continuous Positive Airway Pressure Reduces Risk of Motor Vehicle Crash among Drivers with Obstructive Sleep Apnea; Systematic Review and Meta-analysis. Sleep. 2010; 33:1373-1380.
4. http://www.fmcsa.dot.gov/rules-regulations/topics/mep/mep-reports.htm.

Otolaryngology office-based treatment of obstructive sleep apnea-hypopnea syndrome with titratable and nontitratable thermoplastic mandibular advancement devices. Friedman M, Pulver T, Wilson MN, Golbin D, Leesman C, Lee G, Joseph NJ. *Otolaryngol Head Neck Surg. 2010 Jul;143(1):78-84.*

How effective is thermoplastic mandibular advancement device therapy in persons with obstructive sleep apnea?

Subjects	Methods	Outcomes
Subjects with OSA who either refused or failed CPAP or surgical therapy	Cohort study Subjects were provided with MADs, including: • Nontitratable Snore Guard: n = 38 • Nontitratable SomnoGuard 2.0: n = 8 • Titratable SomnoGuard AP: n = 41 Assessments: • Objective response • Subjective response • Adherence • ESS • Snoring level • PSG Definitions: • Objective response: ≥ 50% decrease in AHI and an AHI < 20 • Overall success rate: objective response plus adherence at two months follow-up	Overall success rate was 38.6% Objective response was achieved in 62.1% of subjects • Overall mean AHI reduction: 39.96 ± 23.70 to 14.86 ± 13.46* • Adherence at two months: 58.5% • No difference in objective response or adherence in difference types of MADs • Improvements in AHI and minimum SaO_2 were better for titratable than nontitratable devices

AHI: apnea hypopnea index; CPAP: continuous positive airway pressure; ESS: Epworth sleepiness scale; MAD: mandibular advancement device; OSA: obstructive sleep apnea; PSG: polysomnography; SaO_2: arterial oxygen saturation; *P = 0.000

Conclusion
Thermoplastic mandibular advancement device therapy for persons with obstructive sleep apnea was associated with an overall success rate of less than 40%.

Commentary

Successful treatment of any disease is always dependent on the interplay of a multitude of factors. Although treatment efficacy is important and always an essential component in the selection of any intervention, it may not be the major factor determining overall success. Compliance with treatment recommendations can significantly affect the ultimate goal of disease control. Poor compliance is a known factor for all chronic diseases and OSAHS is no exception. Studies on CPAP compliance suggest variable, but relatively low, levels of compliance. Further, it is likely that the population of patients who are compliant represents those with moderate/severe disease. Based on our experience, the vast majority of patients with mild disease avoid diagnosis because of the decision to avoid CPAP. Obviously, if patients are not diagnosed they cannot be successfully treated.

Our study in otolaryngology-based mandibular advancement devices (MADs) was prompted by a need that was apparent during our care of sleep apnea patients. Patients with sleep apnea often are subjected to fractured, uncomfortable, and sometimes conflicting recommendations for treatment. Many patients come to us after experiencing this type of care. If they see a "sleep specialist" they are offered CPAP. If they are part of the unfortunate subset of patients who cannot or will not use CPAP, many are offered no other options, and often feel as if the sleep center has "no use for them." At this point many patients seek consultation with an otolaryngologist who may offer surgery as an option, but more often than not will warm the patient of the "horrors of surgery" and poor results.

In search of help, sleep apnea patients often respond to widespread dental marketing that offers "non-CPAP" treatment with dental appliances. Although many dentists will recommend a polysomnogram to titrate a MAD and confirm its value, often patients are given a device without PSG evidence of efficacy. Because of these needs, we routinely referred patients to a dental specialist for a MAD and attempted to coordinate care. However, in spite of our encouragement the vast majority of patients failed to follow-up and never obtained a MAD. The most common reasons for avoiding MAD included: 1) inconvenience of seeing yet another specialist; 2) frustration over the fractionated care of being sent from one specialist to another; 3) financial concerns because the significant cost; and 4) reluctance of some dentists to participate in preferred provider insurance plans. Compliance with our MAD recommendations hovered around 20%, which is what drove us to incorporate in-office specialized dental care for the treatment of OSA.

As an otolaryngology practice that treats most patients with CPAP and some with a wide variety of minimally-invasive and traditional procedures, we felt the need to integrate the availability of MADs into our practice. As we stated in our article: "*Due largely to their smaller size and intraoral application, MADs offer several advantages over CPAP, including noiselessness and superior portability...Thermoplastic MADs are designed for simplified, on-site office-based molding and can easily be incorporated into an otolaryngology practice with an interest in sleep medicine.*"

When disease is mild, patients are often not accepting of CPAP. In this circumstance, MADs can be an efficacious alternative given the right environment to foster compliance. Moreover, MADs can be especially beneficial for those patients with mild disease and those with adverse or unfavorable anatomy (Friedman Tongue Position III or IV) who are very poor candidates for

158

surgery. In addition to these patients, we have hundreds of patients with moderate or incomplete relief from surgery who need options beyond CPAP and traditional surgery.

Our current policy is to educate our sleep apnea patients about all of their available treatment options so that they can make an informed decision regarding their care. The results have been staggering. Since our integration of a dental specialist within our ENT practice, compliance with MAD therapy has jumped to over 80%. It is important for our patients to know that one center will provide the entirety of their care regardless of their treatment choice, which has gone a long way in improving compliance and better overall treatment outcomes. We encourage patients to try CPAP as their first-line therapy, as CPAP remains the gold standard for treatment of OSAHS. If they fail CPAP, dental appliances are offered in parallel to surgical options and most patients are encouraged to exhaust non-surgical options first. We have recently expanded our MAD services to include custom-made mandibular advancement devices made through our office. With the expertise of a dentist who comes to our office on a regular basis, we can offer both the types of management and devices needed to cover the entire spectrum of treatment under one roof – a significant convenience for patients that yields greatly improved levels of treatment compliance.

Michael Friedman
Section of Otolaryngology
Advocate Illinois Masonic Medical Center, Chicago
Department of Otolaryngology – Head and Neck Surgery
Section of Sleep Surgery
Rush University Medical Center

Kanwar Kelley
Section of Otolaryngology
Advocate Illinois Masonic Medical Center, Chicago

Outcomes of home-based diagnosis and treatment of obstructive sleep apnea. Skomro RP, Gjevre J, Reid J, McNab B, Ghosh S, Stiles M, Jokic R, Ward H, Cotton D. *Chest. 2010 Aug;138(2):257-63.*

Are there any significant differences in outcomes with continuous positive airway pressure therapy for obstructive sleep apnea diagnosed in the sleep laboratory or home?

Subjects	Methods	Outcomes
102 subjects • Age: 47.4 ± 11.4 yrs • Gender: 62% male • BMI: 32.3 ± 6.3 • ESS: 12.5 ± 4.3	Randomized trial Subjects were randomized to either: • HM level 3 followed by 1 week of APAP and fixed-pressure CPAP based on 95% pressure derived from APAP • In-laboratory split night PSG with CPAP titration Assessments (at 4 weeks): • BP • CPAP adherence • Daytime sleepiness: ESS • QOL: SAQLI, SF-36 • Sleep quality: PSQI • Patient preference	Significant improvements in ESS, PSQI, BP, and QOL compared to baseline were seen in both groups Results after 4 weeks of CPAP therapy included: • No differences in ESS* 1. PSG: 6.4 ± 3.8 2. HM: 6.5 ± 3.8 • No difference in PSQI** 1. PSG: 5.4 ± 3.1 2. HM: 6.2 ± 3.4 • No difference in SAQLI*** 1. PSG: 4.5 ± 1.1 2. HM: 4.6 +/- 1.1 • No difference in SF-36 vitality[#] 1. PSG: 62.2 ± 23.3 2. HM: 64.1 ± 18.4 • No difference in SF-36 HM[##] 1. PSG: 84.0 ± 10.4 2. HM: 81.3 ± 14.9 • No difference in BP[###] 1. PSG: 129/84 ± 11/0 2. HM: 125/81 ± 13/9 • No difference in CPAP adherence[^] 1. PSG: 5.6 ± 1.7 hrs/night 2. HM: 5.4 ± 1.0 hrs/night 76% of subjects preferred HM over PSG

APAP: automated positive airway pressure; BMI: body mass index; BP: blood pressure; CPAP: continuous positive airway pressure; ESS: Epworth sleepiness scale; HM: home monitoring;

OSA: obstructive sleep apnea; PSG: polysomnography; PSQI: Pittsburgh sleep quality index; QOL: quality of life; SAQLI: Sleep apnea quality of life index; SF 36: 36-Item Short-form health survey; *P = .71 ; **P = .30; ***P = .85; #P = .79; ##P = .39; ###P = .121; ^P = .49

Conclusion

Home-based and sleep laboratory-based diagnosis and treatment of obstructive sleep apnea resulted in comparable benefits in sleepiness, sleep quality, blood pressure and quality of life as well as similar continuous positive airway pressure therapy adherence.

Commentary

OSA is one of the most common chronic conditions and its prevalence is on a rise. As obesity rates and recognition of OSA increase so does the demand for in-lab PSG, which has long been considered a "gold standard" for the diagnosis of OSA.

Untreated OSA is associated with an increased risk of mortality, cardiovascular morbidity, MVA crashes and occupational accidents, yet most OSA patients remain undiagnosed. In many countries lack of access to in-lab PSG constitutes significant barrier to early diagnosis and therapy. Thus a simplified home-based approach, if proven as effective as in-lab PSG, could improve access to sleep apnea diagnosis and could potentially be more cost-effective than full in-lab PSG.

The application of limited cardio-respiratory (AASM classification type III) monitors in the diagnosis of OSA has been of significant interest to Sleep Medicine physicians, patients, health care organizations and home care companies for some time. In many areas the implementation of type III monitors in the diagnosis of OSA has preceded scientific evidence that would justify such an approach.

Early studies of portable monitors (PM) focused on the validation of a variety of devices and demonstrated reasonable utility in the in-patient setting (i.e. in the sleep lab), but not in the out-patient (home) setting. Outcome studies using an integrated approach to home-based OSA diagnosis and management were lacking until recently. Furthermore early studies were criticized because of low patient enrollment, methodological weaknesses and limited external validity.

In the last 4 years the evidence from three RCTs provided scientific basis for limited use of portable monitoring in selected patients with OSA. Mulgrew et al demonstrated in that home management of OSA using oximetry and CPAP in selected patients with AHI > 15 leads to similar outcomes after three months of therapy.[1]

Antic et al, demonstrated that in very selected group of OSA patients the use of oximetry and auto-CPAP supervised by experienced specialist nurses was associated with CPAP adherence and outcomes which were similar to those in the traditional approach (physician led in-lab PSG) but were more cost-effective.[2] Similarly Berry et al showed that CPAP adherence, FOSQ scores and daytime sleepiness were no different between HM and in-lab pathways.[3]

Our study confirms and extends these findings by demonstrating that the potential number of OSA patients treated in this fashion may be higher than previously thought (only 58 out of 270 or 21.5% patients in our study did not meet the inclusion criteria because of co-morbidity), that the cut-off RDI for type III PM monitors in symptomatic OSA patients can be lowered to 5 (previous investigators enrolled patients with RDI > 15) and that patients may prefer to be tested at home.

There are however significant limitations of this study: it was performed in a single tertiary care sleep clinic, in a population with high pre-test probability of OSA and no significant co-morbidities. The results of type III PM and auto CPAP titrations were evaluated by experienced PSG technologists and Sleep Medicine physicians. Back up PSG was readily available. Finally the cost-effectiveness of this approach was not evaluated in our study. These factors have to be taken into consideration when applying our results to other populations.

Medicine knows countless examples of clinical scenarios where the "gold standard" is not necessarily the first test applied to rule in or rule out the diagnosis. It is well known that not every patient presenting with suspected VTE will have to undergo CT PE, not all patients with a solitary pulmonary nodule will be subjected to a lung biopsy, and not all presenting with acute coronary syndrome will need to undergo a coronary angiography. Similarly not all patients suspected to have OSA need to undergo a PSG.

The challenge facing our field therefore is not necessarily how to diagnose our OSA patients but rather how to diagnose them efficiently, accurately and cost-effectively, particularly in regions with high prevalence rates and limited PSG access.

PM devices have already been incorporated in clinical algorithms of OSA management, further studies however, are needed to define the role of PM in primary practice, in pediatric population and in those patients with co-morbidities.

Robert Skomro
Division of Respiratory, Critical Care and Sleep Medicine
Department of Medicine
University of Saskatchewan

References
1. Mulgrew AT et al. Diagnosis and initial management of obstructive sleep apnea without polysomnography: a randomized validation study. Ann Inter Med. 2007; 146(3):157-66.
2. Antic NA et al. A randomized controlled trial of nurse-led care for symptomatic moderate-severe obstructive sleep apnea. AJRCCM. 2009; 179(6):501-8.
3. Berry RB et al. Portable monitoring and autotitration versus polysomnography for the diagnosis and treatment of sleep apnea. Sleep. 2008; 31(10):1423-31.

Plasma levels of MCP-1 and adiponectin in obstructive sleep apnea syndrome. Kim J, Lee CH, Park CS, Kim BG, Kim SW, Cho JH. *Arch Otolaryngol Head Neck Surg. 2010 Sep;136(9):896-9.*

Does obstructive sleep apnea alter levels of proinflammatory cytokines?

Subjects	Methods	Outcomes
59 subjects with OSA	Assessments: • Radioimmunoassay analyses of serum proinflammatory cytokines: MCP-1, adiponectin, IL-6, IL-8 and TNF • BMI • PSG: AHI and lowest SaO_2	Compared with normal controls, subjects with OSA had: • Increased MCP-1* • Decrease in adiponectin (in severe OSA)** • No difference in IL-6, IL-8 and TNF Correlation coefficients were: • 0.62 between MCP-1 and AHI • 0.66 between adiponectin and AHI

AHI: apnea hypopnea index; BMI: body mass index; IL-6: interleukin 6; IL-8: interleukin 8; MCP-1: monocyte chemotactic protein 1; OSA: obstructive sleep apnea; PSG: polysomnography; SaO_2: arterial oxygen saturation; TNF: tumor necrosis factor; *P < .001; **P = .006

Conclusion
Obstructive sleep apnea was associated with increased levels of monocyte chemotactic protein 1 and decreased adiponectin.

Commentary
Kim et al conducted a study looking at levels of pro-inflammatory and anti-inflammatory markers in three groups of patients: i) normal controls without Obstructive Sleep Apnea (OSA), ii) moderate OSA (AHI between 5 and 20), and iii) severe OSA (AHI >20). Specifically they determined levels of the pro-inflammatory cytokines interleukin 6 (IL-6), interleukin 8 (IL-8), and tumor necrosis factor (TNF). They also examined the levels of monocyte chemotactic protein 1 (MCP-1) which is involved in the migration of leukocytes to inflammatory tissue, as well as levels of adiponectin, an adipocytokine with anti-inflammatory and anti-atherogenic properties. They found that MCP-1 levels were significantly higher in subjects with OSA compared to the control subjects, and those with severe OSA had the highest levels. The adiponectin level was higher in the normal group compared to the severe OSA group but not between the normal group and the moderate OSA group. Both MCP-1 and adiponectin were positively correlated with the apnea hypopnea Index (AHI) and body mass index (BMI). They did not find a difference among the groups in the other measurements. The authors concluded that in the OSAS patients, serums levels of adiponectin tend to be lower whereas that of MCP-1 tend to be higher.

Studying the levels of adiponectin in those with OSA is important because it has anti-inflammatory and anti-atherogenic properties and hypoadiponectinemia has been linked to endothelial dysfunction and cardiovascular morbidity in clinical studies.[1,2] Also, leukocyte migration to inflamed tissue is an integral part of the process in atherosclerosis.[3] In order for the leukocytes to adhere to microvascular endothelium, pro-inflammatory mediators, such as MCP-1, play an active role. Therefore, studies that show a higher level of pro-inflammatory markers (such as MCP-1 in this study) and lower level of anti-inflammatory markers (such as adiponectin) can give us a potential biological plausibility of the link between OSAS and cardiovascular disease.

Previous studies examining the relationship between OSA and adiponectin have yielded conflicting results. Makino et al[4] studied 200 Japanese men and found that hypoadiponectinemia was strongly related to visceral adiposity and insulin resistance. However, they found no association with AHI, minimum oxygen saturation, or duration of oxygen saturation less than 90%. Sharma et al[5] studied Indian men, and also found that adiponectin levels were not correlated with AHI or sleep hypoxemia, but did correlate with obesity. In a BMI-matched case controlled study, McArdle et al[6] found no difference in adiponectin levels between OSA and non OSA patients.

Other researchers have found a significant association between AHI and adiponectin levels. Masserini et al[7] found a trend of decreasing adiponectin levels in 3 groups of subjects with increasing severity of OSA. Two similar studies[8,9] also reported reduced adiponectin levels in subjects with severe OSA, compared with subjects without OSA. However, a randomized controlled trial[10] failed to show any change in adiponectin levels after four weeks of CPAP treatment.

In terms of MCP-1 and OSA, previous studies by Hayashi et al and Ohga et al[11,12] showed that levels are increased in patients with higher AHI. Ohga et al[11] and more recently Tamaki et al[13] have shown promising results with nasal CPAP in reducing MCP-1 pro-inflammatory cytokines.

In our opinion, Kim et al have conducted a study that adds to the growing body of literature *suggesting* that OSA is associated with an inflammatory state. Although, the current study excluded patients with diabetes, hypertension and other co morbidities, this study is limited by the fact that it cannot determine whether the changes noted are separate from the changes that can be attributed to obesity alone. In addition, adiponectin exists in different complexes in the circulation and the high-molecular-weight (HMW) form is thought to be the more biologically active form of adiponectin.[14,15] For example, the relative proportion of HMW adiponectin, rather than the total adiponectin level, is strongly correlated with a lower risk of coronary artery disease (CAD).[15,16] The effects of OSA on the biologically active form of adiponectin remain to be determined.

Imran Iftikhar
Division of Pulmonary, Allergy, Critical Care, and Sleep Medicine
The Ohio State University Medical Center

Meena Khan
Division of Pulmonary, Sleep, Critical Care, and Allergy
Division of Neurology
The Ohio State University Medical Center

References

1. Kumada M et al. Association of hypoadiponectinemia with coronary artery disease in men. Arterioscler Thromb Vasc Biol. 2003; 23(1):85-9.
2. Zoccali C et al. Adiponectin, metabolic risk factors, and cardiovascular events among patients with end-stage renal disease. J Am Soc Nephrol. 2002; 13(1):134-41.
3. Springer TA. Adhesion receptors of the immune system. Nature. 1990; 346(6283):425-34.
4. Makino S et al. Obstructive sleep apnoea syndrome, plasma adiponectin levels, and insulin resistance. Clin Endocrinol (Oxf). 2006; 64(1):12-9.
5. Sharma SK et al. Obesity, and not obstructive sleep apnea, is responsible for metabolic abnormalities in a cohort with sleep-disordered breathing. Sleep Med. 2007; 8(1):12-7.
6. McArdle N et al. Metabolic risk factors for vascular disease in obstructive sleep apnea: a matched controlled study. Am J Respir Crit Care Med. 2007; 175(2):190-5.
7. Masserini B et al. Reduced levels of adiponectin in sleep apnea syndrome. J Endocrinol Invest. 2006; 29(8):700-5.
8. Takahashi K et al. Plasma thioredoxin, a novel oxidative stress marker, in patients with obstructive sleep apnea before and after nasal continuous positive airway pressure. Antioxid Redox Signal. 2008; 10(4):715-26.
9. Nakagawa Y et al. Nocturnal reduction in circulating adiponectin concentrations related to hypoxic stress in severe obstructive sleep apneahypopnea syndrome. Am J Physiol Endocrinol Metab. 2008; 294(4):E778-84.
10. Kohler M et al. Effects of continuous positive airway pressure on systemic inflammation in patients with moderate to severe obstructive sleep apnoea: a randomised controlled trial. Thorax. 2009; 64(1):67-73.
11. Ohga E et al. Effects of obstructive sleep apnea on circulating ICAM-1, IL-8, and MCP-1. J Appl Physiol. 2003; 94(1):179-84.
12. Hayashi M et al. Hypoxia-sensitive molecules may modulate the development of atherosclerosis in sleep apnoea syndrome. Respirology. 2006; 11(1):24-31.
13. Tamaki S et al. Production of inflammatory mediators by monocytes in patients with obstructive sleep apnea syndrome. Intern Med. 2009; 48(15):1255-62.
14. Kobayashi H et al. Selective suppression of endothelial cell apoptosis by the high molecular weight form of adiponectin. Circ Res. 2004; 94(4):e27-31.
15. Pajvani UB et al. Complex distribution, not absolute amount of adiponectin, correlates with thiazolidinedione-mediated improvement in insulin sensitivity. J Biol Chem. 2004; 279(13):12152-62.
16. Aso Y et al. Comparison of serum highmolecular weight (HMW) adiponectin with total adiponectin concentrations in type 2 diabetic patients with coronary artery disease using a novel enzyme-linked immunosorbent assay to detect HMW adiponectin. Diabetes. 2006; 55(7):1954-60.

Prevalence and clinical characteristics of obesity hypoventilation syndrome among individuals reporting sleep-related breathing symptoms in northern Greece. Trakada GP, Steiropoulos P, Nena E, Constandinidis TC, Bouros D. *Sleep Breath. 2010; 14(4):381-6.*

How common is obesity hypoventilation syndrome among persons with sleep-related breathing disorders in northern Greece, and what are their clinical characteristics?

Subjects	Methods	Outcomes
276 subjects who had PSG for possible OSA	Assessments: • Anthropometric characteristics • Daytime sleepiness • Physical examination • PSG • Sleep characteristics • Spirometry • Wake ABG Definition of OHS used in the study: • Daytime hypercapnia ($PaCO_2 \geq 45$ mmHg) • Obesity (BMI $\geq$ 30) • SRBD • Without any other cause of hypoventilation	OHS was identified in 13.8% of subjects (38 of 276) Characteristics of OHS subjects (compared to non-OHS): • Older • More obese: greater neck, waist and hip circumference, and larger WHR • More somnolent • Lower average and minimum SpO_2 during sleep; greater time with $SpO_2 < 90\%$ • No significant difference in wake PFT No differences in anthropometric measures were noted between OHS+OSA vs. OHS without OSA groups, although the former had higher AHI and lower SpO_2 Greater prevalence of CHF in subjects with OHS vs. those with OSA Most commonly reported comorbidities in subjects with OHS+OSA were HTN and DM

ABG: arterial blood gas; AHI: apnea hypopnea index; BMI: body mass index; CHF: congestive heart failure; DM: diabetes mellitus; HTN: arterial hypertension; OHS: obesity hypoventilation syndrome; OSA: obstructive sleep apnea; $PaCO_2$: partial pressure of carbon dioxide; PaO_2: partial pressure of oxygen; PFT: pulmonary function testing; PSG: night polysomnography; SpO_2: oxygen saturation; SRBD: sleep-related breathing disorders; WHR: waist-hip ratio

Conclusion
Approximately one in every seven persons with sleep-related breathing disorders in northern Greece met diagnostic criteria for obesity hypoventilation syndrome.

Commentary
This study aimed to examine the prevalence, clinical data, reported comorbidities, pulmonary function test results and polysomnographic characteristics of patients with Obesity Hypoventilation Syndrome (OHS) and to compare them with those of patients with Obstructive Sleep Apnea Syndrome (OSAS) and those of controls. All of them where recruited by a larger population of individuals who were referred to the sleep unit of the pulmonary clinic of a university hospital in northern Greece.

The present study determined the prevalence of OHS among this large number of patients reporting sleep- related breathing symptoms. OHS was identified in 13.8% of the examined individuals. Although the prevalence of OHS in the general population remains unknown, the prevalence of OHS among OSAS patients has been estimated in previous studies between 9% and 20%.[1-9] Our findings are consistent with these results, and are even closer to those reported in other Mediterranean countries in Europe (France, Italy, Spain) where OHS among OSAS patients ranges between 10% and 17%.[1,5-8] Additional analysis revealed that in 13.2% of our OHS patients, no apneic events occurred during sleep but only nocturnal hypoventilation. This percentage is similar to the approximately 10% that was previously reported in literature.[1,4,10]

An outcome of importance is the high prevalence of comorbidities. Arterial hypertension was reported by more than half of the recruited OHS patients, followed by diabetes mellitus, both conditions associated with obesity. It is also remarkable that the prevalence of congestive heart failure was found to differ, in a statistically significant way, between OHS and OSAS patients (13.2% vs. 2.9% respectively, $P = 0.026$).

OHS is a condition, associated with impaired quality of life, increased medical payments, and poor prognosis, therefore the estimation of the prevalence and the description of the features of the syndrome is certainly clinically useful. It is well-accepted that the optimal management of patients with OHS requires multidisciplinary approach combining different medical and surgical subspecialties.[11] This approach, which initially requires a high index of clinical suspicion, should be followed by referral of the patient for polysomnography, in order to apply noninvasive positive pressure ventilation, the established treatment which enhances long-term survival.[12] As obesity becomes a global epidemic, OHS is certainly a condition that should be born in mind of all clinicians.

Georgia Trakada
Medical School
Democritus University of Thrace

Paschalis Steiropoulos
Medical School
Democritus University of Thrace

Evangelia Nena
Medical School
Democritus University of Thrace

References

1. Kessler R et al. The obesity hypoventilation syndrome revisited: a prospective study of 34 consecutive cases. Chest. 2001; 120:369-376.
2. Berg G et al. The use of health-care resources in obesity-hypoventilation syndrome. Chest. 2001; 120:377-383.
3. Tsara V et al. Greek version of the Epworth Sleepiness Scale, Sleep Breath. 2004; 8:91-95.
4. Mokhlesi B et al. Obesity hypoventilation syndrome: prevalence and predictors in patients with obstructive sleep apnea. Sleep Breath. 2007; 11:117-124.
5. Laaban JP et al. Daytime hypercapnia in adult patients with obstructive sleep apnea syndrome in France, before initiating nocturnal nasal continuous positive airway pressure therapy. Chest. 2005; 127:710-715.
6. Resta O et al. Hypercapnia in obstructive sleep apnoea syndrome. Neth J Med. 2000; 56:215-222.
7. Verin E et al. Prevalence of daytime hypercapnia or hypoxia in patients with OSAS and normal lung function. Respir Med. 2001; 95:693-696.
8. Golpe R et al. Diurnal hypercapnia in patients with obstructive sleep apnea syndrome. Chest. 2002; 122:1100-1101.
9. Littleton SW et al. The pickwickian syndrome-obesity hypoventilation syndrome. Clin Chest Med. 2009; 30:467-478.
10. Rapoport DM et al. Hypercapnia in the obstructive sleep apnea syndrome. A reevaluation of the "Pickwickian syndrome." Chest. 1986; 89:627-635.
11. Al Dabal L et al.Obesity hypoventilation syndrome. Ann Thorac Med. 2009; 4:41-49.
12. Budweiser S et al.Mortality and prognostic factors in patients with obesity-hypoventilation syndrome undergoing noninvasive ventilation. J Intern Med. 2007; 261:375-83.

Randomized controlled trial comparing flexible and continuous positive airway pressure delivery: effects on compliance, objective and subjective sleepiness and vigilance. Bakker J, Campbell A, Neill A. *Sleep. 2010 Apr 1;33(4):523-9.*

Can reducing pressure during expiration enhance compliance to continuous positive airway pressure therapy for obstructive sleep apnea?

Subjects	Methods	Outcomes
76 subjects with severe OSA • AHI: 60.2 ± 32.9 • ESS: 13.6 ± 4.5 • BMI: 35.6 ± 7.8 • No cardiac, respiratory, psychiatric or sleep disorders	Double-blind, parallel-arm randomized controlled (3-month) trial Subjects were randomized to: • C-Flex* (dip level 2) • CPAP Assessments (baseline and after 1 and 3 months): • Modified MWT • PVT • Questionnaires	Median compliance** • C-Flex: 5.51 hrs per night • CPAP: 5.89 hrs per night No significant differences between groups in • PVT reaction time • Subjective sleepiness • Sleep quality • HRQOL • Treatment comfort • Modified MWT SOL

AHI: apnea hypopnea index; BMI: body mass index; CPAP: continuous positive airway pressure; ESS: Epworth sleepiness scale; HRQOL: health-related quality of life; MWT: Maintenance of wakefulness test; OSA: obstructive sleep apnea; PAP: positive airway pressure; PVT: Psychomotor vigilance task; SOL: sleep onset latency; *Philips Respironics, PA, USA; **P = 0.82

Conclusion

Reducing pressure during expiration failed to alter compliance to therapy for obstructive sleep apnea compared to continuous positive airway pressure.

Commentary

The first-line treatment for obstructive sleep apnea (OSA) is continuous positive airway pressure (CPAP) therapy, which has been shown to eliminate obstructive respiratory events while improving daytime symptoms[1] and long-term cardiovascular health.[1-3] However, the effectiveness of treatment is limited by sub-optimal compliance and high rejection rates.[4] Several modifications of pressure delivery have been developed in recent years, including flexible pressure, with the overall aim of improving comfort and therefore compliance to treatment. Flexible pressure reduces incoming air pressure during early-exhalation, returning to therapeutic pressure for late-exhalation and subsequent inhalation. The first flexible pressure device was marketed by Philips Respironics (PA, USA) using the brand name 'C-Flex'; this technology reduces pressure proportional to expiratory flow, and can be set to one of three dip settings.[5] After a promising initial report of an incompletely blinded study indicating a beneficial effect of C-Flex on compliance[6], subsequent double-blinded randomized controlled trials including our own pilot[7] failed to replicate this finding[8-12], suggesting a placebo effect.

We therefore aimed to evaluate the effectiveness of C-Flex in increasing objectively-measured compliance compared with standard CPAP, with key secondary outcome measures including objective sleepiness (modified Maintenance of Wakefulness Test), vigilance (Psychomotor Vigilance Task reaction time), subjective sleepiness (Epworth Sleepiness Scale and Stanford Sleepiness Scale), sleep quality (Pittsburgh Sleep Quality Index and Functional Outcomes of Sleep Questionnaire), health-related quality of life (Short-Form 36 Health Survey), and treatment comfort evaluated using an in-house questionnaire. Treatment efficacy was assessed using the residual AHI metric recorded by the devices. Seventy-six consecutive patients with severe OSA (mean ± SD apnea hypopnea index (AHI) 60.2 ± 32.9 events/hour) underwent full-night manual titration on their randomized device (CPAP or C-Flex; mean pressure 11.6 cmH$_2$O). The aforementioned outcome measures were completed at baseline, and one and three months following titration. Median compliance to C-Flex at three months was 5.51 hours/night, which was not significantly different from the CPAP group (median 5.89 hours/night; p=0.82). This trend persisted when patients using treatment ≥ 1 and ≥ 4 hours/night were analyzed separately (n = 71 and n = 54 respectively), and when patients requiring therapeutic pressure ≥ 12cmH$_2$O and ≥ 14cmH$_2$O were analyzed separately (n = 31 and n = 18 respectively). There were no significant differences between groups in terms of vigilance, subjective sleepiness, sleep quality, health-related quality of life, or treatment comfort at one or three months. There was no significant difference between the treatment groups regarding the change in modified Maintenance of Wakefulness Test sleep latency, and no significant difference in machine-interpreted residual AHI at three months.

Our results are in agreement with other randomized controlled trials reporting no significant difference in compliance between CPAP and C-Flex.[7-12] These trials, as well as the current study, have subsequently been incorporated into a meta-analysis, which reached the same conclusion.[13] However, there may still be patient sub-groups that might benefit from a switch to C-Flex after attempting CPAP, such as those suffering from nasal congestion or aerophagia, or patients having trouble becoming compliant. It is also worth considering that the real appeal of flexible pressure may lie in allowing patients to vary their dip setting, giving them a sense of control over their treatment that is denied them with standard CPAP. This question has not yet been addressed.

In conclusion, this study found no significant difference between CPAP and C-Flex in terms of compliance to treatment, objective or subjective sleepiness, and vigilance. Given the restriction in device manufacturer and the fact that cheaper devices are available which do not include C-Flex technology, there appears to be no evidence-based rationale for the recommendation of C-Flex over CPAP when initiating treatment. However, there is no indication that C-Flex is a less effective treatment than CPAP and both modes led to significant improvements in secondary outcome measures over one and three months, so physicians can be reasonably confident that C-Flex and CPAP are both highly effective treatments of severe OSA.

This clinical trial was funded by Philips Respironics, the manufacturer of the C-Flex device under investigation. C-Flex devices used for the previously published pilot study were provided by Care Medical, New Zealand.

Jessie P. Bakker
WellSleep Sleep Investigation Centre
Department of Medicine
University of Otago

References

1. Montserrat JM et al. Effectiveness of CPAP treatment in daytime function in sleep apnea syndrome: a randomized controlled study with an optimized placebo. AJRCCM. 2001; 164:608-13.

2. Young T et al. Sleep disordered breathing and mortality: eighteen-year follow-up of the Wisconsin sleep cohort. Sleep. 2008; 31:1071-8.

3. Martinez-Garcia MA et al. Continuous positive airway pressure treatment reduces mortality in patients with ischemic stroke and obstructive sleep apnea: a 5-year follow-up study. AJRCCM. 2009; 180:36-41.

4. Weaver TE et al. Adherence to continuous positive airway pressure therapy: the challenge to effective treatment. Proceedings of the American Thoracic Society. 2008; 5:173-8.

5. Ruhle KH et al. Analysis of expiratory pressure reduction (C-Flex method) during CPAP therapy Pneumologie. 2007; 61:86-9.

6. Aloia MS et al. Treatment adherence and outcomes in flexible vs standard continuous positive airway pressure therapy. Chest. 2005; 127:2085-93.

7. Marshall NS et al. Randomised trial of compliance with flexible (C-Flex) and standard continuous positive airway pressure for severe obstructive sleep apnea. Sleep & Breathing. 2008; 12:393-396.

8. Nilius G et al. Pressure-relief continuous positive airway pressure vs constant continuous positive airway pressure: a comparison of efficacy and compliance. Chest. 2006; 130:1018-24.

9. Wenzel M et al. Expiratory pressure reduction (C-Flex Method) versus fix CPAP in the therapy for obstructive sleep apnoea. Pneumologie. 2007; 61:692-5.

10. Dolan DC et al. Longitudinal comparison study of pressure relief (C-Flex) vs. CPAP in OSA patients. Sleep & Breathing. 2008; 13:73-77.

11. Leidag M et al. Mask leakage in continuous positive airway pressure and C-Flex. Journal of Physiology & Pharmacology 2008; 59: 401-6.

12. Pepin JL et al. Pressure reduction during exhalation in sleep apnea patients treated by continuous positive airway pressure. Chest. 2009; 136:490-7.

13. Bakker J et al. Flexible pressure delivery modification of continuous positive airway pressure for obstructive sleep apnea does not improve compliance with therapy: Systematic review and meta-analysis. Chest. 2010; in-press.

Randomized controlled trial of variable-pressure versus fixed-pressure continuous positive airway pressure (CPAP) treatment for patients with obstructive sleep apnea/hypopnea syndrome (OSAHS). Vennelle M, White S, Riha RL, Mackay TW, Engleman HM, Douglas NJ. *Sleep. 2010 Feb 1;33(2):267-71.*

Which of the two positive airway pressure modalities - fixed-pressure or variable-pressure - does persons with obstructive sleep apnea prefer?

Subjects	Methods	Outcomes
200 subjects with OSA and EDS • AHI: > 15 • After an attended APAP titration night • CPAP naïve 181 subjects completed the study	Randomized blinded cross-over trial Subjects were randomized to: • Fixed CPAP*: 6 weeks • APAP*: 6 weeks Assessments: • CPAP usage • ESS • HRQOL • Modified OT • Symptoms • Vigilance	Compared to fixed CPAP, APAP was associated with: • No difference in patient preference: APAP (69 subjects) vs. fixed CPAP (72 subjects) • Lower ESS: 9.5 vs. 10.0** • Higher mean CPAP use: 4.2 vs. 4.0 hrs per night***

AHI: apnea hypopnea index; APAP: automated positive airway pressure; CPAP: continuous positive airway pressure; ESS: Epworth sleepiness scale; HRQOL: health-related quality of life; OSA: obstructive sleep apnea; OT: Osler test; *Autoset Spirit; **P = 0.031; ***P = 0.047

Conclusion
There was no difference in user preference between fixed-pressure and variable-pressure positive airway pressure devices.

Commentary
The treatment of choice for obstructive sleep apnea/hypopnea syndrome (OSAHS) is continuous positive airway pressure (CPAP) which initially delivered a preset pressure determined on an overnight titration study. More recently CPAP devices have become available which can vary the pressure delivered according to the patient's requirements. Variable-pressure variable pressure devices tend to be more expensive. Anecdotally some patients have reported preference for variable pressure devices and others for fixed pressure devices.

Consecutive eligible patients were approached with information on the study and asked to consent to participation until 200 patients were recruited. Those agreeing to participate were randomized into the study on the morning after CPAP titration night. Patients received treatment with the same CPAP device (AutoSet Spirit, ResMed, Poway, CA) for 2 periods of 6 weeks, attending for assessment on the last day of each treatment. During one period the CPAP machine was set in fixed-pressure mode at the pressure determined during overnight in-lab CPAP titration, performed using our standard technique of attended in-lab auto-titration without PSG and during the other 6 weeks it was set in variable-pressure mode the order of treatments being randomized. 368 patients with OSAHS were invited to participate in the study (fig 1) and 200 patients (46F) were recruited (mean age 50 SD ± 10 yrs; BMI 34.5 ± 7.8 kg/m^2 ; Epworth Score 14 ± 3). 123 patients had polysomnography with mean AHI 33 ± 18, 77 had a limited sleep study with mean A+H/hr in bed 49 ± 20). The patients who declined to participate were not different from the participants in terms of age, Epworth score or breathing during sleep (P>0.2).19 patients (4 female) did not complete the study of whom 9 were receiving fixed and 10 variable pressure CPAP at the time of drop out; 11 dropped out during the first limb. One patient died from unrelated and non vascular causes during the first limb.

The primary result of the study was that after 6 weeks treatment with each form of therapy, patients with OSAHS expressed no preference between fixed-pressure and variable-pressure CPAP. Overall on variable pressure CPAP, there was greater CPAP use (4.2 SEM 0.2, 4.0 SEM 0.2 hrs/night; P = 0.047) and patients reported being less sleepy (Epworth 9.5 SEM 0.4, 10.0 SEM 0.3; P = 0.031) than on fixed pressure CPAP but there were no significant differences between the treatments in terms of objective sleepiness or quality of life. There was a significant time order effect in preference, more patients preferring the first treatment they received.

Although variable pressure CPAP produced better outcomes in terms of Epworth Sleepiness score and CPAP use, the advantages were marginal. The difference in Epworth scores between the treatments was 0.6 and the difference in CPAP use was only 0.2 hrs/night (5%) over the 4 week period analyzed on each treatment. Whether these differences are sufficient to influence choice of therapy will depend on the healthcare system and the differences in CPAP machine prices locally. The fact that there were no significant differences in objective sleepiness, vigilance, quality of life or nocturnal symptoms indicates there is no compelling advantage of variable over fixed pressure CPAP in unselected patients.

Limitations of this study include the fact that 10% of the patients enrolled in the study dropped out. Dropout rates were similar between the 2 devices and this is therefore unlikely to have skewed the findings of the study. Drop outs are inevitable with CPAP and the rate we observed in this study is not unusual. Another limitation is the relatively short battery of tests that could be fitted in at follow up while minimizing patient inconvenience. The shortened Osler test might have masked a real difference had more sleep opportunities been studied. Another limitation is that unselected patients requiring CPAP were recruited, not sub-groups who may have particularly benefited from variable pressure CPAP.

It must be stressed that our results reflect our patient population and will not be generalizeable to all settings. Similarly they were obtained on a single CPAP device and cannot be extended to other devices.

The marked order effect with greater benefit from the first form of CPAP used not only complicated the analysis but also may be of real concern in clinical practice. Eighty six patients preferred the first type of CPAP they received compared to 55 who preferred the second form of CPAP. Some centers have adopted a practice of titrating CPAP by giving patients variable devices for a week or more at home, reading the level of CPAP pressure required and then issuing cheaper fixed pressure devices at that pressure. The current study raises concerns that such practice might result in worse outcomes and possibly lower CPAP use on the subsequent fixed pressure CPAP compared with those put on fixed pressure CPAP immediately after an overnight titration with a variable device.

Marjorie Vennelle
Department of Sleep Medicine
Royal Infirmary of Edinburgh
University of Edinburgh

Residual sleep apnea on polysomnography after 3 months of CPAP therapy: clinical implications, predictors and patterns. Mulgrew AT, Lawati NA, Ayas NT, Fox N, Hamilton P, Cortes L, Ryan CF. *Sleep Med. 2010 Feb;11(2):119-25.*

How commonly does obstructive sleep apnea persist following CPAP titration, whether performed in the sleep laboratory or at home using an automated positive airway pressure device?

Subjects	Methods	Outcomes
61 sleepy subjects with high risk of moderate to severe OSA	Post hoc secondary analysis of data from a previous randomized trial Subjects were randomized to: • Standard CPAP titration during PSG: 30 subjects • Ambulatory titration using APAP and HSAT: 31 subjects Assessments (3 months on fixed-pressure CPAP therapy): • AHI on CPAP during PSG • ESS • SAQLI • CPAP pressure • CPAP compliance (objective)	15 (25%) subjects had AHI > 10 on CPAP • PSG group: 7 subjects • APAP group: 8 subjects Compared with fully treated OSA, residual OSA was associated with: • Worse compliance: 4.6 vs. 5.7 hrs • Periodic breathing: 12 of 15 subjects with residual OSA • Higher ESS: 9 vs. 5 • Poorer SAQLI: 4.6 vs. 5.6

AHI: apnea hypopnea index; APAP: automated positive airway pressure; BMI: body mass index; CPAP: continuous positive airway pressure; ESS: Epworth sleepiness scale; HSAT: home sleep apnea testing; OSA: obstructive sleep apnea; PSG: polysomnography; RDI: respiratory disturbance index; SAQLI: Sleep apnea quality of life index

Conclusion
Residual sleep apnea was common even after ambulatory or laboratory titration of continuous positive airway pressure therapy, and was associated with worse clinical outcomes.

Commentary
This study was prompted by the unexpected finding of frequent residual respiratory events on full overnight PSG in patients with a high probability of OSA after 3 months of CPAP therapy, despite rigorous CPAP titration. In the previously reported randomized trial[1], patients with a high probability of moderate to severe OSA had CPAP therapy titrated either by conventional PSG or by an ambulatory strategy using auto-CPAP and overnight oximetry. Despite careful titration and 3 months of treatment, 25% of patients had a residual AHI > 10/h.

The prevalence and clinical significance of RSA on CPAP therapy have been the subject of some controversy.[2,3] The true prevalence of RSA remains unclear since few studies have followed titrated patients for prolonged periods. Various studies, including our own, have estimated the prevalence of RSA as ranging between 13 to 25%.[4-9] A recent retrospective study, however, suggested that RSA improves over time.[10] Nonetheless, the findings of worse outcomes in patients with RSA after 3 months of treatment is a cause for concern because of the potential for poorer long term CPAP adherence and lower overall treatment success in these patients.

Previous studies of RSA have been based on retrospective data and have not looked specifically at clinical outcomes. Our data were collected prospectively and included information on important clinical outcomes. Patients with RSA were sleepier and had poorer quality of life and lower compliance with CPAP therapy compared with fully treated patients. These differences could not be explained by differences in CPAP pressure or mask leak, or by differences in age, gender, body weight, sleepiness, sleep apnea clinical scores or severity of OSA at baseline. These poorer outcomes are probably clinically significant and may reflect the consequences of partially treated OSA, in a manner similar to mild OSA which has been shown to predispose to adverse cardiovascular events, failure to lower blood pressure and increased risk for motor vehicle crashes.[11-14]

The cause of RSA remains unclear. Possible explanations include under-titration of CPAP resulting in residual obstructive events; over-titration of CPAP leading to the emergence of central events; or underlying ventilatory control instability either as a primary abnormality or as a consequence of severe OSA.[15,16] Due to the difficulty in differentiating between central and obstructive hypopneas without a quantitative assessment of ventilatory effort[17], we suspect that many central events, including periodic breathing, were misclassified as obstructive hypopneas. Failure to recognize this misclassification can lead to over-titration of CPAP, potentially compounding the problem of RSA and leading to poorer outcomes. By analyzing compressed PSG tracings (300sec/page), we identified a high prevalence of periodic breathing in patients with RSA, likely reflecting ventilatory control instability.

In terms of the frequency of RSA, conventional CPAP titration using PSG was no better than the ambulatory strategy using auto-CPAP and oximetry. This suggests that neither approach can be relied upon to ensure that all patients are fully treated. Nevertheless, the majority of patients are unlikely to require further PSG to confirm ongoing CPAP efficacy, regardless of whether CPAP is initially titrated conventionally in the sleep laboratory or by a validated ambulatory strategy. We are not aware of any other studies that have compared RSA on CPAP machine downloads with PSG. CPAP machine recorded residual respiratory events alone had relatively low sensitivity (55%) for RSA, but together with evidence of residual sleepiness (ESS) had a high positive likelihood ratio for RSA. Therefore, careful attention should be paid to patients who have residual respiratory events on data downloaded from their CPAP machines, together with residual sleepiness or poor treatment compliance. Our findings raise the interesting possibility that in future follow-up PSG in patients with OSA who are not responding optimally to treatment could be used mainly to reassess the efficacy of CPAP and ensure a correct diagnosis, rather than for initial CPAP titration. This could promote expedited treatment for patients and potential savings to the health care system.

Our study has several limitations that warrant consideration. First, the analysis was not predefined and the results should be considered descriptive. Second, the patients were a highly selected group and the results may not be generalizeable to routine clinical care. Third, we did not investigate the mechanisms for the RSA. Prospective studies with accurate measurement of ventilatory effort and a prolonged follow up period are required to answer that question.

Our results suggest that patients with RSA have worse outcomes. We recommend that patients with evidence of RSA, poor treatment compliance or suboptimal improvements in sleepiness and quality of life on CPAP should be reevaluated by PSG to ensure a correct and complete diagnosis and an effective positive airway pressure titration. For patients who have evidence of persistent or emergent ventilatory control instability on CPAP, consideration should be given to more advanced forms of positive airway pressure therapy such as adaptive servo-ventilation.

Frank Ryan
Respiratory Division
Department of Medicine
University of British Columbia

Alan Mulgrew
Bon Secours Hospital, Tralee

References

1. Mulgrew AT et al. Diagnosis and initial management of obstructive sleep apnea without polysomnography: a randomized validation study. Ann Intern Med. 2007; 146:157-166.
2. Gay PC. Complex sleep apnea: it really is a disease. J Clin Sleep Med. 2008; 4:403-405.
3. Malhotra A et al. Complex sleep apnea: it isn't really a disease. J Clin Sleep Med. 2008; 4:406-408.
4. Baltzan MA et al. Prevalence of persistent sleep apnea in patients treated with continuous positive airway pressure. Sleep. 2006; 29:557-563.
5. Lehman S et al. Central sleep apnea on commencement of continuous positive airway pressure in patients with a primary diagnosis of obstructive sleep apnea-hypopnea. J Clin Sleep Med. 2007; 3:462-466.
6. Pack AI et al. Modafinil as adjunct therapy for daytime sleepiness in obstructive sleep apnea. Am J Respir Crit Care Med. 2001; 164:1675-1681.
7. Pittman SD et al. Follow-up assessment of CPAP efficacy in patients with obstructive sleep apnea using an ambulatory device based on peripheral arterial tonometry. Sleep Breath. 2006; 10:123-131.
8. White DP et al. Evaluation of the Healthdyne NightWatch system to titrate CPAP in the home. Sleep. 1998; 21:198-204.
9. Morgenthaler TI et al. Complex sleep apnea syndrome: is it a unique clinical syndrome? Sleep. 2006; 29:1203-1209.
10. Kuzniar TJ et al. Natural course of complex sleep apnea--a retrospective study. Sleep Breath. 2008; 12:135-139.
11. Pepperell JC et al. Ambulatory blood pressure after therapeutic and subtherapeutic nasal continuous positive airway pressure for obstructive sleep apnoea: a randomised parallel trial. Lancet. 2002; 359:204-210.

12. Shahar E et al. Sleep-disordered breathing and cardiovascular disease: cross-sectional results of the Sleep Heart Health Study. Am J Respir Crit Care Med. 2001; 163:19-25.

13. Young T et al. Sleep-disordered breathing and motor vehicle accidents in a population-based sample of employed adults. Sleep. 1997; 20:608-613.

14. Young T et al. Population-based study of sleep-disordered breathing as a risk factor for hypertension. Arch Intern Med. 1997; 157:1746-1752.

15. Weitzman ED et al. Quantitative analysis of sleep and sleep apnea before and after tracheostomy in patients with the hypersomnia-sleep apnea syndrome. Sleep. 1980; 3:407-423.

16. Younes M et al. Chemical control stability in patients with obstructive sleep apnea. Am J Respir Crit Care Med. 2001; 163:1181-1190.

17. Iber I et al. Manual for the Scoring of Sleep and Associated Events: Rules, Terminology and Technical Specifications. Westchester, Illinois: American Academy of Sleep Medicine, 2007.

Shift in sleep apnoea type in heart failure patients in the CANPAP trial. Ryan CM, Floras JS, Logan AG, Kimoff RJ, Series F, Morrison D, Ferguson KA, Belenkie I, Pfeifer M, Fleetham J, Hanly PJ, Smilovitch M, Arzt M, Bradley TD; CANPAP Investigators. *Eur Respir J. 2010 Mar;35(3):592-7.*

Does improvement in heart function during continuous positive airway pressure therapy of central sleep apnea in persons with heart failure lead to conversion of respiratory events into obstructive apneas?

Subjects	Methods	Outcomes
98 subjects with HF and CSA • Age: 18-79 yrs • NYHA class: II-IV • LVEF: < 40% • AHI: ≥ 15 (> 50% central apneas) • Stable on medical therapy for 4 weeks Exclusion criteria: • Pregnancy • MI or cardiac surgery within previous 3 months • OSA	Sub-analysis of the control arm of CANPAP randomized controlled trial Assessments: • PSG (either at 3 months or 2 yrs) • LVEF • Assessment of dyspnea • Medications • Body position • BMI • LECT Definitions • Non-converter: > 50% of events remained central at follow-up • Converter: ≥ 50% of events were obstructive at follow-up	Number of converters at follow-up: 18 subjects • 18% converters • 82% non-converters Compared with nonconversion, conversion was associated with: • Greater increase in the LVEF* • Greater fall in LECT** • Lower dyspnea score*** • Younger age • Greater obesity*** Conversion was associated with • Improvement in LVEF • No change in medication use • No change in BMI • No change in %TST in supine position

AHI: apnea hypopnea index; CANPAP: Canadian Continuous Positive Airway Pressure for Patients with Central Sleep Apnea and Heart Failure trial; CSA: central sleep apnea; HF: heart failure; LECT: lung-to-ear-circulation time; LVEF: left ventricular ejection fraction; MI: myocardial infarction; NYHA: New York Heart Association class; OSA: obstructive sleep apnea; TST: total sleep time; *2.8% vs. -0.07%; **7.6 s vs. 0.6 s; ***P < 0.05.

Conclusion
Improvement in left ventricular systolic function and reduction in lung-to-ear-circulation time led to conversion from predominantly central to obstructive sleep apnea in 18% of persons with heart failure.

Commentary

There is a high prevalence of both OSA and CSA in HF patients.[1-3] OSA may contribute to the development and progression of HF[4] and untreated, is associated with increased cardiovascular mortality.[5] In contrast, CSA is probably a consequence of HF[6] but is also associated with increased mortality risk.[7]

Despite the differences in pathogenesis of OSA and CSA, previous studies have demonstrated the presence of both sleep-breathing disorders during the same night in patients with HF. In fact, we demonstrated in a small study of 12 subjects a shift from predominantly obstructive to predominantly central events occurring over one night and another study demonstrated a shift in sleep apnea type occurring over a period of one or more months.[8,9] In both these studies, the shift from OSA to CSA occurred in association with a reduction in the nocturnal PCO_2 and a prolongation of the LECT, indicating worsening cardiac function.

Following cardiac transplant CSA resolved in the majority of subjects and conversion to OSA occurred in a small minority.[10] However, it has been unclear whether or not this shift in sleep apnea type in HF patients over time is as a result of changes in cardiac function or other factors.

Therefore, we analysed patients in the control arm of the CANPAP study which was a multicentre randomized controlled trial to determine whether treatment of CSA in HF patients by continuous positive airway pressure (CPAP) would improve heart transplant free survival. We compared polysomnographic data, LVEF, medications and dyspnea assessments (NYHA class and chronic heart failure questionnaire dyspnea scores) from the last follow-up (either 3 months or 2 years) in which all relevant data were available to the baseline data. The study demonstrated, prospectively, that in a cohort of subjects with HF and CSA, 18% converted from predominantly CSA to predominantly OSA. This conversion occurred in HF subjects who were younger, more overweight and more dyspneic than their counterparts with persistent CSA on follow-up. There were no differences in the etiology of HF, presence of arrhythmias or medications between those subjects who converted and those who did not. Furthermore, the switch from CSA to OSA was accompanied by a significant improvement in the LVEF and the LECT.

Our study suggests that in some subjects with HF, OSA and CSA may be part of a spectrum of sleep-related breathing disorders whose predominant nature may change over time in association with alterations in cardiac function. A recent study by our group demonstrating greater fluid retention and rostral fluid shifts in CSA rather than OSA subjects with HF may be a common pathogenetic mechanism linking both sleep apnea types.[11] If so, then it is possible that with improved cardiac function, conversion from CSA to OSA may have been related to a reduction in fluid retention, and in overnight rostral fluid displacement from the legs.

Clodagh Ryan
University of Toronto
Toronto General Hospital

T. Douglas Bradley
University of Toronto
Toronto General Hospital

References

1. Yumino D et al. Prevalence and physiological predictors of sleep apnea in patients with heart failure and systolic dysfunction. J Card Fail. 2009; 15:279-285.
2. Javaheri S. Sleep disorders in systolic heart failure: A prospective study of 100 male patients. The final report. Int J Cardiol. 2006; 106:21-28.
3. Schulz R et al. Sleep apnoea in heart failure. Eur Respir J. 2007; 29:1201-1205.
4. Shahar E et al. Sleep-disordered breathing and cardiovascular disease: Cross-sectional results of the sleep heart health study. Am J Respir Crit Care Med. 2001; 163:19-25.
5. Wang H et al. Influence of obstructive sleep apnea on mortality in patients with heart failure. J Am Coll Cardiol. 2007; 49:1625-1631.
6. Bradley TD et al. Sleep apnea and heart failure: Part ii: Central sleep apnea. Circulation. 2003; 107:1822-1826.
7. Javaheri S et al. Central sleep apnea, right ventricular dysfunction, and low diastolic blood pressure are predictors of mortality in systolic heart failure. J Am Coll Cardiol. 2007; 49:2028-2034.
8. Tkacova R et al. Overnight shift from obstructive to central apneas in patients with heart failure: Role of pco2 and circulatory delay. Circulation. 2001; 103:238-243.
9. Tkacova R et al. Night-to-night alterations in sleep apnea type in patients with heart failure. J Sleep Res. 2006; 15:321-328.
10. Mansfield DR et al. The effect of successful heart transplant treatment of heart failure on central sleep apnea. Chest. 2003; 124:1675-1681.
11. Yumino D et al. Nocturnal rostral fluid shift: A unifying concept for the pathogenesis of obstructive and central sleep apnea in men with heart failure. Circulation. 2010; 121:1598-1605.

Sleep disordered breathing is associated with appropriate implantable cardioverter defibrillator therapy in congestive heart failure patients. Tomaello L, Zanolla L, Vassanelli C, LoCascio V, Ferrari M. *Clin Cardiol. 2010 Feb;33(2):E27-30.*

Does sleep disordered breathing affect the frequency of discharges from implantable cardioverter defibrillators in persons with heart failure?

Subjects	Methods	Outcomes
22 subjects with systolic CHF and ICD • LVEF < 27± 5% • NYHA class: II-III	Retrospective study Assessment: • In home cardio-respiratory monitoring • Analysis of ICD memory	77.2% (n = 17) had AHI ≥ 10 • OSA: 50% • CSA: 22% After controlling for LVEF and NYHA class, ICD discharges correlated with: • AHI* • Severity of hypoxia during sleep**

AHI: apnea hypopnea index; CHF: congestive heart failure; CSA: central sleep apnea; ICD: implantable cardioverter defibrillator; LVEF: left ventricular ejection fraction; NYHA: New York Heart Association class; OSA: obstructive sleep apnea; PSG: polysomnography; SDB: sleep disordered breathing; *r = 0.718; P < .001; **r = - 0.619; P = .003

Conclusion
Sleep disordered breathing was common among persons with heart failure and implantable cardioverter defibrillators, and increased the frequency of appropriate discharges by the latter.

Commentary
In recent years there has been great interest in Sleep Disordered Breathing (SDB) possibly being related to malignant ventricular arrhythmia in patients affected by congestive heart failure (CHF).

Central and obstructive sleep apnea (CSA/OSA) are characterized by recurrent cycles of hypoventilation, hypoxia, hypercapnia, hyperventilation and arousals from sleep that contribute to autonomic disturbance resulting in myocardial electric instability.[1,2]

The autonomic derangements associated with SDB are not limited to sleep: daytime muscle sympathetic nerve activity (MSNA) is higher in CHF patients affected by OSA than in controls, a phenomenon that may suggest an independent excitatory effect of OSA on central sympathetic outflow.[3] Obstructive sleep apnea causes repetitive forced inspiration against occluded pharynx (Mueller maneuver) that generates negative pressure in the chest cavity resulting in augmented venous return, impaired diastolic filling and increased right and left ventricular afterload[4]; both direct mechanical stretch on atrial/ventricular wall and stimulation of pulmonary veins filling receptors may influence cardiac efferent sympatho-vagal activity potentially triggering arrhythmia.[5,6]

Patients with left ventricular dysfunction and CSA have evidence for greater arrhythmic risk compared with patients without CSA and high levels of resting sympathetic drive increase even further during episodes of central apnea.[7,8]

The involvement of SDB in cardiac electric instability has been recently assessed by evaluating T Wave Alternans (TWA), a risk marker for Sudden Cardiac Death (SCD)[9], in CHF patients. Takasugi et al. observed that apnea hypopnea index (AHI) was an independent predictor of peak nocturnal TWA elucidating a mechanism by which sleep apnea may be proarrhythmic.[10] Moreover TWA was positively correlated to the frequency and severity of oxygen desaturation episodes during sleep. Apnea associated hypoxemia may induce myocardial ischemia leading to repolarization heterogeneity especially in conjunction with structurally abnormal, scarred myocardium as in ischemic CHF.[11] In a large scale prospective observational study Yumino et al. have shown that sleep apnea is associated with a significantly increased incidence of SCD in patients with ischemic CHF but not in those with non ischemic etiology.[12] In our study we found a correlation between both AHI and degree of nocturnal oxygen desaturation and appropriate implantable cardioverter defibrillator (ICD) therapies in CHF patients with mainly ischemic etiology (about 70%).

Previous work by Gami et al has found that severity of obstructive sleep apnea correlated directly with the risk of nighttime sudden death from cardiac causes.[13] Moreover in a large cohort study the incidence of cardiac events wasn't significantly higher in subjects with AHI between 5 and 30 events/hour suggesting that only patients with severe OSA (e.g. AHI > 30 events/h) may be at risk.[14] Similarly Lanfranchi et al. described a higher incidence of ventricular arrhythmias and a worse prognosis among patients with CHF and severe CSA. [8,15] Our study involved too of a small number to detect differences in terms of event-free survival in patients with OSA or CSA but our observation essentially agrees with the cited works supporting the hypothesis that severe SDB, especially if associated with ischemic etiology, represent a risk factor for malignant arrhythmia in CHF.

Recent contributions from well designed large-scale prospective studies add important evidence to the relationship between sudden cardiac death and sleep apnea in CHF patients who received an ICD. By following for 6 months 71 patients with CHF, Serizawa et al found a fourfold increased risk of appropriate ICD discharge due to SDB. Of these 66% were found to have SDB with an AHI of ≥ 10 events/h. Thirty patients (64%) were implanted with an ICD in secondary prevention, no distinction was made between OSA and CSA and no association between severity of SDB and arrhythmic risk was reported.[16]

In our study we examined ICD recipients for primary SCD prevention showing a correlation between SDB severity and appropriate device discharges in subjects at lower risk for arrhythmia than those studied by Serizawa. Moreover we found a similar prevalence of SDB.
Bitter et al. performed the largest prospective study to date revealing an independent association between OSA and CSA with an increased risk of appropriate ICD discharge after a follow up of 48 months in 169 CHF patients. Different OSA/CSA diagnostic thresholds (AHI more than 5 or 15 events/h) did not present with different hazard ratios and no significant difference in event free survival between OSA and CSA was shown.[17]

Despite these two landmark studies a number of critical questions still remain unanswered: which is (or does even exist) the AHI threshold to be considered to start treatment? Can a patient with minimal AHI but severe nocturnal hypoxia and ischemic CHF be left untreated? Can electrophysiological and neurophysiological tests (e.g. TWA and sleep fragmentation analysis)[18] help to distinguish among CSA or OSA patients those at higher risk for SCD?

These uncertainties are a matter of great concern since definite data from randomized intervention trials are still lacking while increasing evidence demonstrates that sleep apnea is a risk factor for malignant ventricular arrhythmia in heart failure.

Luca Tomaello
Department of Medicine
University of Verona

Luisa Zanolla
Department of Medicine
University of Verona

Daniela Lanza
Department of Medicine
University of Verona

Marcello Ferrari
Department of Medicine
University of Verona

References
1. Somers VK et al. Sympathetic neural mechanisms in obstructive sleep apnea. J Clin Invest. 1995; 96: 897-1904.
2. Spicuzza L et al. Autonomic modulation of heart rate during obstructive versus central sleep apneas in patients with sleep disordered breathing. Am J Resp Crit Care Med. 2003; 167:902-910.
3. Spaak J et al. Muscle sympathetic nerve activity during wakefulness in heart failure patients with and without sleep apnea. Hypertension. 2005; 46:1327-1332.
4. Somers VK et al. Autonomic and hemodynamic responses and interactions during the Mueller maneuver in humans. J Auton Nerv Syst. 1993; 44:253-259.
5. Hakumaki MO. Seventy years of the Bainbridge reflex. Acta Physiol Scand.1987; 130:177-185.
6. Bradley TD et al. Augmented sympathetic neural response to simulated obstructive apneas in heart failure. Clin Sci. 2003; 104:231-238.
7. Van de Borne P et al. Effects of Cheyne-Stokes respiration on muscle symapathetic nerve activity in severe congestive heart failure secondary to ischemic or idiopathic dilated cardiomyopathy. Am J Cardiol. 1998; 81: 432-436.
8. Lanfranchi PA et al. Central sleep apnea in left ventricular dysfunction: prevalence and implications for arrhythmic risk. Circulation. 2003; 107:727-732.

9. Stein PK et al. Ambulatory ECG- based T wave alternans predicts sudden cardiac death in high risk post-MI patients with left ventricular dysfunction in the EPHESUS study. J Cardiovasc Electrophysiol. 2008 ; 19 :1037-1042.

10. Takasugi N et al. Sleep apnea induces cardiac electrical instability assessed by T-wave alternans in patients with congestive heart failure. Eur J Heart Fail. 2009; 11:1063-1070.

11. Nearing BD et al. Quantification of ischaemia induced vulnerability by precordail T wave alternans analysis in dog and human. Cardiovasc Res. 1994; 28:1440-1449.

12. Yumino D et al. Relationship between sleep apnoea and mortality in patients with ischeamic heart failure. Heart. 2009; 95:819-824.

13. Gami AS et al. Day night pattern of sudden cardiac death in obstructive sleep apnea. N Engl J Med.2005; 352: 1206-1214.

14. Marin JM et al. Long term cardiovascular outcomes in men with obstructive sleep apnea-hypopnea with and without treatment with continuous positive airway pressure: an observational study. Lancet. 2005; 365:1046-1053.

15. Lanfranchi PA et al. Prognostic role of Cheyne-Stokes respiration in chronic heart failure. Circulation. 1999; 99:1435-1440.

16. Serizawa N et al. impact of sleep disordered breathing on life-threatening ventricular arrhythmia in heart failure patients with implantable cardioverter defibrillator. Am J Cardiol. 2008; 102:1064-1068.

17. Bitter T et al.Cheyne –Stokes respiration and obstructive sleep apnea are independent risk factors for malignant ventricular arrhythmias requiring appropriate cardioverter defibrillator therapies in patients with congestive heart failure. Eur Heart J. 2011; 32:61-74.

18. Mc Ginty D. Neurobiology of sleep. In: Saunders NA; Sullivan CE (eds): Sleep and breathing 2nd ed., vol 71. New York: Marcel Dekker, 1994.

Sustained hyperoxia stabilizes breathing in healthy individuals during NREM sleep. Chowdhuri S, Sinha P, Pranathiageswaran S, Safwan Badr M. *J Appl Physiol. 2010 Nov;109(5):1378-83.*

Does sustained hyperoxia alter apneic threshold, carbon dioxide reserve and hypocapnic ventilatory response during non-rapid eye movement sleep?

Subjects	Methods	Outcomes
9 healthy subjects • Age: 23.6 ± 3.8 yrs • Gender: 45% males • BMI: 23.6 ± 3.0 • Neck circumference: 34.2 ± 4.3 cm	Subjects were placed on nasal NIMV and randomized to: • Normoxic condition (RA) • Hyperoxic condition (PiO_2 > 250 mmHg for > 20 min) NIMV was adjusted to induce hypocapnia and CA during stable NREM (N2 or N3) sleep Assessments (before and after the exposure to hyperoxia): • AT • CO2 reserve • Eupneic $PetCO_2$ • Hypocapnic ventilatory response Definitions: • AT: $PetCO_2$ of the apnea closest to eupnea; absolute measured $PetCO_2$ demarcating the central apnea following NIMV • CO_2 reserve: minimal change in $PetCO_2$ between eupnea and hypocapnic central apnea; difference between the AT and the eupneic $PetCO_2$ • Eupneic $PetCO_2$: average of breaths during control room air period	Compared with RA, hyperoxia was associated with: • Reduction in eupneic $PetCO_2$* • Widening of CO_2 reserve** • Decrease in AT*** • Decline in hypocapnic ventilatory response[#] • Higher eupneic MV[##]

	immediately prior to the onset of NIMV • Hypocapnic ventilatory response: change in ventilation below eupnea for each change in $PetCO_2$	

AT: apneic threshold; BMI: body mass index; CA: central apnea; CO_2: carbon dioxide; F_1O_2: fraction of inspired oxygen; MV: minute ventilation; NIMV: noninvasive mechanical ventilation; NREM: non-rapid eye movement sleep; $PetCO_2$: end-tidal partial pressure of carbon dioxide; PiO_2: partial pressure of inspired oxygen; PSG: polysomnography; RA: room air; *37.5 ± 0.6 vs. 41.1 ± 0.6 Torr, P = 0.001; **-3.8 ± 0.8 vs. -2.0 ± 0.3 Torr, P = 0.03; ***33.3 ± 1.2 vs. 39.0 ± 0.7 Torr; P = 001; #2.5 ± 0.5 vs. 3.7 ± 0.5 L/min/mmHg; P = 0.008; ##7.2 ± 0.6 vs. 5.9 ± 0.9 L/min; P < 0.05

Conclusion
Sustained hyperoxia was associated with reduced apneic threshold and hypocapnic ventilatory response as well as widening of the carbon dioxide reserve, and, thus, may stabilizing breathing during non-rapid eye movement sleep.

Commentary
Hyperoxic hyperventilation was noted in our study starting at least after 10-15 minutes of hyperoxia.[1] Multiple animal and human studies have shown hyperoxic hyperventilation, after an initial transient hypoventilation.[2,3] While an initial hypoventilation due to peripheral chemoreceptor inhibition, has not been demonstrated consistently[4,5], subsequent hyperventilation has been noted, probably via central mechanisms.[5,6]

Potential mechanisms underlying hyperoxic hyperventilation include increased brain tissue PCO_2 via cerebral vasoconstriction[7-10], the Haldane effect[8] or alternatively, a direct stimulatory effect on chemosensitive respiratory neurons[9] via production of reactive oxygen species. The potential mechanisms of hyperoxic hyperventilation in sleeping humans were not addressed by our study protocol.

In our study there was a decline in the hypocapnic chemoreflex sensitivity likely by blunting of the peripheral responsiveness to hypocapnia, resulting in lower hypocapnic ventilatory response. In addition, the development of hyperoxic hyperventilation and the concomitant decrease in eupneic $P_{ET}CO_2$ suggest reduced "plant gain"[11], as a greater change in minute ventilation was required for a given decrease in eupneic $P_{ET}CO_2$. In turn, the CO_2 reserve was widened by lowering the eupneic CO_2, thus stabilizing respiratory control. Thus, hyperoxia promoted breathing stability during NREM sleep.

The above findings are clinically significant as these explain the mechanism for hyperoxia as potential therapy for treating central sleep apnea. However, long-term safety and efficacy of hyperoxia have not been established, especially given the potential for production of reactive oxygen species upon prolonged oxygen use in patients with central apnea without evidence of hypoxemia. Other safety concerns associated with high F_IO_2 include hypercarbia in patients with ventilatory limitation and alveolar atelectasis. Further studies are needed to determine the lowest effective dose and to ascertain long-term safety.

In conclusion, hyperoxia stabilizes breathing in healthy individuals during NREM sleep by stimulating hyperventilation. Our findings provide a mechanistic explanation for the reported therapeutic effect of supplemental oxygen in patients with central sleep apnea, associated with high altitude, congestive heart failure, and idiopathic central apnea.[12,13] Potential mechanisms include decreased plant gain or reduced CO_2 chemoreflex sensitivity.[5,14] Our findings are consistent with both mechanisms, as well as increased baseline ventilatory motor output, resulting in widening of the CO_2 reserve.

Susmita Chowdhuri
John D Dingell VA Medical Center
Wayne State University

Sukanya Pranathiageswaran
Wayne State University

M.Safwan Badr
John D Dingell VA Medical Center
Wayne State University

References
1. Chowdhuri S et al. Sustained hyperoxia stabilizes breathing in healthy individuals during NREM sleep. J Appl Physiol. 2010; 109(5):1378-83.
2. Becker H et al. Ventilatory response to isocapnic hyperoxia. J Appl Physiol. 1995; 78:696-701.
3. Miller MJ et al. Hyperoxic hyperventilation in carotid deafferented cats. Respir Physiol. 1975; 23:23–30.
4. Watt JG et al. Effects of inhalation of 100 per cent and 14 per cent oxygen upon respiration of unanesthetized dogs before and after chemoreceptor denervation. Am J Physiol. 1943; 138:610–617.
5. Gautier H et al. Ventilatory response of the conscious or anesthetized cat to oxygen breathing. Respir Physiol. 1986; 65:181–196.
6. Lahiri S et al. Carotid body chemosensory function in prolonged normobaric hyperoxia in the cat. J Appl Physiol. 1987; 62:1924–1931.
7. Kety SS et al. The effects of altered arterial tensions of carbon dioxide and oxygen on cerebral blood flow and oxygen consumption of normal young men. J Clin Invest. 1948; 27:484–486.
8. Loeppky JA et al. Quantitative description of whole blood CO2 dissociation curve and Haldane effect. Respir Physiol. 1983; 51:167–181.
9. Mulkey DK et al. Hyperbaric oxygen and chemical oxidants stimulate CO2/H_ sensitive neurons in rat brain stem slices. J Appl Physiol. 2003; 95:910–921.
10. Dempsey JA et al. Pathophysiology of sleep apnea. Physiol Rev. 2010; 1:47–112.
11. Dempsey JA. Crossing the apnoeic threshold: causes and consequences. Exp Physiol. 2010; 90:13–24.

12. Franklin KA et al. Reversal of central sleep apnea with oxygen. Chest. 1997; 111:163–169.
13. Gold AR et al. The effect of chronic nocturnal oxygen administration upon sleep apnea. Am Rev Respir Dis. 1986; 134:925–929.
14. Xie A et al. Influence of arterial O2 on the susceptibility to posthyperventilation apnea during sleep. J Appl Physiol. 2006; 100:171–177.

The effects of posterior fossa decompressive surgery in adult patients with Chiari malformation and sleep apnea. Botelho RV, Bittencourt LR, Rotta JM, Tufik S. *J Neurosurg. 2010 Apr;112(4):800-7.*

What are the effects on respiration during sleep of surgical posterior fossa decompression in persons with Chiari malformation?

Subjects	Methods	Outcomes
25 subjects with symptomatic craniovertebral junction malformations (Chiari malformation and basilar invagination) • 68% had sleep apnea (AHI > 5) preoperatively • Gender: 44% males • Age: 43 ± 13 yrs • BMI: 25 ± 3.9	Prospective study Assessments (before and after surgical decompression of the cranial posterior fossa): • PSG • Bindal questionnaire • ESS • Craniocervical MR imaging	Surgical decompression of the cranial posterior fossa was associated with: • Decrease in mean number of respiratory events: 180.70 vs. 69.29* • Decrease in mean number of obstructive events: 107.37 vs. 60.58** • Decrease in mean number of central events: 38.45 vs. 8.05*** • Decrease in mean AHI: 26.68 vs. 12.98[#] • Decrease in mean central apnea index: 13.81 vs. 1.68[##] • No change in minimal SaO_2: 79 ± 11 vs. 81 ± 10[###] • No change in ESS in 12/17 persons with AHI > 5[^] • Decrease in microarousal index : 24 ± 14 vs. 17 ±11[^^] • Decrease in Bindal score: 80 ± 32 vs. 56 ± 32[^^^]

AHI: apnea hypopnea index; CAI: central apnea index; CSA: central sleep apnea; ESS: Epworth sleepiness scale; MR: magnetic resonance; OSA: obstructive sleep apnea; PSG: polysomnography; SaO_2: oxygen saturation; *P = 0.005; **P = 0.01; ***P = 0.01; [#]P = 0.06; [##]P = 0.01; [###]P = 0.28; [^]P = 0.10; [^^]P = 0.04; [^^^]P = 0.0009

Conclusion

Decompression of the posterior cranial fossa in persons with Chiari malformation and sleep apnea decreased respiratory events and microarousals during sleep.

Commentary

This is the first systematic study evaluating the effect of posterior fossa surgery in Chiari malformation and sleep respiratory events. In these patients, the associated sleep respiratory disturbances have been described.[1-4]

Systematic studies with polysomnography in patients with Craniovertebral Junction Malformation (CJM) have shown the prevalence of sleep respiratory disturbances to be between 59%[4] and 70%.[5] In this study the prevalence was 68%. These data confirm a greater prevalence of sleep-disordered breathing in patients with CJM.

The mechanisms of apneas are partly shared by both events obstructive and central.[6] In patients with predominantly obstructive events probably craniofacial factors are in rule, particularly those related to the volume capacity of the pharyngeal airway (This fact deserves particular attention in regard to other craniofacial factors, particularly those related to the volume capacity of the pharyngeal airway). In patients with predominantly central events alterations in the local reflex control of breathing could occurs as a result of the oropharynx hyperexcitability reflex, thereby inhibiting the inspiratory drive.

The main issue addressed in this work is the improvement in respiratory dysfunction obtained by surgery. This effect was observed for all respiratory events, although more pronounced in patients with central apnea. Several isolated case reports of severe respiratory dysfunctions that were improved by surgery have been described.[7] To our knowledge, only 1 other paper has described the results of a more systematic study regarding the effects of surgery on sleep respiratory dysfunction in patients with CJM.[8] Recently prospective observational studies showed that sleep apnea need be treating considering the higher morbidity and mortality rates comparing with subjects without disease or treated patients.[9]

Ricardo Vieira Botelho
Disciplina de Medicina e Biologia do Sono
Departamento de Psicobiologia
Universidade Federal de São Paulo
Hospital do Servidor Público do Estado de São Paulo

References

1. Bokinsky GE et al. Impaired peripheral chemosensitivity and acute respiratory failure in Arnold– Chiari malformation and syringomyelia. N Engl J Med. 1973; 288:947-948.
2. Alvarez D et al. Acute respiratory failure as the first sign of Arnold–Chiari malformation associated with syringomyelia. Eur Respir J. 1995; 8:661-663.
3. Botelho RV et al. Apnéia do sono central em paciente com malformação de Chiari tipo I e siringomielia: tratamento com cirurgia descompressiva. Relato de caso. J Bras Neurocir. 1998; 9:111-114.

4. Botelho RV et val. Prospective controlled study of sleep respiratory events in patients with craniovertebral junction malformation. J Neurosurg. 2003; 99:1004-1009.
5. Dauvilliers Y et al. Chiari malformation and sleep related breathing disorders.J Neurol Neurosurg Psychiatry. 2007; 78:1344-1348.
6. Rabec C et al. Central sleep apnoea in Arnold–Chiari malformation: evidence of pathophysiological heterogeneity. Eur Respir J. 1998; 12:1482-1485.
7. Zolty P et al. Chiari malformation and sleep-disordered breathing: a review of diagnostic and management issues. Sleep. 2000; 23:637–643.
8. Gagnadoux F et al. Sleepdisordered breathing in patients with Chiari malformation: improvement after surgery. Neurology. 2006; 66:136-138.
9. Nathaniel S et al. Sleep Apnea as an Independent Risk Factor for All-Cause Mortality: The Busselton Health Study. Sleep. 2008; 31:1079-1085.

Circadian Neurobiology and Circadian Rhythm Sleep Disorders

A compromise circadian phase position for permanent night work improves mood, fatigue, and performance. Smith MR, Fogg LF, Eastman CI. *Sleep. 2009 Nov 1;32(11):1481-9.*

Does reducing the misalignment between circadian rhythms and night work shift alter mood, fatigue and performance?

Subjects	Methods	Outcomes
39 subjects Degree of circadian realignment • Not re-entrained: n = 12 • Partially re-entrained: n = 21 • Completely re-entrained: n = 6	Subjects were assigned to either: • Experimental group: interventions to delay and partially align circadian clocks to night shift schedule 1. Intermittent bright light pulses during night shifts 2. Dark sunglasses outside 3. Sleep episodes in the dark 4. Late sleep schedule on days off 5. Light "brake" in the afternoons • Control group: no interventions Protocol • Blocks of simulated night shifts alternated with days off Assessments: • Computerized test battery every 2 hours during day and night shifts	After about 1 week of night shifts (with a weekend off interspersed), compared to the non-entrained group, those who were partially or completely re-entrained had similarly improved (and close to daytime values) levels of: • Fatigue* • Mood* • Performance*

Conclusion
Partial or complete re-entrainment to permanent night work shift resulted in improved measures of fatigue, mood and performance.

Commentary

The circadian rhythms of most night shift workers do not phase shift enough to align with night work and daytime sleep, and this circadian misalignment leads to immediate decrements in alertness and performance and safety risks as well as long term health risks such as cancer and cardiovascular disease. Sleep specialists have given the label "shift work sleep disorder" to those whose symptoms are the most extreme, which may be necessary for medical systems purposes, but is dangerous and counterproductive when it perpetuates the misconception that it is abnormal to suffer from working nights.

We were able to reduce circadian misalignment using interventions that are feasible for implementation by real night shift workers. One unusual and important finding from our study was that mood, fatigue and performance during night shifts was at or close to daytime levels for subjects that achieved partial alignment (partial re-entrainment). Such vast improvements are not achieved with other common countermeasures, such as stimulants for night work (e.g. caffeine and armodafinil) or sedatives for daytime sleep, which may reduce but not eliminate the circadian low during the night shift.

There were two different routes by which subjects achieved our goal of partial re-entrainment, in which the sleepiest time of day (estimated to be 7 h after the dim light melatonin onset [DLMO]) delayed to between 8:30 am and noon. One was to be in the experimental group and thus receive a balance of phase delaying and phase advancing light combined with a specific pattern of delaying dark (sleep). The experimental subjects slept at home from 8:30 am to 3:30 pm (7 h) after each night shift except for after the last night shift in a series when we had them cut their sleep short and sleep from 8:30 am to 1:30 pm (5 h) in order to build up a little sleep pressure to help them fall asleep earlier on days off. They slept from 3:00 am to noon (9 h) on days off. Experimental subjects got four or five 15 min bright light pulses (~ 4000 lux) once per hour during the night shifts to help delay their circadian rhythms, and wore dark sunglasses (approved for driving) when outside in daylight to attenuate phase advancing morning light on the way home from the night shifts. They were required to go outside for at least 15 min after each sleep episode. The purpose of this advancing bright light exposure was to act as a "light brake" to keep their circadian rhythms from delaying too far. Then, when the sleepiest time of day fell between 8:30 am and noon, it occurred within the sleep episodes after work as well as within the sleep episodes on days off, rather than during the night shifts.

The other route to partial re-entrainment was observed in some control group subjects, who were allowed to sleep whenever they chose, that adopted a sleep pattern that was similar to that of the experimental subjects or even more extremely nocturnal (e.g., see panels G, H, I and J in [1]). These subjects delayed the right amount even without receiving bright light during the night shifts and while only wearing lightly tinted sunglasses when outside in daylight. Most of the control subjects who achieved partial re-entrainment adopted extremely late sleep times on days off, e.g., 6 am to 2 pm. We believe that most real night workers would not want to live such extremely nocturnal lives on their days off. Furthermore, we know that partial re-entrainment was reliably produced in the experimental subjects, so we recommend similar interventions, but tailored to the specific work schedule.

Theoretically, dark sunglasses should only be necessary during the commute home until the day that the sleepiest time, also an estimate for the temperature minimum and the crossover point from delays to advances in the light PRC[2], reaches daytime sleep. Light between the end of night work and the beginning of sleep would then coincide with the phase delay portion of the PRC and facilitate rather than inhibit delays. However, there are several reasons for night workers to wear sunglasses whenever outside in daylight. First, they protect the eyes from ultraviolet (UV) light. Second, they make the individual more sensitive to light at night[3] so that even lower intensity light during the night shift should have a greater phase delaying effect. Third, it's easier to develop a habit of always wearing sunglasses than to have to think about whether or not they are necessary. Our experimental subjects wore inexpensive blue-blocker sunglasses which provide good vision for driving (Uvex black Bandit frames with espresso lenses).

For our system to be implemented in the workplace, the workers, their families and their employers must make changes. The workers must devote all their mornings to sleep, go to bed as soon as possible after night shifts, and sleep late on days off. Families and friends have to be educated about the importance of sleep and this sleep schedule. Employers and workers should cooperate to devise permanent night work schedules or very slowly rotating shift work schedules (e.g. 3-4 weeks of nights) to give workers a chance to adapt to night work. Workers should not be asked to work when it would interfere with their planned sleep time, such as working later than usual or filling in for another shift. Employers should furnish their workers with light boxes or light rooms to use during the night shift and with light boxes to use at home for the light brake when it is inconvenient to go outside. These investments may ultimately pay for themselves with higher productivity, greater worker morale, fewer sick days and reduced health costs.

Charmane I. Eastman
Biological Rhythms Research Lab
Behavioral Sciences Department
Rush University Medical Center

Mark R. Smith
Biological Rhythms Research Lab
Behavioral Sciences Department
Rush University Medical Center

References
1. Smith M et al. Practical interventions to promote circadian adaptation to permanent night shift work: Study 4. Journal of Biological Rhythms. 2009; 24(2):161-172.
2. Revell VL et al. How to trick mother nature into letting you fly around or stay up all night. Journal of Biological Rhythms. 2005; 20:353-365.
3. Hebert M., et al., The effects of prior light history on the suppression of melatonin by light in humans. Journal of Pineal Research. 2002; 33:198-203.

A phase 3, double-blind, randomized, placebo-controlled study of armodafinil for excessive sleepiness associated with jet lag disorder. Rosenberg RP, Bogan RK, Tiller JM, Yang R, Youakim JM, Earl CQ, Roth T. *Mayo Clin Proc. 2010 Jul;85(7):630-8.*

Does armodafinil, a wake-promoting agent, reduce excessive sleepiness associated with jet lag?

Subjects	Methods	Outcomes
427 subjects with a history of jet lag • Age: 18-65 yrs • No history of sleep disorder • MSLT: ≥ 8 min • No medications affecting sleep in previous 7 days • No more than 300 mg daily of caffeine in previous 2 weeks	Double-blind, randomized, parallel-group study Protocol: • 3-day laboratory-based study period • Subjects flew from the US to France (6-hr time zone change) Subjects were randomized to either (each morning at 8 am): • Armodafinil 50 mg: n = 142 • Armodafinil 150 mg: n = 143 • Placebo: n = 142 Assessments (on days 1 and 2): • MSLT SOL • PGIS to jet lag symptoms • KSS • Psychiatric status • Safety • Tolerability	Compared to placebo, armodafinil (150 mg) was associated with: • Improvement in MSLT SOL (days 1-2 mean): 11.7 vs. 4.8 minutes* • Improved PGIS to jet lag symptoms (days 1-2 mean): 1.6 vs. 1.9** 1. Decrease in excessive sleepiness: 4.3 vs. 5.5*** Most common adverse effects related to armodafinil (150 mg) were: • Headache: 27% • Nausea: 13% • Diarrhea: 5% • Circadian rhythm sleep disorder: 5% • Palpitations: 5%

KSS: Karolinska sleepiness scale; MSLT: Multiple sleep latency test; PGIS: Patient global impression of severity; STAI: State and trait anxiety inventory; US: United States; *P < .001; **P < .05; ***P < 0.001

Conclusion
Armodafinil increased wakefulness after eastward travel across six time zones.

Commentary
Jet lag disorder is a circadian rhythm sleep disorder arising from rapid travel through multiple time zones[1] and is characterized by a range of symptoms, including excessive sleepiness,

insomnia, fatigue, and irritability.[2-4] It is surmised that up to two-thirds of all travelers may experience jet lag, resulting in excessive sleepiness during the day, insomnia at night, or both.[2] Furthermore, the symptoms of jet lag tend to be more pronounced when traveling through more time zones and/or when traveling eastward.[5-6]

This was the first study to examine the effect of the wakefulness-promoting agent armodafinil on jet lag disorder. Armodafinil has been shown to significantly improve wakefulness in individuals with excessive sleepiness associated with shift work disorder, obstructive sleep apnea, or narcolepsy. The results of the current study indicate that armodafinil also improves the wakefulness, overall condition, and excessive sleepiness of patients with jet lag disorder who flew eastward across six time zones. Patients receiving placebo had a mean sleep latency time according to the MSLT defined as pathological (< 5 minutes)[7] on the first day of landing at their destination, indicating the presence of jet lag symptoms. Patients with narcolepsy have had similar times as well as untreated OSA patients. Treatment with armodafinil prolonged sleep latency times, although the rate of improvement varied according to dose. Those patients receiving 50 mg/d armodafinil still had moderate sleepiness (MSLT sleep latency: 5-10 minutes) on day 1, whereas 150 mg/d armodafinil improved sleep latency to the point of being near the normal range of > 10 minutes on the first day. As the study progressed, wakefulness improved in all three treatment groups, although mean sleep latency was still less than normal on day 3 in the placebo group.

Armodafinil was generally well tolerated. The most frequently reported adverse events were headache, diarrhea, and nausea and there were no serious adverse events. Discontinuation rates due to adverse events were low and were similar for patients treated with armodafinil or placebo. Nighttime sleepiness was also not significantly affected by treatment as only 3 patients treated with armodafinil reported insomnia.

While other medications have been studied to treat excessive sleepiness or insomnia associated with jet lag disorder, limitations associated with study design affect the applicability of their results to real-world jet lag. For instance, studies have examined the effect of melatonin and tasimelteon on transient insomnia but not excessive sleepiness.[8-9] Slow-release caffeine has been evaluated for the treatment of excessive sleepiness associated with jet lag but it was unknown whether patients had a history of jet lag disorder.[10] In addition, most of the efficacy measures used in these studies were subjective. The current study addressed most of the above limitations. First, efficacy measures in the current study consisted of both objective (MSLT) and subjective (KSS and PGI-S) measures in a larger number of patients (427 adults). Another advantage of the current trial design was its applicability to real-world jet lag disorder. Compared to laboratory-simulated travel, the current study allowed patients to experience conditions that they normally experience on transcontinental flights in coach class (e.g. air pressure, humidity, and restricted movement). The laboratory environment at the study sites in France also controlled for patients' exposure to light, the timing of meals, and their sleep schedules.

The current study demonstrated that armodafinil significantly improved wakefulness and overall condition in patients with jet lag disorder. Currently, there are no FDA-approved medications for the treatment of jet lag disorder. Instead, travelers who experience jet lag rely on a number of over-the-counter, herbal, or dietary options that at best have a modest ability to alleviate jet lag symptoms.

This study was sponsored by Cephalon Inc., Frazer, PA.

Russell P. Rosenberg
NeuroTrials Research and Atlanta School of Sleep Medicine

References

1. American Academy of Sleep Medicine. The International Classification of Sleep Disorders: Diagnostic and Coding Manual. 2nd ed. Westchester, IL: American Academy of Sleep Medicine. 2005:129-30.
2. Arendt J et al. Sleep disruption in jet lag and other circadian rhythm-related disorders. In: Kryger MH et al eds. Principles and Practice of Sleep Medicine. 4th ed. Philadelphia, PA: Elsevier Saunders. 2005:659-72.
3. Rajaratnam SMW et al. Health in a 24-h society. Lancet. 2001;358(92589286):999-1005.
4. Waterhouse J et al. Jet lag: Trends and coping strategies. Lancet. 2007; 369(9567):1117-29.
5. Monk TH et al. Inducing jet-lag in older people: directional asymmetry. J Sleep Res. 2000; 9(2):101-16.
6. Nicholson AN et al. Sleep after transmeridian flights. Lancet. 1986; 328(8517):1205-8.
7. Carskadon MA et al. Guidelines for the multiple sleep latency test (MSLT): A standard measure of sleepiness. Sleep. 1986; 9(4):519-24.
8. Rajaratnam SM et al. Melatonin agonist tasimelteon (VEC-162) for transient insomnia after sleep-time shift: two randomised controlled multicentre trials. Lancet. 2009; 373(9662):482-91.
9. Piérard C et al. Resynchronization of hormonal rhythms after an eastbound flight in humans: Effects of slow-release caffeine and melatonin. Eur J Appl Physiol. 2001; 85(1-2):144-50
10. Beaumont M et al. Caffeine or melatonin effects on sleep and sleepiness after rapid eastward transmeridian travel. J Appl Physiol. 2004; 96(1):50-8.

Caffeine for the prevention of injuries and errors in shift workers. Ker K, Edwards PJ, Felix LM, Blackhall K, Roberts I. *Cochrane Database Syst Rev. 2010 May 12;5:CD008508.*

Does caffeine reduce errors and injuries associated with excessive sleepiness in persons with jet lag or shift work disorder?

Subjects	Methods	Outcomes
13 RCTs on effects of caffeine on injury, error or cognition in persons with JL or SWD	Search and screening by 2 authors of published literature using Cochrane Injuries Group Specialised Register, CENTRAL (The Cochrane Library), MEDLINE, EMBASE, PsycINFO, CINAHL, TRANSPORT, PubMed, Internet, and reference lists Assessments: • Risk of bias • Estimates of treatment effect (OR and SMD) • CI	No RCT measured an injury outcome 2 RCTs measured error • Compared to placebo, caffeine significantly reduced number of errors • In 1 RCT, compared to a nap, caffeine was associated with less errors RCTs on cognitive performance • Compared to placebo, caffeine improved concept formation and reasoning*, memory**, orientation and attention*** and perception# • Caffeine had no beneficial effect on verbal functioning and language skills##

CI: 95% confidence interval; JL: jet lag; NPT: neuropsychological test; OR: odds ratio; RCT: randomized controlled trial; SMD: standardized mean difference; SWD: shift work disorder; *SMD -0.41; 95% CI -1.04 to 0.23; **SMD -1.08; 95% CI -2.07 to -0.09; ***SMD -0.55; 95% CI -0.83 to -0.27; #SMD -0.77; 95% CI -1.73 to 0.20; ##SMD 0.18; 95% CI -0.50 to 0.87

Conclusion
Caffeine reduced the number of errors and improved some measures of cognitive performance in persons with excessive sleepiness due to jet lag or shift work disorder.

Commentary
This is a systematic review and meta-analysis. Caffeine ingestion reigns as the most widely uses sleepiness countermeasure. From a theoretical perspective, caffeination makes perfect sense

when individuals are attempting to temporarily mitigate sleep debt. Increasing brain levels of adenosine occur as a function of sustained wakefulness. Furthermore, recover sleep reduces adenosine levels in certain brain areas. This oscillation produced by wakefulness and sleep is posited by some as a major endogenous underpinning of sleep's homeostatic process. Thus, when one curtails sleep, it would follow that adenosine levels remain elevated (inadequately reduced) and sleepiness would ensue. Caffeine, as an adenosine antagonist, would seem the logical antidote and has long been used to assist "waking up" in the morning by individuals after a night of insufficient sleep. However, shift workers, especially night shift workers, face a more complex problem and caffeine's efficacy requires close scrutiny.

Reduced performance during night shift work involves both circadian misalignment and possible accumulated sleep deprivation. The circadian wakefulness generators presumably decrease or cease activity overnight and reactivate in the morning. Sleep difficulties during the day can produce sleep debt. Alertness difficulties at night can arise from increasing homeostatic sleep drive in the face of reduced circadian alertness drive. These factors, if severe enough or when afflicting a susceptible individual, may provoke Shift Work Sleep Disorder. However, many shift workers do not have a disorder. Nonetheless, we know from other published literature that sleepiness, whether induced via homeostatic or circadian mechanism, impedes performance and increases the risk of injury. The question remains - Can caffeine offset the deficits and risks affecting shift workers? The Cochrane Collaboration embodies a group of professionals providing systematic literature reviews concerning health-related interventions. Established in 1992, they have provided scientific work using an evidence-based medicine approach. Their work provides hard information for patients, clinicians, and policy makers. In some cases, as it is here, little or no high-level evidence does not exist for the primary question. Nonetheless, knowing what one does not know is the first step toward discovery. In this particular case, "injury" may be too rare an event to determine if it is reduce by caffeine using a randomized controlled trial methodology. A derivative question, however, cognitive or performance error reduction by caffeine among individuals with Shift Work Sleep Disorder or Jet-lag was formulated, with the expectation that findings could be extrapolated or generalized.

The review provides a marvelous example of evidence-based meta-analysis and includes Forest Plots for studies meeting inclusion criteria. These "plots" graphically represent results from multiple research studies allowing the reader to grasp the state-of-the-science in a glance. Not only is the relationship between caffeine and performance in shift workers reviewed but studies comparing napping and napping plus caffeine round out the assessment. While it may come as no surprise that caffeine "may be an effective intervention for improving performance in shift workers…", the authors also found no difference between caffeine and some of the other countermeasures they targeted (including, napping, bright light, and modafinil). Unfortunately, there exists insufficient evidence of the type meeting their rigorous inclusion criteria to draw conclusions about injury or on-the-job error reduction. Consequently, we are left to rely on our experience and judgment, however biased it may be.

Max Hirshkowitz
Department of Medicine & Menninger Department of Psychiatry
Baylor College of Medicine
Sleep Disorders & Research Center
VA Medical Center, Houston

Lack of short-wavelength light during the school day delays dim light melatonin onset (DLMO) in middle school students. Figueiro MG, Rea MS. *Neuro Endocrinol Lett. 2010;31(1):92-6.*

What is the effect of eliminating morning short-wavelength (blue) light on dim light melatonin onset in adolescents?

Subjects	Methods	Outcomes
11 8th-grade students	Assessments (before and after wearing orange glasses during a 5-day school week): • DLMO *Note*: orange glasses eliminated short-wavelength light	Wearing orange glasses significantly delayed DLMO (30 minutes)

DLMO: dim light melatonin onset

Conclusion
In middle-school children, elimination of morning short-wavelength blue light by wearing orange glasses delayed circadian rhythms.

Commentary
Patterns of light and dark in today's built environment are often inconsistent with the natural 24-hour rhythm of sunset and sunrise. Electric light in buildings can pale in comparison to outdoor light levels during the day - even under cloud cover or during the winter. Light exposures in buildings may be low enough to induce "circadian darkness" during the day, but some sources of light in the evening may be bright enough to prolong daytime into the night. Moreover, these bright and dark light exposures may not be regular or consolidated across the 24-hour day. Measurement of actual light exposures is then a key consideration for our evolving understanding of how light entrains or disrupts our circadian rhythms.

Lack of regular exposure to morning light, or exposure to too much light in the evening, can delay the brain's clock, thereby delaying sleep onset and, if a person needs to rise early on a fixed schedule, create chronic sleep restriction or circadian disruption. Long-term effects of sleep restriction or circadian disruption will likely have negative impacts on our health, well-being, and performance. In fact, recent studies using animal models showed that circadian disruption by irregular light/dark patterns are associated with increased mortality, higher risks for developing diabetes, obesity, cardiovascular disease, and even cancer. Epidemiological studies in humans suggest that shift workers, who are more likely to experience sleep restriction and circadian disruption, are at higher risks for diseases, including cancer.

This irregular light/dark pattern exposure may be particularly important when it comes to teenagers. Sleep restriction is common in adolescents and has received growing attention. Pubertal changes in sleep regulation mechanisms are believed to underlie their tendencies toward later bed and rise times[1]. Rigid school schedules require teens to be in class early in the morning, yet schools may provide adequate daylight to stimulate their circadian system. Since the circadian system responds to short-wavelength ("blue") light, the electric light in classrooms may be insufficient for stimulating the brain's clock even though it is perfectly adequate for reading. As teenagers spend more time indoors, they may miss out on essential morning light needed to stimulate their circadian system. Moreover, if they spend more time outdoors in the late spring, the brain's clock may be over-stimulated in the evening.

In the first phase of the study we examined how restriction of short-wavelength, circadian light exposure impacted dim light melatonin onset (DLMO) in the evening, a marker of circadian time.[2] This field study was conducted at a Middle School in North Carolina with unusually high levels of daylight in the classrooms. When the teenage subjects wore special orange glasses in the morning to remove short-wavelength, circadian light, their DLMO was delayed by about 30 minutes compared to the previous week, when they did not wear the glasses. The orange glasses allowed them to see well enough to perform their visual tasks, but their circadian clock was not receiving enough stimulation in the morning.

In the second phase of this study, 22 students participated before and during school hours for a week in 2009.[3] Half the students studied wore the orange glasses, while a control group did not wear them. DLMO was significantly delayed (approximately 30 minutes) for those students who wore orange glasses compared to the control group. Sleep durations were slightly, but not significantly, curtailed in the orange-glasses group. Performance scores on a brief, standardized psychomotor vigilance test and self-reports of well-being were not significantly different between the two groups.

In another related study, 17 teenage students participated in a seasonal study. Evening melatonin onset was measured one winter evening and one spring evening in the same subjects. We found that melatonin onset as well as sleep onset was delayed about 17 minutes in the spring relative to that in the winter.[4] In all studies, the student subjects wore a circadian light dosimeter, the Daysimeter[5] which measured actual circadian light exposures for the study weeks. The delays in melatonin onset in both studies were consistent with the measured differential circadian light exposures. Namely, restricting circadian light in the morning and extending circadian light exposure in the evening will delay melatonin onset in the evening.

Putting it all together then, to help minimize sleep restriction and possibly circadian disruption, teenagers should receive higher levels of morning daylight in schools and lower levels of evening daylight at home. The present results demonstrate, in real-life applications, well-founded concepts of circadian physiology and human response to light from laboratory studies.

The studies were funded by the US Green Buildings Council and the Trans-National Institutes of Health Genes, Environment and Health Initiative.

Mariana G. Figueiro
Lighting Research Center
Rensselaer Polytechnic Institute

References

1. Carskadon, M.A., et al., Adolescent sleep patterns, circadian timing, and sleepiness at a transition to early school days. Sleep. 1998; 21(8):871-81.
2. Figueiro M et al. Lack of short-wavelength light during the school day delays dim light melatonin onset (DLMO) in middle school students. NeuroEndocrinology Letters. 2010; 31(1): in press.
3. Figueiro M et al. Measuring circadian light and its impact on adolescents. Lighting Research and Technology, 2010.
4. Figueiro M et al. Evening daylight may cause adolescents to sleep less in spring than in winter. Chronobiol Int. 2010; 27(6):1242-1258.
5. Bierman A et al. The Daysimeter: A device for measuring optical radiation as a stimulus for the human circadian system. Measurement Science and Technology. 2005; 16:2292-2299.

Melatonin treatment for eastward and westward travel preparation. Paul MA, Miller JC, Gray GW, Love RJ, Lieberman HR, Arendt J. *Psychopharmacology (Berl). 2010 Feb;208(3):377-86.*

What is the appropriate dosing of melatonin for facilitating adaptation to phase shifts in circadian rhythms?

Subjects	Methods	Outcomes
13 subjects in experiment 1 9 subjects in experiment 2	Testing was conducted in the laboratory from Tuesday evenings until Thursday Protocol: • Phase advance: administration of melatonin or placebo at 1600 hrs Wednesday, and DLMO assessments on Tuesday and Thursday • Phase delay: drug administration at 0600 hrs, and Wednesday, with DLMO assessments on Tuesday and Wednesday, and MelOff on Thursday morning Assessments: • Evaluation of efficacy for circadian phase advance and delay of 3 formulations of melatonin (RR 3 mg, SR 3 mg and SSR 3 mg) using: 1. DLMO 2. MelOff	Phase advances (using 1.0 pg/ml DLMO) were: • Placebo: 0.73 hr • RR: 1.23 hr* • SR: 1.44 hr** • SSR: 1.16 hr*** *Note*: No difference between formulations Phase delay (using 1.0 pg/ml MelOff) for RR compared to placebo by 1.12 hr[#] *Note*: Phase shifts for SR and SSR could not be determined

DLMO: dim light melatonin onset; MelOff: dim light melatonin offset; RR: regular release; SR: sustained release; SSR: surge-sustained release (1 mg RR and 2 mg SR); *P < 0.003; **P < 0.0002; ***P < 0.012; [#]P < 0.012

Conclusion
Melatonin administration, when timed appropriately, hastened adaptation to circadian rhythm phase shifts.

Commentary

The most appropriate timing of oral melatonin treatment to optimize circadian phase shifts can be derived from a phase response curve (PRC).[1-4] The goal of the two studies in our paper[5] was to compare the ability of 3 formulations of melatonin: a 3 mg regular release dose, a 3mg sustained release (SR) (with an 8-hour linear release profile) and a surge-sustained formulation (SSR) of 3 mg (made up of 1 mg regular release and 2 mg sustained release (also with an 8-hour linear release profile)), to both advance and delay the circadian system. For our phase advance study, melatonin treatment time (1600 h) was based on the data of Lewy et al.[6] For our phase delay study, melatonin treatment time (0600 h) was based on a compromise between the PRC of Lewy et al.[6] based on a 0.5 mg regular release melatonin dose and the PRC reported by Burgess et al.[1] based on a 3-mg regular release melatonin dose.

Using Dim Light Melatonin Onset (DLMO) as the phase marker, we found that all three melatonin formulations resulted in similar phase advances whether we used a 1.0 pg/ml threshold or a threshold defined as the time at which values exceeded the mean baseline concentration by 2 SD. For our phase delay study, we could not employ DLMO as the phase marker because it was masked by high residual levels of exogenous melatonin 12 hours after ingestion, for all 3 formulations. We were however able to use Dim Light Melatonin Offset (MelOff) as the phase marker to compare the 3 mg regular release formulation against placebo.

We could not establish a phase delay attributable to either the SR or SSR formulations since even MelOff was still masked by endogenous melatonin from these two formulations 31 hours after ingestion. While it is possible that the SR and SSR formulations might have produced an unrecognized phase delay, it is also possible that the elevated levels of exogenous melatonin provoked by these two formulations might have "spilled over"[7] into the phase advance portion of the PRC resulting in minimal or no net phase change. It is also possible that a 0.5 mg dose of melatonin would have avoided this potential "spill over" effect. For prophylaxis against jetlag, preflight use of 0.5 mg and post-flight use of higher doses to facilitate sleep during recovery from jetlag have been recommended.[8]

Since humans produce between 0.025 and 0.035 mg per day at the rate of about 0.003 to 0.005 mg per h during physiologic night[9,10], even a 0.5 mg dose is about 20 times the normal daily endogenous melatonin production. However, endogenous melatonin is continuously trickled into the circulation during physiologic night whereas regular release melatonin can produce an initial large supraphysiologic spike in circulating melatonin levels, although the work of Deacon and Arendt[11] indicates that a 0.05 dose of regular release melatonin did not produce supraphysiologic levels in circulating melatonin. Nevertheless, to limit concerns about bioavailability of exogenous melatonin, one possibility would be to evaluate a 0.1 mg dose (made up of 0.05 mg regular release along with 0.05 mg of sustained release with a release profile as close to "physiologic release kinetics" as possible) for efficacy in circadian phase shifting by advance and delay.

Michel A. Paul
Performance Group
Individual Readiness Section
Defence R&D Canada

References

1. Burgess HJ et al. A three pulse phase response curve to three milligrams of melatonin in humans. J Physiol. 2008; 586.2:639-647

2. Burgess HJ et al. Human Phase Response Curves to 3 Days of Daily Melatonin: 0.5 mg versus 3.0 mg. Journal of Clinical Endocrinlology and Metabolism. 2010; doi:10.1210/jc.2009-2590.

3. Eastman CI et al. Advancing circadian rhythms before eastward flight: a strategy to prevent or reduce jet lag. Sleep. 2005; 28:33-44.

4. Lewy AJ et al. Melatonin shifts human circadian rhythms according to a phase-response curve. Chronobiol Int. 1992; 9:380-92.

5. Paul MA et al. Melatonin treatment for eastward and westward travel preparation. Psychopharmacology. 2010; 208:377-387.

6. Lewy AJ et al. The human phase response curve (PRC) to melatonin is about 12 hours out of phase with the PRC to light. Chronobiol Int. 1998; 15:71-83.

7. Lewy AJ et al. Low, but not high, doses of melatonin entrained a free-running blind person with a long circadian period. Chronobiol Int. 2002; 19:649-58.

8. Arendt J. Managing jet lag: Some of the problems and possible new solutions. Sleep Medicine Reviews. 2009; 13:249-256.

9. Fourtillan JB et al. Melatonin secretion occurs at a constant rate in both young and older men and women. Am J. Physiol Endocrinol Metab. 2001; 280(1):E11-22.

10. Lane EA et al. Pharmacokinetics of melatonin in man: first pass hepatic metabolism. J Clin Endocrinol Metab. 1985; 61:1214-6.

11. Deacon S et al. Melatonin-induced temperature suppression and its acute phase-shifting effects correlate in a dose-dependent manner in humans. Brain Research. 1995; 688:77-85.

Movement Disorders

Acute dopamine-agonist treatment in restless legs syndrome: effects on sleep architecture and NREM sleep instability. Ferri R, Manconi M, Aricò D, Sagrada C, Zucconi M, Bruni O, Oldani A, Ferini-Strambi L. *Sleep. 2010 Jun 1;33(6):793-800.*

Is restless legs syndrome associated with changes in cyclic alternating pattern, and, if so, is the latter affected by administration of a dopamine agonist?

Subjects	Methods	Outcomes
34 subjects with RLS 13 normal controls	Subjects were given either: • Pramipexole 0.25 mg: n = 19 • Placebo: n = 15 Assessments: • PSG (at baseline and after either pramipexole or placebo administration) 1. Sleep stages 2. CAP 3. Leg movements	At baseline, compared to normal controls, subjects with RLS had: • Longer REM SL • Higher PLMSI • Increase in CAP rate Administration of pramipexole in subjects with RLS resulted in: • Increase in number of stage shifts per hour, SE and %N2 sleep • Decrease in WASO • Lower PLMSI • No change in CAP

CAP: cyclic alternating pattern; %N2: percentage of sleep stage 2; PLMSI: periodic leg movement during sleep index; PSG: polysomnography; REM SL: rapid eye movement sleep latency; RLS: restless legs syndrome; SE: sleep efficiency; WASWO: wake time after sleep onset

Conclusion
Sleep instability was noted in restless legs syndrome, and cyclic alternating pattern was unaffected by acute administration of pramipexole.

Commentary
Even if one of the most often reported symptoms of restless legs syndrome (RLS) is insomnia, with difficulty in falling asleep, sleep maintenance and sleep duration, only few studies have analyzed the objective polysomnographic (PSG) features of RLS.[1-6] Moreover, beside the amount of arousals, no specific data have been reported on sleep microstructure in RLS. It is also known that dopamine agonists are effective in reducing both subjective symptoms and periodic leg movements during sleep (PLMS) in RLS patients but their effects on objective PSG-derived measures seem to be less evident.[2-6] However, sleep problems may persist even after an effective treatment of RLS symptoms and PLMS by means of dopamine-agonists.[7,8] For these reasons, the aim of this investigation was to analyze, in detail, the eventual baseline differences

in Cyclic Alternating Pattern (CAP), a powerful method to evaluate sleep microstructure[9], between normal controls and RLS patients and the eventual changes in sleep architecture and instability induced by the acute administration of a standard low dose of pramipexole in idiopathic RLS patients.

A prospective single-blind placebo-controlled study was carried out on 34 patients with RLS, free of drug medication at the time of the study, and never treated before for RLS (including dopaminergic agents, benzodiazepines, opioids and anticonvulsants). All subjects underwent 2 nocturnal polysomnographic recordings, after one adaptation night, and were randomly subdivided into pramipexole (19 patients) and placebo (15 patients) subgroups. Before the 2nd night recording, one group received a single oral dose of 0.25 mg pramipexole at 9.00 p.m., while the other group received a placebo (single blind procedure). A group of normal controls was also arranged undergoing only one nocturnal baseline polysomnographic recording, after one adaptation night.

At baseline, only REM sleep latency was significantly longer in RLS patients than in normal controls; also PLMS index was significantly higher in the patient group, as expected. While subjective pre-sleep RLS symptoms improved significantly in the pramipexole group, but not in the placebo group, after treatment, the self-reported quality of nocturnal sleep was not improved in the majority of patients in both subgroups. Regarding sleep architecture and PLMS, patients treated with pramipexole showed: a moderate increase in number of stage shifts/hour, an increase in sleep efficiency, an increase in percentage of sleep stage 2, a decrease of wakefulness after sleep onset and a marked suppression of the PLMS index. On the contrary, RLS patients treated with placebo did not show any significant change in sleep architecture parameters and PLMS index.

Several baseline CAP parameters were significantly different in normal controls and RLS patients with an increase in CAP (percentage of NREM sleep occupied by CAP). RLS patients also showed a significantly different parameters related to CAP A phase subtypes, with a decrease in those characterized by predominant slow waves (A1) and an increase in those corresponding to arousals (A2 and A3); moreover, the mean duration of CAP sequences was significantly longer in RLS patients than in normal controls. Finally, no treatment effects were observed on CAP after the first administration of either pramipexole or placebo.

This study demonstrates that patients with RLS show a higher NREM sleep instability than controls, with approximately 75% of this sleep stage occupied by CAP sequences. There is increasing evidence that CAP might have a role in sleep-related cognitive processing.[10-12] Thus, it is possible to speculate that CAP alterations might play a role in the mechanisms of cognitive dysfunction reported in RLS patients which, in turn, seems to be similar to that expected as a consequence of a general sleep loss.[13,14] Differently from CAP, classical sleep architecture parameters do not seem to be able to support this view, being similar to those of controls.

This study confirms once again that the first administration of pramipexole is followed by a dramatic decrease of PLMS and a subjective amelioration of RLS symptoms; however, it is followed only by minor changes in objective sleep architecture parameters and by no changes in sleep microstructure, which continues to show a high amount of sleep instability/discontinuity. Moreover, the significant decreased in pre-sleep RLS subjective severity was not accompanied by a similar improvement of the subjective quality of nocturnal sleep; thus, CAP parameters correlated better than the classical sleep architecture parameters with the patient subjective perception of sleep.

Our study demonstrates that the acute administration of pramipexole seems to exert a very limited action on the central sleep microstructure mechanisms and the moderate effects seen on sleep architecture might be interpreted as the beneficial consequence of the removal of pre-sleep RLS symptoms and PLMS.

Future studies on the effects of long-term therapy with dopamine agonists might be potentially able to provide information useful for developing new therapeutic strategies in RLS, possibly with a combination of drugs, in order to modify not only subjective RLS symptoms and PLMS but also sleep microstructure abnormalities and to normalize CAP in these patients.

Raffaele Ferri
Sleep Research Centre
Department of Neurology IC
Oasi Institute for Research on Mental Retardation and Brain Aging IRCCS, Troina

References

1. Allen RP et al. Restless legs syndrome: diagnostic criteria, special considerations, and epidemiology. A report from the restless legs syndrome diagnosis and epidemiology workshop at the National Institutes of Health. Sleep Med. 2003; 4:101-19.
2. Montplaisir J et al. Clinical, polysomnographic, and genetic characteristics of restless legs syndrome: a study of 133 patients diagnosed with new standard criteria. Mov Disord. 1997; 12:61-5.
3. Saletu B et al. Sleep laboratory studies in restless legs syndrome patients as compared with normals and acute effects of ropinirole. 1. Findings on objective and subjective sleep and awakening quality. Neuropsychobiology. 2000; 41:181-9.
4. Saletu M et al. Acute placebo-controlled sleep laboratory studies and clinical follow-up with pramipexole in restless legs syndrome. Eur Arch Psychiatry Clin Neurosci. 2002; 252:185-94.
5. Manconi M et al. First night efficacy of pramipexole in restless legs syndrome and periodic leg movements. Sleep Med. 2007; 8:491-7.
6. Manconi M et al. Defining the boundaries of the response of sleep leg movements to a single dose of dopamine agonist. Sleep. 2008; 31:1229-37.
7. Montplaisir J et al. Persistence of repetitive EEG arousals (K-alpha complexes) in RLS patients treated with L-DOPA. Sleep. 1996; 19:196-9.
8. Montplaisir J et al. Restless legs syndrome improved by pramipexole: a double-blind randomized trial. Neurology. 1999; 52:938-43.
9. Terzano MG et al. Atlas, rules, and recording techniques for the scoring of cyclic alternating pattern (CAP) in human sleep. Sleep Med. 2001; 2:537-53.
10. Ferri R et al. The slow-wave components of the Cyclic Alternating Pattern (CAP) have a role in sleep-related learning processes. Neurosci Lett. 2008; 432:228-31.
11. Bruni O et al. Sleep architecture and NREM alterations in children and adolescents with Asperger syndrome. Sleep. 2007; 30:1577-85.
12. Ferini-Strambi L et al. Increased periodic arousal fluctuations during non-REM sleep are associated to superior memory. Brain Res Bull. 2004; 63:439-42.

13. Pearson VE et al. Cognitive deficits associated with restless legs syndrome (RLS). Sleep Med. 2006; 7:25-30.
14. Durmer JS et al. Neurocognitive consequences of sleep deprivation. Semin Neurol. 2005; 25:117-29.

Intravenous iron dextran for severe refractory restless legs syndrome. Ondo WG. *Sleep Med. 2010 May;11(5):494-6.*

How effective is high-dose intravenous iron dextran therapy for restless legs syndrome?

Subjects	Methods	Outcomes
25 subjects with RLS • Refractory to conventional treatments • Age: 53.2 ± 11.9 • Gender: 28% male • Age of RLS onset: 32.6 ± 13.0 yrs • FH of RLS: 15 subjects • Baseline ferritin: 5 to 248 ng/ml (mean 43.5 ± 58.0)	Retrospective review of subjects who received IV iron (1 g of HMW iron dextran over 5 hrs)	Improvements of RLS symptoms included: • Complete amelioration of all symptoms – n = 2 • Marked improvement – n = 11 • Moderate improvement – n = 2 • Mild improvement – n = 3 • No improvement – n = 6 Improvement in symptoms, when present, ranged in duration from 1-60 weeks (mean 15.8 ± 17.7 weeks) 12 subjects had multiple infusions 2 subjects did not complete their entire infusion because of anaphylactic type symptoms

FH: family history; HMW: high molecular weight; IV: intravenous; RLS: restless legs syndrome

Conclusion

Intravenous iron dextran therapy was effective in improving symptoms in some, but not all, subjects with refractory restless legs syndrome.

Commentary

Restless legs syndrome (RLS) is a common neurological condition clinically defined by: 1) an urge to move the legs, 2) improvement during movement, 3) worsening while at rest, and 4) worsening in the evening and night.[1] The most consistent pathologic finding in RLS is reduced brain iron, and alterations in iron related proteins.[2,3,4] This has been found in the striatum and in the choroid plexus in autopsied brains. The pattern is not fully understood, but suggests alteration in homeostatic mechanisms within the brain rather than just reduced availability across the blood brain barrier, as transferrin receptors are reduced. In system iron deficiency they should be increased.

System iron deficiency is not a consistent finding in RLS but is associated with "secondary" RLS, especially in those with an older age of onset and who lack a family history.[5, 6] Serum iron levels only crudely correlate with brain levels so one cannot assess brain iron by simply measuring serum iron indices. Interestingly, in rodents that are iron deprived, the spinal cord looses iron much more dramatically than the brain.[7] Spinal cord iron has never been assessed in humans with RLS but has long been postulated to be the anatomic substrate for RLS.

Given the apparent reluctance for brain iron to change as a function of systemic iron stores in RLS, and the intense regulation of iron at the blood brain barrier, it is unlikely that modest increases in systemic iron would dramatically increase CNS iron, and presumably improve RLS symptoms. Oral iron supplements have been reported to help RLS but controlled trials showed no benefit.[8] It is more likely that the aberrant iron regulatory mechanisms would require massive amounts of iron to overwhelm them. This would require high dose intravenous iron.

In our study, we retrospectively identified 25 subjects (age 53 ± 12, 7 male) that received 1 gm of intravenous high molecular weight iron dextran for their medically refractory RLS.[9] The age of RLS onset was 33 ± 13 years and 15 had a positive family history. Inclusion was not based on the presence of serum iron deficiency. Baseline ferritin ranged from 5 to 248 ng/ml, with a mean of 44 ± 58. Overall, 2 subjects reported complete amelioration of all RLS symptoms, 11 reported marked improvement, 2 moderate improvement, 3 mild improvement, 6 reported no improvement, and 2 were unable to complete the infusion. The duration of effect was highly variable, mean 16 ± 18 weeks, range 1-60 weeks. Twelve subjects have had multiple infusions. We concluded that some patients with severe refractory RLS could benefit from intravenous iron dextran but were not able to predict who would respond, based on patient demographics, RLS severity, or baseline ferritin levels.

Single open label reports of intravenous iron dextran for idiopathic RLS [10] and uremic associated RLS [11] have showed benefit. Iron dextran is also proven to increase brain iron based on imaging studies.[12] Recent controlled trials of intravenous iron sucrose did not significantly improve RLS symptoms.[13, 14] This may have a biological basis, as iron dextran is retained longer by macrophages compared with other preparations. This may be necessary to allow for the greater time needed to push the iron into the CNS. Anecdotally, patients usually report a delay of at least three days before achieving any benefit. The downside of high molecular weight iron dextran compared to other iron preparations is its higher rate of anaphylaxis.[15] A low molecular iron dextran preparation is available and we currently use this preparation. Our sample size with this preparation is too small to compare efficacy against the high molecular weight drug, but others who use it have anecdotally reported similar results. Controlled trials of low molecular weight iron dextran are needed.

William G Ondo
Baylor College of Medicine

References

1. Allen RP et al. Montplaisi J. Restless legs syndrome: diagnostic criteria, special considerations, and epidemiology. A report from the restless legs syndrome diagnosis and epidemiology workshop at the National Institutes of Health. Sleep Med. 2003; 4(2):101-119.

2. Connor JR. Pathophysiology of restless legs syndrome: evidence for iron involvement. Current Neurology & Neuroscience Reports. 2008; 8(2):162-166.
3. Connor JR et al. Neuropathological examination suggests impaired brain iron acquisition in restless legs syndrome. Neurology. 2003; 61(3):304-309.
4. Connor JR et al. Decreased transferrin receptor expression by neuromelanin cells in restless legs syndrome. Neurology. 2004; 62(9):1563-1567.
5. Earley CJ et al. Ferritin levels in the cerebrospinal fluid and restless legs syndrome: effects of different clinical phenotypes. Sleep. 2005; 28(9):1069-1075.
6. Ondo WG et al. Exploring the relationship between Parkinson disease and restless legs syndrome. Arch Neurol. 2002; 59(3):421-424.
7. Qu S et al. Locomotion is increased in a11-lesioned mice with iron deprivation: a possible animal model for restless legs syndrome. J Neuropathol Exp Neurol. 2007; 66(5):383-388.
8. Davis BJ et al. A randomized, double-blind placebo-controlled trial of iron in restless legs syndrome. European Neurology 2000;43(2):70-75.
9. Ondo WG. Intravenous iron dextran for severe refractory restless legs syndrome. Sleep Med. 2010; 11(5):494-496.
10. Earley CJ et al. Repeated IV doses of iron provides effective supplemental treatment of restless legs syndrome. Sleep Med. 2005; 6(4):301-305.
11. Sloand JA et al. A double-blind, placebo-controlled trial of intravenous iron dextran therapy in patients with ESRD and restless legs syndrome. Am J Kidney Dis. 2004; 43(4):663-670.
12. Earley CJ et al. The treatment of restless legs syndrome with intravenous iron dextran. Sleep Med. 2004; 5(3):231-235.
13. Grote L et al. A randomized, double-blind, placebo controlled, multi-center study of intravenous iron sucrose and placebo in the treatment of restless legs syndrome. Mov Disord. 2009; 24(10):1445-1452.
14. Earley CJ et al. A randomized, double-blind, placebo-controlled trial of intravenous iron sucrose in restless legs syndrome. Sleep Med. 2009; 10(2):206-211.
15. Chertow GM et al. Update on adverse drug events associated with parenteral iron. Nephrol Dial Transplant. 2006; 21(2):378-382.

Long-term maintenance treatment of restless legs syndrome with gabapentin enacarbil: a randomized controlled study. Bogan RK, Bornemann MA, Kushida CA, Trân PV, Barrett RW; XP060 Study Group. *Mayo Clin Proc. 2010 Jun;85(6):512-21.*

How effective is gabapentin therapy for moderate to severe primary restless legs syndrome?

Subjects	Methods	Outcomes
Subjects with moderate to severe primary RLS Single blind phase • 221 of 327 subjects completed Double blind phase • 168 of 194 subjects completed • Responders from the single blind phase Definition: • Responder: improvements on IRLS CGI-Improvement scale at week 24	Protocol • 24-week, single-blind phase (gabapentin enacarbil 1200 mg) • Followed by 12-week randomized double-blind phase (once daily administration at 5 pm): 1. Gabapentin 1200 mg: n = 96 2. Placebo: n = 98 Assessments (during double blind phase): • IRLS • CGI • Study withdrawal due to lack of efficacy	Compared to placebo, gabapentin was associated with: • Less relapse: 23% vs. 9%* • Common adverse effects included somnolence and dizziness • No clinically relevant changes in laboratory values, vital signs or ECG

CGI: Clinical Global Impression; CI: confidence interval; ECG: electrocardiography; IRLS: International Restless Legs Scale; OR: odds ratio; RLS: restless legs syndrome; *OR, 0.353; 95% CI, 0.2-0.8; P = .02

Conclusion
Gabapentin administration improved symptoms of restless legs syndrome.

Commentary
This 36 week study examines the efficacy and safety of gabapentin enacarbil (Gen) (1200mg) in the treatment of moderate to severe primary restless legs syndrome (RLS) in a long-term maintenance of effect study. Gabapentin enacarbil is a gabapentin prodrug absorbed at carboxylate intestinal sites and metabolized to gabapentin resulting in enhanced absorption due to broad active intestinal transport. Gabapentin has variable, limited absorption with nonlinear pharmacokinetics.

Restless legs syndrome is typically treated with dopamine agonists. However, tolerance, rebound, augmentation and adverse side effects may limit their use. Gabapentin has shown benefit in small RLS studies but as noted has variable absorption.

Double blind (DB) placebo controlled pivotal trials with gabapentin enacarbil have shown efficacy in the treatment of primary RLS. This is a 36 week maintenance of effect study conducted as a single blind (SB) maintenance of effect for 24 weeks followed by a double blind placebo controlled randomized 12 week withdrawal paradigm. The primary endpoint was the proportion of patients relapsing during the DB phase measured by worsening of the International Restless Legs Study Scale and investigator Clinical Global Impression (CGI) of change. Additional measures included time to relapse, responder analysis at week 36, CGI and Patient Global Impression of symptoms as well as Medical Outcomes Sleep Scale, and an investigator-designed Post Sleep Questionnaire. IRLS, CGI and patient global impression data in the single blind period are also presented.

The study corroborates the previous pivotal studies demonstrating the effectiveness of gabapentin enacarbil for treatment of primary RLS for 36 weeks. There was a significant improvement in RLS symptoms as well as sleep complaints associated with RLS. Some of the exploratory findings are unique in the demonstration of change in time of day onset of symptoms using a 24 hour diary pre and post therapy. The time course and intensity of symptom recurrence in the placebo group after 24 weeks of single blind therapy raises questions as to the pharmacodynamics of gabapentin enacarbil. There may be an enduring therapeutic effect upon withdrawal unlike dopamine agonists. The compound was well tolerated with the most common side effects of drowsiness and dizziness.

In conclusion, this report provides important clinical insight into the long-term maintenance of efficacy and tolerability of GEn in adults with moderate-to-severe primary RLS.

Richard K. Bogan
University of South Carolina
School of Medicine
SleepMed Incorporated

References
1. Allen RP et al. Restless legs syndrome prevalence and impact: REST general population study. Arch Intern Med. 2005; 165(11):1286-1292.
2. Winkelman JW et al. Augmentation and tolerance with long-term pramipexole treatment of restless legs syndrome (RLS). Sleep Med. 2004; 5(1):9-14.
3. Bogan RK et al. Ropinirole in the treatment of patients with restless legs syndrome: a US-based randomized, double-blind, placebo-controlled clinical trial. Mayo Clin Proc. 2006; 81(1):17-27.
4. Trenkwalder C et al. Ropinirole in the treatment of restless legs syndrome: results from the TREAT RLS 1 study, a 12 week, randomised, placebo controlled study in 10 European countries. J Neurol Neurosurg Psychiatry. 2004; 75(1):92-97.
5. Walters AS et al. Ropinirole is effective in the treatment of restless legs syndrome. TREAT RLS 2: a 12-week, double-blind, randomized, parallel-group, placebo-controlled study. Mov Disord. 2004; 19(12):1414-1423.
6. Winkelman JW et al. Efficacy and safety of pramipexole in restless legs syndrome. Neurology. 2006; 67(6):1034-1039.

7. Garcia-Borreguero D et al. Treatment of restless legs syndrome with gabapentin: a double-blind, cross-over study. Neurology. 2002; 59(10):1573-1579.

8. Happe S et al. Gabapentin versus ropinirole in the treatment of idiopathic restless legs syndrome. Neuropsychobiology. 2003; 48(2):82-86.

9. Stewart BH et al. A saturable transport mechanism in the intestinal absorption of gabapentin is the underlying cause of the lack of proportionality between increasing dose and drug levels in plasma. Pharm Res. 1993; 10(2):276-281.

10. Cundy KC et al. XP13512 [(+/-)-1-([[alpha-isobutanoyloxyethoxy)carbonyl] aminomethyl)-1-cyclohexane acetic acid], a novel gabapentin prodrug: I. Design, synthesis, enzymatic conversion to gabapentin, and transport by intestinal solute transporters. J Pharmacol Exp Ther. 2004; 311(1):315-323.

11. Cundy KC et al. Clinical pharmacokinetics of XP13512, a novel transported prodrug of gabapentin. J Clin Pharmacol. 2008; 48(12):1378-1388.

12. Kushida CA et al. Randomized, double-blind, placebo-controlled trial of XP13512/GSK1838262 in patients with RLS. Neurology. 2009(5); 72:439-446.

13. Allen RP et al. Psychometric evaluation and tests of validity of the Medical Outcomes Study 12-item Sleep Scale (MOS sleep). Sleep Med. 2008; 10(5):531-539.

14. Montplaisir J et al. Ropinirole is effective in the long-term management of restless legs syndrome: a randomized controlled trial. Mov Disord. 2006; 21(10):1627-1635.

15. Kushida CA et al. A randomized, double-blind, placebo-controlled, crossover study of XP13512/GSK1838262 in the treatment of patients with primary restless legs syndrome. Sleep. 2009; 32(2):159-168.

Proposed dose equivalence between clonazepam and pramipexole in patients with restless legs syndrome. Shinno H, Oka Y, Otsuki M, Tsuchiya S, Mizuno S, Kawada S, Innami T, Sasaki A, Hineno T, Sakamoto T, Inami Y, Nakamura Y, Horiguchi J. *Prog Neuropsychopharmacol Biol Psychiatry. 2010 Apr 16;34(3):522-6.*

How does clonazepam compare to pramipexole as therapy of restless legs syndrome and how does one convert from one agent to the other?

Subjects	Methods	Outcomes
26 subjects with RLS • Age (mean): 69.2 ± 11.0 yrs • Treated with clonazepam (≤ 2 mg per day • No other sleep disorders	Prospective, open-label study Protocol • Subjects were rapidly switched from clonazepam to pramipexole (conversion factor of 4:1) • Daily pramipexole dose was increased or decreased by 0.125mg at each examination Assessments: • IRLS • CGI-S • ESS	Results following conversion from clonazepam to pramipexole included: • Decrease in IRLS* • Decrease in ESS** • Improved CGI scores Adverse effects of pramipexole: • Somnolence • Sensation of oppression in the lower limbs • Diarrhea, nausea

CGI-I: Clinical Global Impression-Improvement; ESS: Epworth sleepiness scale; IRLS: International Restless Legs Syndrome severity rating scale; RLS: restless legs syndrome; *16.3 ± 8.7 to 9.1 ± 6.3; **6.5 ± 4.2 to 4.4 ± 3.2

Conclusion
A conversion factor of 4:1 for clonazepam to pramipexole was effective in improving symptoms of restless legs syndrome and sleepiness.

Commentary
Restless legs syndrome (RLS) is a neurological disorder characterized by an urge to move, and usually associated with uncomfortable leg sensations. The National Institutes of Health RLS workshop has defined the diagnostic criteria. The four essential criteria are: 1) An urge to move, usually accompanied or caused by uncomfortable and unpleasant sensations in the legs; 2) The urge to move or unpleasant sensations begin or worsen during periods of rest or inactivity such as lying and sitting; 3) The urge to move or unpleasant sensations are partially or totally relieved by movement, such as walking or stretching, at least as long as activity continues; and 4) The urge to move or unpleasant sensations are worse in the evening or night than during the day or occur only in the evening or night. Most RLS patients report difficulties falling asleep. It is also

difficult for patients with RLS to maintain their sleep because they awaken with unpleasant sensations shortly after sleep onset. As a consequence of frequent arousals from nocturnal sleep, patients often experience excessive daytime fatigue and somnolence. It is, therefore, mandatory to treat RLS adequately.

Dopaminergic medications are now widely prescribed for RLS treatment. Initially, the short-term efficacy of L-dopa was well documented. Polysomnographic studies showed that L-dopa administration induced a significant reduction in RLS symptoms present at bedtime as well as reducing periodic limb movements (PLM) throughout the night. Varying degrees of long-term benefit from L-dopa, however, have been found, ranging from 85 % to 31 % after a few years. Several adverse effects have been reported in patients treated with L-dopa, such as nausea, vomiting, tachycardia, orthostatic hypotension, hallucinations, and insomnia. Morning rebound and RLS augmentation are known as more specific adverse effects. Dopaminergic agonists are now considered the first-line treatment for RLS because they are more effective and produce fewer adverse effects. The Movement Disorder Society (MDS) commissioned a task force to perform an evidence-based review of current treatment strategies, and non-ergot-derived dopamine agonists were indicated to be efficacious treatment for RLS. In this decade, pramipexole, non-ergoline derivative agonists for dopamine D2/D3 receptor, have been studied for RLS treatment. Results from several double-blind, placebo-controlled studies have demonstrated the superiority of pramipexole for the broad range of RLS symptoms. There have also been several long-term studies demonstrating sustained efficacy of pramipexole in RLS.

Several studies have shown that benzodiazepines such as clonazepam improve the quality of sleep and reduce periodic limb movements during sleep (PLMs) as well as PLMs-associated arousals in patients with RLS, as has been reported its acute therapeutic efficacy regarding insomnia. Clonazepam is prescribed to improve sleep continuity and used as an adjunct treatment because dopaminergic agents sometimes worsen insomnia. However, regarding subjective RLS symptoms, sufficient studies demonstrating the effects of clonazepam have not been conducted, even though clonazepam prescription is prevalent in some countries of Asia and Europe.

To date, there have not been any studies on the conversion to non-ergot dopamine agonists in patients with RLS, although several articles have reported the conversion from ergot to non-ergot dopamine agonists in patients with advanced Parkinson's disease. Furthermore, there have not been any studies examining equivalent doses of pramipexole and clonazepam. The aim of this study is to evaluate equivalent doses of pramipexole and clonazepam in Japanese patients with RLS, using efficacy and tolerability after switching from clonazepam to pramipexole as indications of dose equivalence.

Periodic limb movements during sleep (PLMs) is most often associated with RLS, while a frequent comorbidity with other sleep disorders, such as sleep apnea, narcolepsy, parasomnia, has also been reported. Disturbances with a significant impact on the quality of life as well as increased PLM indices (number of PLM per hour of time in bed) are common in RLS. Some studies have reported that clonazepam is prescribed to improve sleep continuity in patients with RLS because dopaminergic agents sometimes worsen insomnia. There is, however, no clear evidence that subjective or objective PLM measures of therapeutic benefit have been achieved. These studies did not measure or discuss daytime somnolence, although clonazepam has a very prolonged effect and may cause such somnolence. Although dopamine agonists such as pramipexole may cause daytime sleepiness, previous studies in patients with RLS demonstrated that there was no significant difference in ESS score between pramipexole and placebo. As indicated in an evidence-based review established by the MDS-commissioned task force, the therapeutic effect of clonazepam on RLS may be investigational, although patients with subjective and/or objective sleep disturbances may indeed require treatment such as clonazepam. The strategy for conversion from clonazepam to dopaminergic agents should, therefore, be considered, when clonazepam fails to improve RLS symptoms sufficiently, or induces adverse effects.

It remains controversial whether rapid switch is preferable to slow titration. There have been several studies on switching protocol in patients with Parkinson's disease, although switching protocol has not been investigated in patients with RLS. Reports have shown that rapid conversion was safer, and that some patients with slow titration experienced enhanced Parkinsonism. Based on these findings, we rapidly switched to pramipexole in principle and pramipexole dose was calculated using a daily milligram conversion of 1:4 for clonazepam dose. However, in patients pretreated with higher doses of clonazepam (over 1mg/day), half daily doses of clonazepam were administered for a week instead of rapid discontinuation because it was necessary to prevent withdrawal symptoms. In the present study, a smaller proportion of subjects (4 of 26: 15.4%) exhibited adverse events. We consider that conversion to pramipexole may be relatively safe, although the lower percentage of adverse effects may be due to the lower daily doses of pramipexole prescribed for patients with RLS.

To our knowledge, there have not been any studies that investigated the switchover from clonazepam to pramipexole in patients with RLS. The present study demonstrates the important and practical findings that had not been investigated in patients with RLS. First, the comparison of efficacy and safety between pramipexole and clonazepam seems to be meaningful because there have been no comparative trials to agents other than placebo. We have demonstrated that conversion to pramipexole resulted in improvements of RLS symptoms and daytime somnolence. We consider that pramipexole may be preferable to clonazepam. Second, we have defined a conversion ratio to facilitate switching from clonazepam to pramipexole in a simple, safe, and effective manner for patients with RLS. Statistical analysis confirmed that a 4:1 conversion ratio for clonazepam to pramipexole is appropriate. Our study, however, has some limitations since it is an open-label trial and includes only 26 patients. Further studies using a double-blind design or a crossover design are recommended.

Hideto Shinno
Department of Neuropsychiatry
Kagawa University

References
1. Allen RP et al. Restless legs syndrome: diagnostic criteria, special considerations, and epidemiology. A report from the restless legs syndrome diagnosis and epidemiology workshop at the National Institutes of Health. Sleep Med. 2003; 4:101-19.
2. Allen RP et al. Restless legs syndrome prevalence and impact: REST general population study. Arch Intern Med. 2005; 165(11):1286-92.

3. Earley CJ et al. Pergolide and carbidopa/levodopa treatment of the restless legs syndrome and periodic leg movements in sleep in a consecutive series of patients. Sleep. 1996; 19(10):801-10.

4. Ferini-Strambi L et al. Effect of pramipexole on RLS symptoms and sleep: A randomized, double-blind, placebo-controlled trial. Sleep Med. 2008; 9(8):874-81.

5. Goetz CG et al. Switching dopamine agonists in advanced Parkinson's disease. Neurology. 1999; 52(6):1227-9.

6. Hanna PA et al. Switching from Pergolide to pramipexole in patients with Parkinson's disease. J Neural Transm. 2001; 108(1):63-70.

7. Johns MW. A new method for measuring daytime sleepiness: the Epworth sleepiness scale. Sleep. 1991; 14(6):540-5.

8. Matthews WB. Treatment of the restless legs syndrome with clonazepam. Br Med J. 1979; 1(6165):751.

9. Montplaisir J et al. Restless legs syndrome improved by pramipexole: a double-blind randomized trial. Neurology. 1999; 52(5):938-43.

10. Oertel WH et al. The Pramipexole RLS Study Group. Efficacy of pramipexole in restless legs syndrome: A six-week, multicenter, randomized, double-blind study. Mov Disord. 2007; 22(2):213-9.

11. Partinen M et al. Efficacy and safety of pramipexole in idiopathic restless legs syndrome: A polysomnographic dose-finding study- The PRELUDE study. Sleep Med. 2006;7:407-17.

12. Read DJ et al. Clonazepam: effective treatment for restless legs syndrome in uremia. Br Med J 1981; 283(6296): 885-6.

13. Silber MH et al. Pramipexole in the management of restless legs syndrome. Sleep 2003; 26(7): 819-21.

14. The International Restless Legs Syndrome Study Group. Validation of the International Restless Legs Syndrome Study Group rating scale for restless legs syndrome. Sleep Med 2003; 4(2): 121-32.

15. Trenkwalder C et al. Why do restless legs occur at rest? –pathophysiology of neuronal structures in RLS. Neurophysiology of RLS (part 2). Clin Neurophysiol 2004; 115: 1975-88.

16. Trenkwalder C et al. The German RLS-Pramipexole Study Group. Controlled withdrawal of pramipexole after 6 months of open-label treatment in patients with restless legs syndrome. Mov Disord 2006; 21(9):1404-10.

17. Trenkwalder C et al. Treatment of restless legs syndrome: an evidence-based review and implications for clinical practice. Mov Disord 2008; 23(16): 2267-302.

18. Winkelman JW et al. Efficacy and safety of pramipexole in restless legs syndrome. Neurol 2006; 67(6): 1034-9.

Parasomnias

Cognitive-behavioral treatment for chronic nightmares in trauma-exposed persons: assessing physiological reactions to nightmare-related fear. Rhudy JL, Davis JL, Williams AE, McCabe KM, Bartley EJ, Byrd PM, Pruiksma KE. *J Clin Psychol. 2010 Apr;66(4):365-82.*

Does cognitive behavioral therapy for chronic nightmares reduce nightmare-related fear?

Subjects	Methods	Outcomes
40 subjects	Randomized controlled study of CBT for chronic nightmares Subjects were randomized to: • Treatment group: n = 19 • Waitlist control group: n = 21 Assessments of reactions to personally relevant nightmare imagery (at pretreatment and at post treatment [1 week, 3 months and 6 months]) • Physiological responses: skin conductance, HR and facial EMG • Subjective responses: displeasure, fear, anger, sadness and arousal	CBT reduced physiological (skin conductance, HR and facial EMG) and subjective (displeasure, fear, sadness and arousal) reactions to nightmare imagery • Benefits were generally maintained at 6 months of follow-up

CBT: cognitive behavioral therapy; EMG: electromyography; HR: heart rate

Conclusion
Cognitive behavioral therapy for chronic nightmares decreased both physiological and subjective responses, including fear.

Commentary
Nightmares are a symptom of posttraumatic stress disorder [PTSD], are reported frequently by trauma-exposed individuals, and are associated with distress[1] and poor long-term functioning.[2] Increasingly, it is suggested that nightmares may be more than a symptom of PTSD, and may contribute to the initiation and/or maintenance of PTSD.[3] Nightmares are also resistant to psychological and pharmacological interventions that broadly target PTSD[4-5], but appear to respond well to cognitive behavioral interventions in which they are directly targeted.[6-7]

The fear associated with the experiences of nightmares and nightmare-related imagery may promote and maintain not only the chronicity and severity of the nightmares themselves, but related distress (e.g., anxiety, depression, sleep quality). Indeed, studies have found that sleep-onset insomnia may be driven by the fear associated with anticipating nightmares.[8] Levin and Nielsen[9] have argued that distressing posttraumatic nightmares reflect a failure of fear extinction processes that would normally occur during dreaming. It has been suggested that the chronicity of nightmares may reflect that the nightmares themselves become a significant fear stimulus[10], a part of the pathological fear network.[11-12] The heightened physiological arousal subsequent to nightmare related thoughts may significantly interfere with ability to go to sleep, quality of sleep, and return to sleep following a nightmare.[13] Stimuli related to the nightmares [e.g., sleep, bedroom environment] may become conditioned to elicit the fear response over time, further maintaining distress. Lack of sleep and nightmare-related fear may also promote other psychological problems, such as posttraumatic stress, anxiety, and depression. Reducing nightmare related fear may then reduce the frequency and severity of nightmares, depression, and anxiety, and may increase sleep quality. This is the first study to determine the effect of a direct nightmare intervention on physiological and subjective indices of nightmare-related fear.

In the present study, a randomized clinical trial was conducted that assessed the efficacy of a direct nightmare intervention to reduce nightmare-related fear (i.e., *Exposure, Relaxation, and Rescripting Therapy*, ERRT). We assessed participants' responses to script-driven imagery [nightmare imagery and non-personally-relevant fear imagery] utilizing physiological (SC, HR, facial EMG) and subjective (displeasure, fear, anger, sadness, arousal) measures before and after treatment, or at equivalent times for control participants. The overall findings were that physiological and subjective reactions to nightmare imagery were reduced following treatment, and these gains were maintained at the six month follow up. This study is the first to demonstrate that a direct treatment for nightmares is associated with decreased physiological and subjective responses to nightmare-related imagery. The fact that changes were not noted in the control group suggests that the decreased response was not due to habituation related to exposure to the personal nightmare script.

We suggest that physiological arousal due to nightmare-related fear and subsequent sleep problems are primary conditions driving other psychological problems in some trauma-exposed persons. If this proposition is true, then reducing that arousal and promoting sleep should decrease those other psychological problems. Indeed, previous studies have found *Exposure, Relaxation, and Rescripting Therapy* decreases the frequency and severity of nightmares, improves sleep quality and quantity, and improves symptoms of PTSD and depression, even though it does not directly address the traumatic event or other PTSD symptoms.[6]

The findings of the present study have clinical implications in the area of sleep medicine. First, the data in the nightmare literature appears to be converging on the idea that for some trauma-exposed individuals, nightmares are a primary condition that requires direct intervention efforts. We do not know at this point, however, how to distinguish these individuals from those for whom nightmares may be a secondary condition. Determining this will be important for guiding treatment planning for trauma-exposed individuals suffering from nightmares and sleep problems. Second, the findings suggest new considerations for a possible mechanism of change for the treatment. Reduction of physiological arousal may be a primary mechanism of change by means of relaxation efforts, subsequently promoting both quality and quantity of sleep, and decreasing distress and impaired functioning associated with sleep deprivation. Alternatively, the process of written exposure to and rescripting of the nightmares, which are components of ERRT, may reduce fear and subsequently reduce physiological arousal to nightmare-related thoughts and images.

Joanne L. Davis
Department of Psychology
University of Tulsa

Jamie L. Rhudy
Department of Psychology
University of Tulsa

Christopher C. Cranston
Department of Psychology
University of Tulsa

References

1. Kilpatrick DG et al. The posttraumatic stress disorder field trial: Evaluation of the PTSD construct: Criteria A through E. In: Widiger TA, A.J. Frances, H.A. Pincus, M.B. First, R. Ross, & W. Davis, ed. DSM-IV sourcebook (Volume IV). Washington, D.C.: American Psychiatric Press, 1998.
2. Harvey AG et al. The relationship between acute stress disorder and posttraumatic stress disorder: a prospective evaluation of motor vehicle accident survivors. Journal of Consulting and Clinical Psychology. 1998; 66:507-12.
3. Ross R et al. Sleep disturbance as the hallmark of posttraumatic stress disorder. Am J Psychiatry. 1989; 146:697-707.
4. Clark RD et al. Cyproheptadine treatment of nightmares associated with posttraumatic stress disorder. Journal of Clinical Psychopharmacology. 1999; 19:486-7.
5. Forbes D et al. The validity of the PTSD checklist as a measure of symptomatic change in combat-related PTSD. Behaviour Research and Therapy. 2001; 39:977-86.
6. Davis JL et al. Randomized clinical trial for treatment of chronic nightmares in trauma-exposed adults. Journal of Traumatic Stress. 2007; 20:123-33.
7. Krakow B et al. Imagery rehearsal therapy for chronic nightmares in sexual assault survivors with posttraumatic stress disorder: A randomized controlled trial. JAMA. 2001; 286:537-45.
8. Neylan TC et al. Sleep disturbances in the Vietnam generation: Findings from a nationally representative sample of male Vietnam veterans. Am J Psychiatry. 1998; 155:929-33.
9. Levin R et al. Disturbed dreaming, posttraumatic stress disorder, and affect distress: A review and neurocognitive model. Psychol. Bull. 2007; 133:482-528.
10. Davis JL. Treating post-trauma nightmares: a cognitive behavioral approach. New York, NY: Springer Publishing Company, 2009.
11. Levin R et al. Disturbed dreaming, posttraumatic stress disorder, and affect distress: a review and neurocognitive model. Psychological Bulletin. 2007; 133:482-528.
12. Foa EB et al. Emotional processing of fear: exposure to corrective information. Psychological Bulletin. 1986; 99:20-35.
13. Rhudy JL et al. Physiological-emotional reactivity to nightmare-related imagery in trauma-exposed persons with chronic nightmares. Behavioral Sleep Medicine. 2008; 6:158-77.

Controlled clinical, polysomnographic and psychometric studies on differences between sleep bruxers and controls and acute effects of clonazepam as compared with placebo. Saletu A, Parapatics S, Anderer P, Matejka M, Saletu B. *Eur Arch Psychiatry Clin Neurosci. 2010 Mar;260(2):163-74.*

What are the main clinical, polysomnographic and psychometric features of sleep bruxism, and how are these features affected by administration of clonazepam?

Subjects	Methods	Outcomes
21 subjects with bruxism 21 age- and sex-matched controls	Subjects with bruxism and controls spent 3 and 2 nights in the sleep laboratory, respectively Acute effects of clonazepam (1 mg) and placebo were compared Assessments: • Symptoms • Objective and subjective sleep and waking quality • PSG • Psychometry	Characteristics of subjects with bruxism included: • Deteriorated PSQI, SAS, SDS and IRLSSG measures • PSG features: 1. Impaired sleep maintenance 2. Increased movement time 3. Higher stage shift index 4. Greater PLMs and arousals • Psychometry features: 1. Deteriorated subjective sleep and awakening quality, evening/morning well-being, drive, mood, drowsiness, attention variability, memory, and fine motor activity Compared with placebo, clonazepam was associated with significantly reduced SB index (-42 ± 15%)

AI: arousal index; N1: sleep stage 1; PLM: periodic leg movement; PSG: polysomnography; PSQI: Pittsburg sleep quality index; SB: sleep bruxism; SE: sleep efficiency; SL: sleep latency

Conclusion
The severity of sleep bruxism, which was associated with several adverse clinical, polysomnographic and psychometric consequences, was attenuated by administration of clonazepam.

Commentary
Sleep bruxism is a condition that may or may not be associated with painful jaw and facial muscles, even headache. Bite splints are known to help and in some cases eliminate the pain

associated with the bruxism but not the sleep bruxism itself. What is not well known is the association with micro-arousal and the possible symptoms of daytime sleepiness. Therefore the main form of treatment is simply with a bite splint. The use of adjunctive medication is primarily muscle relaxers and analgesics if there is pain. Dentists with advanced training in orofacial pain may elect to use other medications such as amitriptyline or nortriptyline.

The incidence of sleep bruxism is cited at 8% with typically higher percentages in the younger population and lower percentages as we age. Therefore the use of medication such as clonazepam may be restricted to a limited number of people and may be restricted further to those who have associated pain or where the sounds due to grinding disturb the bed partner, much like snoring.

Sleep bruxism is potentially made worse by medications, substances and drugs that can cause an increase in the bruxism. The SSRI medications, amphetamines, alcohol, nicotine and cocaine are some examples. In these instances other measures should be utilized such as limiting the use of these substances as opposed to adding another medication in an attempt to control the bruxing.

In the absence of other contributing factors clonazepam may have significant benefit as it helps with anxiety (a contributing factor to bruxing and clenching), is a muscle relaxer and helps with mood by improving sleep.

Because sleep bruxism has been shown to occur in those who snore or are at risk for sleep apnea the improvement in sleep seen with the use of clonazepam needs to be considered in light of these findings. A careful assessment for snoring and for being at risk for sleep apnea should be considered prior to the use of clonazepam for bruxing.

The results of the use of clonazepam for bruxism were also shown to improve PLMD. This is not surprising since it has been proposed that RLS, PLMD and sleep bruxism all have the same central nervous system origin.

The individual using a medication such as clonazepam for the management of bruxism needs to understand the actions, side effects and long-term nature of using this medication. The dentist is often times the main provider when it comes to bruxism and needs to have a full knowledge of the various means by which this condition can be managed, especially when a bite splint is not optimally effective. Since the incidence of bruxism tends to diminish as we age the use of clonazepam may be more applicable in the younger age group (20s to 50s) as opposed to those over the age of 60.

Dennis Bailey
Dental Sleep Medicine Mini-Residency
School of Dentistry
University of California Los Angeles
Los Angeles, California

Effect of botulinum toxin injection on nocturnal bruxism: a randomized controlled trial. Lee SJ, McCall WD Jr, Kim YK, Chung SC, Chung JW. *Am J Phys Med Rehabil. 2010 Jan;89(1):16-23.*

Does botulinum toxin type A have any salutary effects on nocturnal bruxism?

Subjects	*Methods*	*Outcomes*
12 subjects with nocturnal bruxism	Double-blind, randomized clinical trial Subjects were randomized to one of two groups: • Botulinum: botulinum toxin was injected in both masseters (n = 6) • Saline: saline was injected in both masseters (n = 6) Assessments: • Questionnaires about bruxism symptoms • Nocturnal EMG activity (masseter and temporalis muscles) before injection, and at 4, 8, and 12 wks after injection	Compared to saline injection, botulinum toxin injection was associated with: • Significantly decreased bruxism events in the masseter muscles* • No difference in temporalis muscle bruxism events Compared to baseline, subjective symptoms of bruxism decreased in both groups after injection**

EMG: electromyography; NB: nocturnal bruxism; *P = 0.027; **P < 0.001

Conclusion
Injection of botulinum toxin type A in both masseter muscles reduced the number of bruxism events.

Commentary
There problems with this study, not the least of which are the small "N" and the assumption that finding decreased EMG activity in masseter muscles paralyzed by botulinum toxin was indicative of overall decrease in bruxism. The fact that there was a negligible reduction in temporalis muscle activity after the masseter muscle injections is actually an indication that bruxing behavior did not decrease since temporalis muscle activity was unchanged. Both the temporalis and masseter muscles are jaw closers and contract together during closing, mastication or bruxing events.

The authors were measuring reduced masseter muscle activity during bruxing events, not overall reduction in bruxism. Using botulinum toxin in cases of persistent and refractory muscle pain may be beneficial for pain that does not respond to physical therapy. However, this paper does not support the hypothesis that botulinum toxin will reduce bruxism, although, as expected, it will reduce the muscle activity of the injected muscle during bruxing events.

Robert L. Merrill
School of Dentistry
University of California, Los Angeles

Medical, Neurological and Psychiatric Disorders

Effects of salmeterol on sleeping oxygen saturation in chronic obstructive pulmonary disease.
Ryan S, Doherty LS, Rock C, Nolan GM, McNicholas WT. *Respiration. 2010;79(6):475-81.*

Does inhaled salmeterol, a long-acting beta agonist, improve sleep-related oxygen saturation and sleep quality in persons with moderate to severe stable chronic obstructive pulmonary disease?

Subjects	Methods	Outcomes
15 subjects with moderate to severe stable COPD 12 subjects completed the trial • Age (median): 69 yrs • FEV_1: 39%	Randomized, double-blind, placebo-controlled, crossover study Subjects were randomized to either (4 weeks of treatment): • Salmeterol: 50 mcg twice daily • Placebo Assessments: • PSG (at baseline, 4 weeks and 8 weeks) • PFT	Compared to placebo, salmeterol administration was associated with: • Improved mean SaO_2* 1. Salmeterol: 92.9% 2. Placebo: 91.0% • Less % of sleep with SaO_2 < 90%** 1. Salmeterol: 1.8% 2. Placebo: 25.6% • Better static lung volumes • No difference in PSG sleep quality

COPD: chronic obstructive pulmonary disease; FEV_1: forced expiratory volume in 1 s; LABA: long-acting beta(2)-agonist; PFT: pulmonary function testing; PSG: polysomnography; SaO_2: aterial oxygen saturation; *P = 0.016; **P = 0.005

Conclusion
Inhaled salmeterol improved sleep-related oxygen saturation in persons with moderate to severe stable chronic obstructive pulmonary disease.

Commentary
Chronic obstructive pulmonary disease (COPD) is a leading cause of morbidity and mortality worldwide. It is increasingly recognized that sleep may be associated with clinically important adverse effects in patients with COPD such as disordered gas exchange and impaired sleep quality. Hypoventilation and ventilation-perfusion mismatching may lead to significant nocturnal oxygen desaturation (NOD) predisposing to pulmonary hypertension, cardiac arrhythmias during sleep and nocturnal death during exacerbations.[1] Long-acting beta agonists (LABA) are a recommended part of care in patients with moderate to severe COPD, but their effects on NOD and sleep quality are unknown. To investigate this subject, we conducted a

randomized, double-blind, placebo-controlled, crossover study on 15 patients with moderate to severe stable COPD.[2] We performed overnight polysomnography (PSG) and detailed pulmonary function testing at baseline and after 4 weeks of treatment with either the LABA salmeterol or placebo. We found that the addition of salmeterol resulted in significant improvements in NOD, particularly the sleeping time spent with an oxygen saturation below 90%, which averaged only two per cent on salmeterol compared to 25% while on placebo. There was a trend towards improvement in static lung volumes particularly in trapped gas volume with salmeterol suggesting a reduction in hyperinflation as one likely underlying mechanism of the findings. There was no difference in sleep quality between salmeterol and placebo. The magnitude of improvement in nocturnal oxygen saturation with salmeterol in our study is comparable to that previously reported with theophylline and tiotropium treatment.[3,4] The present study findings are also consistent with previous reports that have failed to show a relationship between corrections of hypoxemia and sleep quality in COPD. In a previous study, concerns have been raised of reduced sleep quality with salmeterol.[5] Notably, there was no deterioration in subjective sleep quality with salmeterol in our patient population, and while there appeared to be a trend towards less slow-wave sleep with salmeterol, our study was not sufficiently powered to detect a significant difference; thus further studies would be required to specifically address this point.

We excluded patients with obstructive sleep apnea syndrome (OSAS) from the study to avoid a potentially important confounding disorder that might have compromised the ability to assess the direct effects of salmeterol on oxygen levels in COPD patients while asleep. Nonetheless, we recognize the importance of co-existing COPD and OSAS (commonly referred to as the "overlap syndrome"), which occurs in 1% of the adult population.[6] The degree of NOD is greater in the overlap syndrome than with either disorder alone. We cannot conclude if salmeterol would have a greater or lesser effect on sleep oxygen saturation in such patients, and given the high clinical importance of NOD in the "overlap syndrome" as a driver of systemic inflammation, this question should be addressed in future studies.

Silke Ryan
Respiratory Sleep Disorders Unit
St. Vincent's University Hospital

Walter McNicholas
Respiratory Sleep Disorders Unit
Department of Respiratory Medicine
St. Vincent's University Hospital

References
1. McNicholas WT. Impact of sleep in copd. Chest 2000;117:48S-53S.
2. Ryan S et al. Effects of salmeterol on sleeping oxygen saturation in chronic obstructive pulmonary disease. Respiration. 2010; 79:475-481.
3. McNicholas WT et al. Long-acting inhaled anticholinergic therapy improves sleeping oxygen saturation in copd. Eur Respir J. 2004; 23:825-831.
4. Mulloy E et al. Theophylline improves gas exchange during rest, exercise, and sleep in severe chronic obstructive pulmonary disease. Am Rev Respir Dis. 1993; 148:1030-1036.

5. Jones PW et al. Quality of life changes in copd patients treated with salmeterol. Am J Respir Crit Care Med. 1997; 155:1283-1289.
6. McNicholas WT. Chronic obstructive pulmonary disease and obstructive sleep apnea: Overlaps in pathophysiology, systemic inflammation, and cardiovascular disease. Am J Respir Crit Care Med. 2009; 180:692-700.

Intranasal mometasone furoate therapy for allergic rhinitis symptoms and rhinitis-disturbed sleep. Meltzer EO, Munafo DA, Chung W, Gopalan G, Varghese ST. *Ann Allergy Asthma Immunol. 2010 Jul;105(1):65-74.*

Can inhaled intranasal corticosteroids improve sleep and daytime functioning in persons with nasal congestion related to allergic rhinitis?

Subjects	Methods	Outcomes
29 subjects with perennial AR and RDS	28-day, randomized, double-blind, placebo-controlled, parallel-group, single-center study Subjects were randomized to either (each morning): • Mometasone furoate nasal spray (200 mcg): n = 20 • Placebo: n = 9 Assessments: • AHI (using home sleep study) • Daytime PNIF • ESS • Nighttime FLI • Nighttime symptom score • RQLQ-S score • TNSS • WPAI-AS questionnaire	Compared to placebo, administration of mometasone furoate was associated with: • No difference in AHI • Improvements in: 1. Morning* and evening** TNSS: correlated with improved productivity 2. Morning*** and evening[#] nasal congestion 3. Daily PNIF[##] 4. FLI[###] 5. ESS[^] 6. RQLQ-S score[^^] 7. 2 of 5 WPAI-AS domains

AHI: apnea hypopnea index; AR: allergic rhinitis; BMI: body mass index; ESS: Epworth sleepiness scale; FLI: flow limitation index; INC: intranasal corticosteroids (mometasone furoate); NS: nasal spray; NSS: nighttime symptom score; PNIF: peak nasal inspiratory flow; QOL: quality of life; RDS: rhinitis-disturbed sleep; RQLQ-S: Rhinoconjunctivitis Quality of Life Questionnaire-Standardized score; TNSS: total nasal symptom score; WPAI-AS: Work Productivity and Activities Impairment-Allergy Specific questionnaire; *P = .04; **P = .01; ***P = .049; [#]P = .03; [##]P = .03; [###]P = .02; [^]P = .048; [^^]P = .03

Conclusion
Intranasal mometasone furoate improved nasal symptoms and daytime functioning in persons with perennial allergic rhinitis.

Commentary
Rhinitis-disturbed sleep (RDS) is a prevalent problem with substantial effect on patients' daily lives. Its mechanisms are not fully understood.[1,2] We defined RDS as subjective sleep

impairment coincident with symptomatic allergic rhinitis (AR). Allergic rhinitis can be seasonal (SAR) or perennial (PAR).

In this exploratory study of 29 patients we evaluated the efficacy of mometasone furoate nasal spray (NS) use in patients with moderate to severe PAR and a history of moderate to severe RDS, thought secondary to PAR. The study goal was to assess changes in nasal symptoms, nasal airflow, and airway obstruction during sleep in response to mometasone furoate NS therapy. In addition, the effects of mometasone furoate NS use on daytime somnolence, quality of life (QOL), and daytime functioning were examined.

Mometasone furoate nasal spray is indicated to treat nasal symptoms in seasonal allergic rhinitis and has been found to significantly improve daytime and nighttime total nasal symptom scores (TNSSs) and individual nasal symptoms.[3-6] However, to our knowledge, no studies have reported the efficacy of mometasone furoate NS in improving airway obstruction during sleep in individuals with PAR.

Subjective and objective measures of PAR, sleep quality, and daily functioning were assessed before and after 4 weeks of treatment with mometasone furoate NS or placebo. Post treatment differences between the mometasone furoate NS and placebo groups in apnea hypopnea index (AHI), the primary end point, and snoring events were not significant. However, significant improvements favoring mometasone furoate NS were noted for total nasal symptom scores (TNSS) and 3 of 4 individual nasal symptom scores, objective measures of nasal airflow (PNIF), sleepiness, patient-assessed QOL, and work absenteeism and daily activity level. Mometasone furoate NS therapy thus yields significant and clinically meaningful subjective and objective improvements in AR and RDS.

Pharyngeal obstruction in obstructive sleep apnea syndrome (OSAS) can occur at multiple levels[7] but is primarily related to partial or total collapse of the oropharynx.[8,9] In contrast, airway resistance in allergic congestion occurs primarily in the nasal passages. Mechanical obstruction (with nasal packing) in healthy individuals increased the frequency of apnea and hypopnea episodes[10,11], and it has been suggested that increased nasal airway resistance due to AR may be a risk factor for SDB.[12] However, it is unclear whether AR-related congestion is a risk factor for SDB.

These data do not support a relationship between increased nasal resistance and frequency of airway collapse, suggesting that OSAS and what this article terms RDS are distinct conditions with separate etiologies (oropharyngeal mechanical obstruction in OSAS vs. nasal mucosal inflammation in RDS). Therefore, intranasal corticosteroid treatment in patients with coexisting RDS and OSAS, although improving nasal patency, sleep quality, and daily functioning, would likely have little effect on nonnasal causes of airway obstruction.

In conclusion, this is the first study, to our knowledge, demonstrating the effectiveness of mometasone furoate NS therapy in reducing nasal symptoms in patients with PAR and RDS. The correlation between reduction in nasal symptoms, especially nasal congestion, and improved performance suggests that mometasone furoate NS therapy, through its nasal anti-inflammatory activities, can improve sleep quality, as evidenced by a reduction in daytime sleepiness. Owing to the small sample size, further investigation is warranted to determine whether these improvements translate into meaningful differences in a larger population.

Dominic A. Munafo
Sleep Data, Inc.

Eli O. Meltzer
Allergy & Asthma Medical Group & Research Center

References
1. Shedden A. Impact of nasal congestion on quality of life and work productivity in allergic rhinitis: findings from a large online survey. Treat Respir Med. 2005; 4:439-446.
2. Kakumanu S et al. Poor sleep and daytime somnolence in allergic rhinitis: significance of nasal congestion. Am J Respir Med. 2002; 1:190-200.
3. Hebert JR et al. Once-daily mometasone furoate aqueous nasal spray (Nasonex®) in seasonal allergic rhinitis: an active- and placebo-controlled study. Allergy. 1996; 51:569-576.
4. Gawchik S et al. Relief of cough and nasal symptoms associated with allergic rhinitis by mometasone furoate nasal spray. Ann Allergy Asthma Immunol. 2003; 90:416-421.
5. Mandl M et al. Comparison of once daily mometasone furoate (Nasonex) and fluticasone propionate aqueous nasal sprays for the treatment of perennial rhinitis. Ann Allergy Asthma Immunol. 1997; 79:370-378.
6. Berger WE et al. Mometasone furoate improves congestion in patients with moderate-to-severe seasonal allergic rhinitis. Ann Pharmacother. 2005; 39:1984-1989.
7. Bachar G et al. Laryngeal and hypopharyngeal obstruction in sleep disordered breathing patients, evaluated by sleep endoscopy. Eur Arch Otorhinolaryngol. 2008; 265:1397-1402.
8. Katsantonis GP et al. Determining the site of airway collapse in obstructive sleep apnea with airway pressure monitoring. Laryngoscope. 1993; 103:1126-1131.
9. Malhotra A et al. Obstructive sleep apnoea. Lancet. 2002;360: 237–245.
10. Suratt PM et al. Effect of intranasal obstruction on breathing during sleep. Chest. 1986; 90:324-329.
11. Lavie P et al. The effects of partial and complete mechanical occlusion of the nasal passages on sleep structure and breathing in sleep. Acta Otolaryngol. 1983; 95:161-166.
12. Young T et al. Nasal obstruction as a risk factor for sleep disordered breathing. J Allergy Clin Immunol. 1997; 99:S757-S762.

Nocturnal periodic breathing during acclimatization at very high altitude at Mount Muztagh Ata (7,546 m). Bloch KE, Latshang TD, Turk AJ, Hess T, Hefti U, Merz TM, Bosch MM, Barthelmes D, Hefti JP, Maggiorini M, Schoch OD. *Am J Respir Crit Care Med. 2010 Aug 15;182(4):562-8.*

How do nocturnal breathing pattern and ventilation at very high altitude evolve during acclimatization over several weeks?

Subjects	Methods	Outcomes
34 mountaineers ascending from 3,750 m to the summit of Mt. Muztagh Ata at 7,546 m over 19-20 days • Age (median): 46 yrs • Gender: 79% males • 7 women) climbed from	Assessments: • Nocturnal SaO_2 • Nocturnal RIP • Scores of AMS	Increasing altitude was associated with: • Decrease in nocturnal SaO_2 • Increase in MV • Increase in number of periodic breathing cycles Values at the highest camp (6,850 m) were: • Median nocturnal SaO_2: 64% • Median MV: 11.3 L/min • Median number of periodic breathing cycles: 132.3 cycles per hr Repeated recordings within 5 days (at 4,497 m) and 8 days (at 5,533 m) was associated with: • Increase in SaO_2 • No decrease in periodic breathing Number of periodic breathing cycles positively correlated with days of acclimatization but was not associated with symptoms of AMS

AMS: acute mountain sickness; MV: minute ventilation; PB: periodic breathing; RIP: respiratory inductive plethysmography; SaO_2: arterial oxygen saturation

Conclusion
Increasing altitude was associated with progressive changes in nocturnal oxygen saturation, minute ventilation and periodic breathing.

Commentary

At altitudes greater than 2,500 m, an oscillatory pattern of waxing and waning of ventilation with periods of hyperventilation alternating with central apneas or hypopneas is commonly observed in healthy subjects.[1] Although high-altitude periodic breathing has been known for many years[2-4], several aspects of the respiratory adaptation to hypobaric hypoxia are still incompletely understood since previous studies in a small number of subjects have provided conflicting results on the changes of breathing pattern during acclimatization. In this prospective field study in 34 participants of a high-altitude medical research expedition to Mount Muztagh Ata (7'546 m), China[5], the effects of altitude and acclimatization on nocturnal breathing patterns were investigated.

After baseline examinations in Zurich (490 m) climbers flew to Islamabad, Pakistan, and subsequently travelled by bus on the Karakorum Highway to 3,730 m at the base of Mt. Muztagh Ata. Climbers ascended on skis, led by mountain guides who assured that climbing rate did not exceed 1,036 m/d within 6–8 hours. Polygraphic recordings were performed during several nights at different altitudes using portable equipment including calibrated respiratory inductance plethysmography, pulse oximetry and ECG.[6]

A total of 209 overnight recordings were obtained. There was a significant trend towards a decrease in oxygen saturation with increasing altitude and minute ventilation at 6'865 m reached more than twice the baseline value at 490 m.

To evaluate the effect of acclimatization, recordings obtained twice within a few days at the same altitudes were compared. They revealed a significant increase in oxygen saturation whereas the increase in minute ventilation was not statistically significant. At altitudes > 4,000 m, the mountaineers spent most of the night with periodic breathing. The apnea/hypopnea index increased to very high values of 98.8/h to 151.6/h at the high camps. Periodic breathing was associated with large oscillations in oxygen saturation, with nadirs as low as 60% at > 6,000m. During the second stay at 4,497 m and at 5,533 m, respectively, the apnea/hypopnea index and the time spent with periodic breathing had increased compared to the first time.

To further explore the hypothesis that periodic breathing increased with prolonged acclimatization at altitude, ordinal logistic regression analysis was performed. The quartiles of the apnea/hypopnea index were entered as the dependent variable and acclimatization time (days spent above 3,750 m) as the independent variable, controlled for other, potentially confounding variables, including AMS-c scores. Acclimatization time was highly significantly and positively correlated with the apnea/hypopnea index in multivariate analysis when controlling for confounding variables.

In summary, in this field study performed in a large group of mountaineers for the first time provides quantitative and detailed data on the nocturnal breathing pattern and oxygen saturation at very high altitude up to 6,850 m. Repeated recordings obtained within a few days at base camp (4,497 m) revealed an increase in the apnea/hypopnea index, despite a simultaneous increase in oxygen saturation. This finding, and the progressive rise in minute ventilation over the course of the expedition, is consistent with an increasing gain of the respiratory feedback control system during acclimatization.[7] Thus, a high ventilatory sensitivity to CO_2 and hypoxia in the presence of a reduced CO_2 reserve may have promoted breathing instability with an overshooting response to apnea.[8] Alteration in plant gain related to the major increases in tidal volume that reduced the dead space fraction may have additionally affected the respiratory control stability.

Otto D. Schoch
Pulmonary Divisions
Cantonal Hospital St. Gallen

Konrad E. Bloch
Pulmonary Divisions
University Hospital of Zurich

References

1. Nussbaumer-Ochsner Y et al. Lessons from high-altitude physiology. Breathe. 2007; 4:123-132.
2. West JB et al. Nocturnal periodic breathing at altitudes of 6,300 and 8,050 m. J Appl Physiol. 1986; 61:280-287.
3. Khoo MC et al. Dynamics of periodic breathing and arousal during sleep at extreme altitude. Respir Physiol 1996; 103:33-43.
4. Erba P et al. Acute mountain sickness is related to nocturnal hypoxemia but not to hypoventilation. Eur Respir J 2004; 24:303-308.
5. Bloch KE et al. Effect of ascent protocol on acute mountain sickness and success at Muztagh Ata, 7546 m. High Alt Med Biol 2009; 10:25-32.
6. Clarenbach CF et al. Monitoring of ventilation during exercise by a portable respiratory inductive plethysmograph. Chest 2005; 128:1282-1290.
7. White DP et al. Altitude acclimatization: influence on periodic breathing and chemoresponsiveness during sleep. J Appl Physiol 1987; 63:401-412.
8. Dempsey JA et al. The ventilatory responsiveness to CO(2) below eupnoea as a determinant of ventilatory stability in sleep. J Physiol 2004; 560:1-11.

Short and long sleep are positively associated with obesity, diabetes, hypertension, and cardiovascular disease among adults in the United States. Buxton OM, Marcelli E. *Soc Sci Med. 2010 Sep;71(5):1027-36.*

Does short sleep (< 7 hrs) and long sleep (> 8 hrs) duration affect the risk of obesity, diabetes, hypertension and cardiovascular disease?

Subjects	*Methods*	*Outcomes*
56,507 adult subjects • Age: 18-85 yrs	Analysis of 2004-2005 US National Health Interview Survey data	Sleep duration was strongly associated with risk of obesity, DM, HTN and CVD • 7-8 h sleep duration reduces chronic disease risk

CVD: cardiovascular disease; DM: diabetes mellitus; HTN: hypertension

Conclusion

Daily sleep duration of 7 to 8 hours was associated with reduced risk of obesity, diabetes, hypertension and cardiovascular disease compared to shorter sleep (< 7 hrs) or longer sleep (> 8 hrs) duration.

Commentary

Obesity, diabetes and cardiovascular disease are among the leading causes of death in the United States. Research associates short (and to a lesser extent long) sleep duration with obesity, diabetes, and cardiovascular disease; and although 7-8 h of sleep seems to confer the least health risk, these findings are often based on non-representative data. We hypothesized that short sleep (< 7 h) and long sleep (> 8 h) are positively associated with the risk of obesity, diabetes, hypertension, and cardiovascular disease in US adults.

We analyzed 2004-2005 US National Health Interview Survey data (n = 56,507 observations, adults 18-85) using multilevel logistic regression, simultaneously controlling for individual characteristics (e.g., ethnoracial group, gender, age, education), other health behaviors (e.g., exercise, smoking), family environment (e.g., income, size, education) and geographic context (e.g., census region). Our model correctly classified at least 76% of adults on each of the outcomes studied. Both long sleep duration (> 8 hours/night) and short sleep duration (<7 hours/night) were frequently more strongly associated with these health risks than other covariates.

An important limitation of this study is the cross-sectional design that does not permit a determination on the direction of causality. Arguments for a relationship between short sleep duration and chronic disease using prospective data have been described for obesity[1], diabetes[2], hypertension.[3] Conversely, long sleep duration may be an epiphenomenon of other comorbidities. An important practical limitation of the NHIS dataset is that sleep duration was reported in integer hours, probably substantially degrading the sensitivity of this question, to the extent that self-reports are useful. Finally, the omission of dietary questions from the NHIS dataset is important because it is thought that sleep restriction impacts metabolism in part via changes to dietary choice[4] or extra snacking.[4-5]

These findings emphasize the important role sleep plays in the health of Americans, and indicate that sleep may have a larger influence on these chronic diseases than diet or exercise. These findings suggest a 7-8 h sleep duration directly and indirectly reduces chronic disease risk and appears to be the ideal amount to maximize health benefits and minimize cardiometabolic disease risks. It is also becoming evident that a focus on sleep duration may be important for understanding the long-term health of relatively healthy populations such as foreign-born residents of the U.S.A.[6-8]

Orfeu M. Buxton
Division of Sleep Medicine
Harvard Medical School
Department of Medicine
Brigham and Women's Hospital

Enrico A. Marcelli
Department of Sociology
San Diego State University

References
1. Cappuccio FP et al. Meta-analysis of short sleep duration and obesity in children and adults. Sleep. 2008; 31(5):619-26.
2. Knutson KL et al. Associations between sleep loss and increased risk of obesity and diabetes. Annals of the NY Academy of Science. 2008; 1129:287-304.
3. Stranges S et al. A population-based study of reduced sleep duration and hypertension: the strongest association may be in premenopausal women. J Hypertens. 2010; 28(5):896-902.
4. Buxton OM et al. Sleep adequacy associated with healthier food choices and positive workplace experience in motor freight workers. Am J Public Health. 2009; 99 Suppl 3:S636-43.
5. Nedeltcheva AV et al. Sleep curtailment is accompanied by increased intake of calories from snacks. The American Journal of Clinical Nutrition. 2009; 89(1):126-133.
6. Marcelli E et al. In: Visible (Im)Migrants:The Health and Socioeconomic Integration of Brazilians in Metropolitan Boston. San Diego, CA: San Diego State University, 2009.
7. Marcelli E et al. Permanently Temporary? The Health and Socioeconomic Status of Dominicans in Metropolitan Boston. San Diego, CA: San Diego State University, 2009.
8. Marcelli EA et al. "A Sociogeography of Insufficient Sleep: New Evidence from Legal and Unauthorized Migrants in Metropolitan Boston," Dallas, TX: Population Association of America Annual meeting, 2010.

Sleep disturbance immediately prior to trauma predicts subsequent psychiatric disorder.
Bryant RA, Creamer M, O'Donnell M, Silove D, McFarlane AC. *Sleep. 2010 Jan 1;33(1):69-74.*

Does the extent of sleep disturbance prior to a traumatic event predict subsequent psychiatric disorder?

Subjects	Methods	Outcomes
1033 subjects with traumatic injuries from 4 trauma hospitals across Australia	Prospective cohort study Subjects were assessed initially during hospital admission and again at 3 months after injury Assessments: • Psychiatric disorder (Mini-International Neuropsychiatric Interview) • Sleep disturbance 2 weeks prior to injury (Sleep Impairment Index)	At 3 months, there were 255 (28%) subjects with psychiatric disorder Psychiatric disorder was more likely to develop at 3 months in subjects who had sleep disturbance prior to injury* • The same was also noted in subjects who had never developed a prior disorder**

OR: odds ratio; *OR = 2.44, 95% CI: 1.62-3.69; **OR = 3.16, 95% CI: 1.59-4.75

Conclusion
Pre-trauma disturbed sleep was a risk factor for posttraumatic psychiatric disorder.

Commentary
The major finding from this study was that people who had never suffered a psychiatric diagnosis before in their lives were significantly more likely to develop a disorder following exposure to a traumatic event if they had suffered sleep disturbance in the two weeks prior to the traumatic event. A total of 1033 traumatically injured patients were initially assessed during hospital admission for lifetime psychiatric disorder, as well as sleep disturbance in the two weeks prior to the traumatic event. Three months later 923 were subsequently re-assessed 3 months for current psychiatric disorder. We removed patients who had suffered a prior psychiatric disorder from the analysis because prior sleep disturbance may have occurred as a result of psychiatric disturbance. Although 30% of patients reported a psychiatric disorder for the first time, patients were 3.16 times more likely to have a disorder if they had suffered prior sleep disturbance. Impressively, this pattern held even after controlling for the effects of age, gender, the type of traumatic injury, and severity of injury.

Although there are multiple explanations for this observation, possibly the most intriguing possibility involves the impact of sleep disturbance on memories for trauma. Arguably the most influential model for posttraumatic psychiatric disorders involves fear conditioning, in which excessive fear-inducing arousal at the time of trauma leads to increased noradrenergic activation, which strongly consolidates memories of the trauma.[1] Sleep deprivation contributes to increased levels of arousal immediately prior to the traumatic experience[2], which may in turn render the individual more likely to experiencing greater arousal and expression of stress hormones in the immediate aftermath of the trauma, thereby predisposing them to developing a disorder, and especially posttraumatic stress disorder (PTSD). This possibility converges with evidence that disturbed sleep can impair extinction learning[3], which involves the repeated learning that reminders of a threat are no longer signals of danger, which is regarded as a primary model of psychological recovery from trauma.[4] Interestingly, a recent study found that whereas reactivation of a memory in waking states destabilizes the memory, and permits alteration of the memory, reactivation during slow-wave sleep results in the opposite effect and stabilizes the memory.[5] This raises the interesting possibility that sleep disturbance prior to trauma exposure may result in impaired stabilization of memories following trauma, when successful learning that the threat has passed during waking states may not be consolidated during sleep. Clearly this is not the only possible explanation, however; most models of trauma response implicate resource capacity as an important factor to addressing the consequences of a traumatic event.[6] Sleep deprivation can contribute to depletion of emotional, cognitive, and physical resources, which can compromise one's capacity to manage the demands of the posttraumatic environment.

From an applied perspective, this finding has direct consequences for many populations who are regularly deprived of adequate sleep and are also often exposed to traumatic events. Military personnel, emergency responders, and those involved in sustained efforts following disasters are just some of those who will often be sleep deprived at the time of trauma exposure, thereby placing them at greater risk of developing a psychiatric disorder. The possibility of placing these personnel at greater risk of mental health problems highlights the need for specific attention to enhanced sleep management in specific high-risk populations. This can often be difficult because of the sustained nature of military operations or emergency response activities, or even the disruptive nature of shift work in these organizations. Although this pattern cannot always be altered due to the nature of these events, monitoring the ongoing well-being of those who have been exposed to trauma in the context of sleep deprivation may provide a useful strategy.

Richard A. Bryant
School of Psychology
University of New South Wales

References

1. Rauch SL et al. Neurocircuitry models of posttraumatic stress disorder and extinction: human neuroimaging research-past, present, and future. Biological Psychiatry. 2006; 60: 376-382.
2. Bonnet MH et al. Hyperarousal and insomnia. Sleep Med Rev, 1997; 1:97-108.
3. Pace-Schott EF et al. Sleep promotes generalization of extinction of conditioned fear. Sleep, 2009; 32:19-26.
4. Milad MR et al. Fear extinction in rats: Implications for human brain imaging and anxiety disorders. Biological Psychology. 2006; 73:61-71.
5. Diekelmann S et al. Labile or stable: opposing consequences for memory when reactivated during waking and sleep. Nature Neuroscience. In press

6. Hobfoll SE et al. Five essential elements of immediate and mid-term mass trauma intervention: empirical evidence. Psychiatry. 2007; 70(4):283-315.

Sleep hypoventilation due to increased nocturnal oxygen flow in hypercapnic COPD patients.
Samolski D, Tárrega J, Antón A, Mayos M, Martí S, Farrero E, Güell R. *Respirology.* 2010
Feb;15(2):283-8.

*What happens when nocturnal oxygen flow is increased in hypercapnic persons with chronic
obstructive pulmonary disease on long-term oxygen therapy?*

Subjects	Methods	Outcomes
38 subjects with severe COPD and chronic hypercapnic respiratory failure undergoing LTOT • Age: 68.2 ± 5.5 yrs • BMI: 27.7 ± 4.5 • FEV1%: 22.4 ± 6.2 • GOLD stage: IV • AHI: 7.1 ± 6.4 • Baseline PaO_2: 51.8 ± 6.3 mmHg • Baseline $PaCO_2$: 57.2 ± 6.2 mmHg • Baseline pH: 7.37 ± 0.03 • Baseline HCO_3: 30.7 ± 2.9 • Stable clinical and gas exchange status ≥ 1 month Exclusion criteria: • Thoracic cage abnormalities • Neuromuscular disease • Tracheostomy • Severe comorbidities • OSA	Prospective, cross-over, randomized, single-blind, multicenter trial Subjects were randomized to either: • Daytime O_2 flow rate (to achieve SaO_2 > 90% at rest) on 1 night • Daytime O_2 flow rate plus an additional 1 liter on 1 night Assessments • Nocturnal pulse oximetry • ABG at awakening Definition: • Sleep hypoventilation: > 10 mmHg increase in $PaCO_2$ at awakening (7 am ABG) compared to daytime rest while breathing room air value	Use of oxygen flow at daytime rate failed to correct nocturnal SaO_2 in 8% of subjects Addition of 1 liter more O_2 during the night was associated with: • Improved nocturnal SaO_2* • Improved % sleep time with SaO_2 < 90% • Improved PaO_2 at awakening* • Greater next-morning hypercapnia** and acidosis* Prevalence of sleep hypoventilation: • Using O_2 at daytime rate: 15.7% • Using increased nocturnal O_2 rate: 26.3%

ABG: arterial blood gas; AHI: apnea hypopnea index; BMI: body mass index; COPD: chronic
obstructive pulmonary disease; FEV_1%: forced expiratory volumen in 1 second as percentage of
normal rate; GOLD: Global inititative for COPD; HCO_3: arterial bicarbonate; LTOT: long-term
oxygen therapy; O_2: oxygen; OSA: obstructive sleep apnea; $PaCO_2$: partial pressure of carbon
dioxide; PaO_2: partial pressure of oxygen; SaO_2: arterial oxygen saturation; *P < 0.05

Conclusion
Increasing oxygen flow rate at night compared to daytime values increased both nocturnal
oxygen saturation and next-morning hypercapnia and acidosis in persons with severe chronic
obstructive pulmonary disease and chronic hypercapnic respiratory failure.

Commentary

The main result of this study was that nocturnal SpO_2 was not adequately corrected in 8.1% of patients when they received the oxygen at daytime rate. The increase of this flow in 1 liter more corrected this nocturnal desaturation in all patients. However, this favorable phenomenon was associated with an increase in $PaCO_2$ and a decrease in pH at awakening in a considerable number of patients. Consequently, a higher percentage of SH patients was seen during the "1 liter more" night.

Oxygen can generate potentially detrimental effects, particularly hypercapnia due to different mechanisms.[1-7] Moreover, sleep itself generates ventilatory changes.[8] Consequently, the use of oxygen therapy during sleep in vulnerable individuals with COPD and CHRF could worsen hypoxemia and hypercapnia during the night. The long term of hypercapnia and nocturnal respiratory acidosis seems to be clinically detrimental.[9-11] Our results reinforce the need to evaluate and titrate the nocturnal oxygen flow individually, at least in hypercapnic COPD patients. A longer trial is needed to determine the clinical implications and outcomes of SH in these patients. Also, the appearance of SH as a consequence of nocturnal oxygen therapy could identify a subgroup of patients in whom non-invasive ventilation (NIV) could be potentially beneficial. Prospective studies using nocturnal NIV in this kind of severe COPD patients could confirm or refute this hypothesis.

Daniel Samolski
Respiratory Medicine Dept.
Hospital de la Santa Creu i Sant Pau
Barcelona, Spain

Antonio Antón
Respiratory Medicine Dept.
Hospital de la Santa Creu i Sant Pau
Barcelona, Spain

Mercedes Mayos
Respiratory Medicine Dept.
Hospital de la Santa Creu i Sant Pau
Barcelona, Spain

María Rosa Güell
Respiratory Medicine Dept.
Hospital de la Santa Creu i Sant Pau
Barcelona, Spain

References

1. Standards for the diagnosis and care of patients with COPD. ATS Statement. Am J Respir Crit Care Med. 1995; 152:S77-121.
2. Celli B et al. Standards for the diagnosis and treatment of patients with COPD. ATS/ERS Task Force (Accessed 2004). Available from URL: http://www.copd-ats-ers.org.

3. Robinson T et al. The role of hypoventilation and ventilation-perfusion redistribution in oxygen induced hypercapnia during acute exacerbation of COPD. Am J Respir Crit Care Med. 2000; 161:1524-9.

4. Aubier M et al. Effects of the administration of O2 on ventilation and blood gases in patients with COPD during acute respiratory failure. Am Rev Respir Dis. 1980; 122:747-53.

5. Dunn W et al. Oxygen induced hypercarbia in obstructive pulmonary disease. Am Rev Respir Dis. 1991; 144:526-30.

6. Sassoon CS et al. Hyperoxic indiced hypercapnia in stable COPD. Am Rev Respir Dis. 1987; 135:907-11.

7. Haldane JS et al. The respiratory response to anoxaemia. J Physiol (Lond.). 1919;.52:420-32.

8. Weitzenblum E et al. Sleep and COPD. Sleep Med Rev. 2004;.8:281-94.

9. Fleetham J et al. Sleep, arousals and oxygen desaturation in COPD. The effect of oxygen therapy. Am Rev Respir Dis. 1982; 126:429-33.

10. Jonville S et al. Contribution of respiratory acidosis to diaphragmatic fatigue at exercise. Eur Respir J. 2002; 19:1079-86.

11. Kiely DG et al. Effects of hypercapnia on hemodynamic, inotropic and electrophysiologic indices in humans. Chest. 1996; 109:1215-21.

19. Ohayon MM. Epidemiology of insomnia: what we know and what we still need to learn. Sleep Med Rev. 2002; 6(2):97-111.

20. Ringdahl EN et al. Treatment of primary insomnia. J Am Board Fam Pract. 2004; 17(3):212-9.

21. Bierman EJ et al. The effect of chronic benzodiazepine use on cognitive functioning in older persons: good, bad or indifferent? Int J Geriatr Psychiatry. 2007; 22(12):1194-200.

22. Kripke DF et al. Mortality hazard associated with prescription hypnotics. Biol Psychiatry. 1998; 43(9):687-93.

23. Erman M et al. Zolpidem extended-release 12.5 mg associated with improvements in work performance in a 6-month randomized, placebo-controlled trial. Sleep. 2008; 31(10):1371-8.

24. Krystal AD et al. Long-term efficacy and safety of zolpidem extended-release 12.5 mg, administered 3 to 7 nights per week for 24 weeks, in patients with chronic primary insomnia: a 6-month, randomized, double-blind, placebo-controlled, parallel-group, multicenter study. Sleep. 2008; 31(1):79-90.

25. Neubauer DN. Current and new thinking in the management of comorbid insomnia. Am J Manag Care. 2009; 15 Suppl:S24-32.

26. Morin CM et al. Nonpharmacological interventions for insomnia: a meta-analysis of treatment efficacy. Am J Psychiatry. 1994; 151(8):1172-80.

27. Passos GS et al. Nonpharmacologic treatment of chronic insomnia. Rev Bras Psiquiatr. 2007; 29(3):279-82.

28. Driver HS et al. Exercise and sleep. Sleep Med Rev. 2000; 4(4):387-402.

29. Youngstedt SD. Effects of exercise on sleep. Clin Sports Med. 2005; 24(2):355-65, xi.

30. Youngstedt SD et al. The effects of acute exercise on sleep: a quantitative synthesis. Sleep. 1997; 20(3):203-14.

31. De Mello MT et al. Levantamento Epidemiológico da prática de atividade física na cidade de São Paulo. Rev Bras Med Esporte. 2000; 6:119-24.

32. Morgan K. Daytime activity and risk factors for late-life insomnia. J Sleep Res. 2003; 12(3):231-8.

33. Guilleminault C et al. Nondrug treatment trials in psychophysiologic insomnia. Arch Intern Med. 1995; 155(8):838-44.

34. Reid KJ et al. Aerobic exercise improves self-reported sleep and quality of life in older adults with insomnia. Sleep Med. 2010; 11(9):934-40.

35. King AC et al. Moderate-intensity exercise and self-rated quality of sleep in older adults. A randomized controlled trial. JAMA. 1997; 277(1):32-7.

36. King AC et al. Effects of moderate-intensity exercise on polysomnographic and subjective sleep quality in older adults with mild to moderate sleep complaints. J Gerontol A Biol Sci Med Sci. 2008; 63(9):997-1004.

The effect of pregabalin on pain-related sleep interference in diabetic peripheral neuropathy or postherpetic neuralgia: a review of nine clinical trials. Roth T, van Seventer R, Murphy TK. *Curr Med Res Opin. 2010; 26(10):2411-9.*

Is sleep improved when pregabalin is used in persons with chronic neuropathic pain?

Subjects	Methods	Outcomes
9 randomized double-blind, placebo-controlled clinical trials of pregabalin use in subjects (n = 2399) with painful diabetic peripheral neuropathy and postherpetic neuralgia Subjects were given either pregabalin (75-600 mg per day) or placebo 2-3 times daily	Search using MEDLINE and ISI Web of Knowledge databases through March 2009	No study reported objective measures of sleep Pregabalin was associated with: • Decrease in pain • Improvement in pain-related sleep disturbance

Conclusion
Use of pregabalin in persons with chronic neuropathic pain disorders improved measures of pain and subjective sleep quality.

Commentary
This paper presents the results of a literature search on randomized double blind placebo controlled trials evaluating the effects of pregabalin sleep as well as pain in patients with neuropathic pain. There were 9 such studies evaluating a total of 2,399 patients. The results of these studies are consistent in showing that pregabalin, relative to placebo, was associated with significant improvements in both pain severity and degree of sleep disturbance. These results raise the question as to whether the effects on sleep and the effects on pain are independent parallel effects or alternatively does one effect mediate the other; if the later is true, which effect is primary and which is secondary?

The literature demonstrates an elevated prevalence of sleep disturbances in a variety of acute and chronic pain conditions.[1,2,3] This increased prevalence of sleep disturbances has been demonstrated in both population based samples as well as samples of different pain conditions. Similarly sleep laboratory (i.e. polysomnographic) studies have evaluated, acute pain conditions, neuropathic pain, rheumatologic, headache, and diffuse chronic pain. In these pain populations there have been a variety of sleep findings. Most commonly pain patients show decreased sleep efficiency evidenced by decreased Total Sleep Time, increased Wake Time after Sleep Onset, increased Sleep Latency and increased sleep fragmentation.[4] In addition this sleep fragmentation results in alterations in sleep stage distribution.

Overall pain patients show an increase in "lighter" sleep stage 1 and a parallel decrease in "deeper sleep stages" (i.e. NREM stage 3-4 and REM sleep).[5] In addition to the sleep stage changes there are changes in the frequency of EEG activity. The most notable of these is the presence of alphas delta sleep. Alpha delta refers to the presence of 8-12 cps synchronous activity during NREM. This is felt to be significant as alpha activity is typically seen in individuals when they awake and lying quietly. Thus people have hypothesized that this anomalous EEG activity is associated with patient's reports of poor quality or non-restorative sleep. While alpha delta sleep is most often mentioned in the context of fibromyalgia[6] it is not specific to fibromyalgia patients. It was first reported to be present in patients with depression[7], but has also been reported in other pain conditions, insomniacs and even in normals. Finally, pain patients have a higher prevalence of primary sleep disorders including sleep apnea, Restless Legs Syndrome and Periodic Limb Movement Disorder.[8] However the mechanism for this increased risk for primary sleep disorders is difficult to determine as it is not specific to any pain condition but rather is seen in a variety of pain conditions.

Importantly there is an increasing amount of data on the effect of direct manipulations of sleep on pain sensitivity. Overall sleep deprivation manipulation, including partial sleep deprivation, selective (REM and Stage 3-4) and sleep fragmentation, have all been associated with increased pain reports and decreased pain thresholds.[9] In contrast sleep extension and sleep consolidation have resulted in decreased pain reports and increased pain thresholds.

For example, Roehrs and colleagues demonstrated that both 4 hours of sleep deprivation as well as REM deprivation, without any loss of sleep, increase subjects' sensitivity to thermal pain.[10] In contrast, they showed that in individuals who are sleepy, probably because they have chronic mild sleep restriction as they have no sleep disorder or drug use, show a decrease in pain sensitivity with a 2 hour extension of time in bed for 4 days.[11] This same group recently showed that the use of CPAP in sleep apnea patients reduces sensitivity to thermal pain, and that the removal of CPAP reverts the patients' pain sensitivity to pre CPAP levels.[12]

Turning to pharmacological interventions, the use of gabapentin decreased the frequency of opioid PCA administrations in post operative patients.[13] However, the question remains as to whether this was the result of the analgesic properties of gabapentin or an indirect effect of the sleep promoting effects of gabapentin. In a recent study, zolpidem 10 mg was also able to reduce opioid self administration in post operatively.[14] The importance of this study is that zolpidem has sleep promoting properties but no analgesic properties. In rheumatoid arthritis patients also reporting sleep difficulties, hypnotics (i.e. triazolam and zolpidem) not only improve sleep in these patients but also improved pain related symptoms.[15,16] Taken as a body of work these studies clearly demonstrate that improving sleep by either behavioral or pharmacological interventions positively impacts the management of pain.

Sleep and the experience of pain are two critically important functions necessary for survival. The bidirectional relation between them has profound clinical implications. Many of the circumstances associated with pain such as trauma, hospitalization, and surgical procedures are also associated with sleep disturbances. In addition many analgesics (e.g. opioids) are known to disturb sleep. Clearly these facts highlight the opportunity to better manage pain by addressing sleep habits, sleep disturbances and sleep disorders.

Thomas Roth
Sleep Disorders Center
Henry Ford Hospital

References

1. Pilowsky I et al. Sleep disturbances in clinic patients. Pain. 1985; 23:27-33.
2. Gislason T et al. Somatic diseases and sleep complaints. An epidemiological study of 3201 Swedish men. Acta Med Scand. 1987; 221:475-481.
3. Moffitt PF et al. Sleep difficulties, pain and other correlates. J Int Med. 1991; 230:245-249.
4. Shapiro CM et al. Sleep problems in patients with medical illness Br Med J. 1993; 306:1532-1535.
5. Moldofsky H et al. Musculoskeletal symptoms and non-REM sleep disturbance in patients with "fibrositis syndrome:: and healthy subjects. Psychosomat Med. 1975; 37:341-351.
6. Moldofsky H et al. The relationship of alpha delta EEG frequencies to pain and mood in "fibrositis" patients with chlorpromazine and L-tryptophan. Electroencephal Clin Neurophysiol. 1980; 50:71-80.
7. Hauri P et al. Alpha-delta sleep. Electroencephal Clin Neurophysiol. 1973; 34:233-237.
8. Buchwald DS et al. Sleep disorders in patients with chronic fatigue. Clin Infect Dis. 1994; 18:S568-S572.
9. Kundermann B et al. Sleep deprivation affects thermal pain thresholds but not somatosensory thresholds in healthy volunteers. Psychosom Med. 2004; 66:932-937.
10. Roehrs T et al. Sleep loss and REM sleep loss are hyperalgesic. Sleep. 2006; 29:145-151.
11. Harris E et al. A four-night sleep extension normalizes MSLT in sleepy normals. Sleep. 2009; A410-A411.
12. Khalid I et al. CPAP in severe obstructive sleep apnea reduces pain sensitivity. Sleep. 2010; 33:A170-171.
13. Jesper D et al. A randomzied study of the effects of single-dose gabapetin versus placebo on postoperative pain and morphine consumption after mastectomy. Anesthesiology. 2002; 97:560-564.
14. Tashjian RZ et al. Zolpidem reduces postoperative pain, fatigue and narcotic consumption following knee arthroscopy: a prospective randomized placeb-controlled double-blinded study. J Knee Surg. 2006; 19(2):105-11.
15. Roth T et al. The Effect of Eszopiclone in Patients with Insomnia and Coexisting Rheumatoid Arthritis: A Pilot Study. Prim Care Companion J Clin Psychiatr. 2009; 11(6):292-301.
16. Walsh JK et al. Effects of triazoloam on sleep, daytime sleepiness and morning stiffness in patients with rheumatoid arthritis. J Rheumatol. 1996: 23(2):245-52.

Pediatric Sleep Medicine

Caffeine for Apnea of Prematurity trial: benefits may vary in subgroups. Davis PG, Schmidt B, Roberts RS, Doyle LW, Asztalos E, Haslam R, Sinha S, Tin W; Caffeine for Apnea of Prematurity Trial Group. *J Pediatr. 2010 Mar;156(3):382-7.*

What are the benefits of caffeine therapy for apnea of prematurity?

Subjects	Methods	Outcomes
2006 subjects of the Caffeine for Apnea of Prematurity (CAP) trial	Post-hoc subgroup analyses Assessments: • Indication for drug • PPV at randomization • Timing of initiation of drug (early [≤ 3 days] or late [>3 days])	Starting caffeine early was associated with larger reductions of respiratory support days Effect of caffeine on death or disability based on PPV at randomization* [OR (95% CI)]: • No support: 1.32 (0.81-2.14) • Noninvasive support: 0.73 (0.52-1.03) • ETT: 0.73 (0.57-0.94)

CI: confidence interval; ETT: endotracheal tube; NIV: noninvasive ventilation; OR: odds ratio; PPV: positive pressure ventilation; *P = .03

Conclusion
Earlier administration of caffeine reduced days of respiratory support for apnea of prematurity and improved death or disability in infants receiving positive pressure ventilation.

Commentary
Apnea of prematurity is defined as prolonged central respiratory pauses of 20 seconds or more in duration (or shorter-duration events that include obstructive or mixed respiratory patterns and are associated with a significant physiologic compromise, including decrease in heart rate, hypoxemia, clinical symptoms , or need for nursing intervention) recorded in an infant younger than 37 weeks post conceptional age.[1] It occurs in most infants, to some extent, born at less than 33 weeks.

Respiratory pauses are considered significant when they are associated with hypoxemia or bradycardia. The concerning effect is on the central nervous system, where hypoxia and cerebral hemodynamics can cause neurodevelopmental injury that may or may not be reversible. Its presence is thought due to an "immaturity" of the respiratory control center of the brain. We do not know exactly why the immature infant has such a high propensity for apnea. It may simply resemble the fetal breathing pattern, where breathing can be irregular because its main function is to ensure lung growth.[2] Fetal breathing is diminished if oxygen supply via the placenta is reduced. This is in contrast to adults, who show a sustained increase in ventilation in the presence of hypoxia. This pattern is counterproductive ex utero, but is nevertheless a consistent finding in preterm infants. The switch-over from the fetal to the adult hypoxic ventilatory response occurs at approximately 35 weeks post conceptional age, which correlates well with the clinical course of apnea of prematurity.[3] There is evidence that diaphragmatic fatigue[4] and chemoreceptor resetting[5] also play a role. The closeness between eupneic and apneic threshold responses to CO2 level also destabilizes respiration in neonates.[6] These unique vulnerabilities predispose the neonate to the development of apnea. Precipitating factors for worsening apnea in preterm infants include thermal instability, gastroesophageal reflux, intracranial pathology, drugs, anesthesia, metabolic disturbances, impaired oxygenation and infection.

For most children, long-term outcomes for uncomplicated apnea of prematurity are excellent. However, the prognosis for infants with persistent recurrent apnea spells requiring frequent resuscitation is more guarded and depends on the cause of the apnea and associated comorbidities.[1] During postnatal maturation, as the preterm infant approaches 40 weeks post conceptional age, breathing stability normalizes and apnea of prematurity typically resolves. Even preterm infants with extremely severe apnea and bradycardia usually cease having such events by 43 weeks postconceptional age.[7]

The methylxanthines aminophylline, theophylline and caffeine have been used for decades to treat apnea of prematurity.[8] However, a thorough evaluation of risks and benefits of this medication has been performed only recently. Concerns about impaired growth, lack of neuroprotection during acute hypoxic-ischemic episodes and abnormal behavior has prompted the recent studies.[9] Caffeine citrate was found to be safe and resulted in unexpected benefits. In treated infants, compared with controls, a decreased incidence apneic episodes, rates of bronchopulmonary dysplasia[10] and the need for mechanical ventilation was discovered.[11] It has also been shown to improve the rate of survival without neurodevelopmental disability at 18 to 21 months in infants with very low birth weight. In particular, the incidences of cerebral palsy and cognitive delay were reduced. The rates of death, deafness, and blindness did not differ significantly in the group treated with caffeine as compared with the placebo group. Moreover, growth, as indexed by height, weight, and head circumference, also was not affected by caffeine treatment.[12] A post hoc analysis of a recent report suggests that as much as 55% of the caffeine effect can be explained by reduced needs for respiratory support, supplemental oxygen, postnatal steroids, and surgery to close a patent ductus arteriosus. Still, almost half of the effect of caffeine is unexplained, and other physiological consequences of caffeine administration should be considered as possible contributors to the beneficial effects of caffeine in premature infants.[10]

The mechanisms of action for the methylxanthines are varied; they include primarily stimulation of the respiratory center, adenosine-receptor blockade, increased minute ventilation[13], action as a diuretic and improved function of the respiratory muscles. The persistence of apnea in some infants treated with caffeine also reflects the complex causation of apnea of prematurity and underscores the need to attend to other modifiable causes of apnea, such as airway obstruction and intrinsic lung disease associated with atelectasis.[13]

We know who (infants with birth weights of 500 to 1250 g), when (within 10 days after birth), how (loading dose of 20 mg/kg of caffeine citrate followed by daily maintenance doses of 5 mg/kg, increased to 10 mg/kg if apneas persisted), and how long (until apneas resolve, or to median gestational age of 35 weeks) to treat, and that monitoring of caffeine levels is unnecessary.[14] This report adds that infants receiving respiratory support derived the greatest long-term neurological benefit from caffeine. Earlier discontinuation of any positive airway pressure explained 49% of the beneficial long-term drug effect. This, along with the short-term outcomes from the same trial, lays concerns about adverse effects of caffeine to rest. Infants treated with caffeine were extubated, weaned from continuous positive air pressure, and weaned from supplemental oxygen sooner, and fewer required oxygen at 36 weeks gestation. Because of these data, we now know that our time-honored reliance on methylxanthines for management of apnea of prematurity was not misguided, and in fact appears to be beneficial.[14]

Casey Burg
Division of Sleep Medicine
National Jewish Health

References

1. American Academy of Sleep Medicine. The international classification of sleep disorders : diagnostic and coding manual. 2nd ed. Westchester, Ill.: American Academy of Sleep Medicine, 2005.
2. Poets CF. Apnea of prematurity: What can observational studies tell us about pathophysiology? Sleep Med. 2010; 11(7):701-7.
3. Martin RJ et al. Persistence of the biphasic ventilatory response to hypoxia in preterm infants. J Pediatr. 1998; 132(6):960-4.
4. Heldt GP. Development of stability of the respiratory system in preterm infants. J Appl Physiol. 1988; 65(1):441-4.
5. Fenner A et al. Periodic breathing in premature and neonatal babies: incidence, breathing pattern, respiratory gas tensions, response to changes in the composition of ambient air. Pediatr Res. 1973; 7(4):174-83.
6. Khan A et al. Measurement of the CO2 apneic threshold in newborn infants: possible relevance for periodic breathing and apnea. J Appl Physiol. 2005; 98(4):1171-6.
7. Ramanathan R et al. Cardiorespiratory events recorded on home monitors: Comparison of healthy infants with those at increased risk for SIDS. JAMA. 2001; 285(17):2199-207.
8. Kuzemko JA et al. Apnoeic attacks in the newborn treated with aminophylline. Arch Dis Child. 1973; 48(5):404-6.
9. Millar D et al. Controversies surrounding xanthine therapy. Semin Neonatol. 2004; 9(3):239-44.
10. Schmidt B et al. Caffeine therapy for apnea of prematurity. N Engl J Med. 2006; 354(20):2112-21.
11. Henderson-Smart DJ et al. Methylxanthine treatment for apnoea in preterm infants. Cochrane Database Syst Rev. 2010; 12:CD000140.
12. Schmidt B et al. Long-term effects of caffeine therapy for apnea of prematurity. N Engl J Med. 2007; 357(19):1893-902.
13. Yaffe SJ et al. Neonatal and pediatric pharmacology : therapeutic principles in practice. 4th ed. Philadelphia: Wolters Kluwer/Lippincott Williams & Wilkins Health, 2010.

14. Benitz WE. Use of caffeine for apnea of prematurity also has long-term neurodevelopmental benefits. J Pediatr. 2008; 152(5):740-1.

High exercise levels are related to favorable sleep patterns and psychological functioning in adolescents: a comparison of athletes and controls. Brand S, Gerber M, Beck J, Hatzinger M, Pühse U, Holsboer-Trachsler E. *J Adolesc Health. 2010 Feb;46(2):133-41.*

Does vigorous exercise affect sleep and psychological functioning?

Subjects	Methods	Outcomes
434 adolescent subjects • Athletes: n = 258 1. Exercise hrs weekly: 17.69 hrs • Controls: n = 176 1. Exercise hrs weekly: 4.69 hrs • Age (mean): 17.2 yrs • Gender: 36% males	Assessments: • Sleep log for 7 days • Questionnaires on exercise • Mood • Daytime tiredness • Daytime concentration • Psychological functioning (depression, state-trait-anxiety, everyday stress and sleep related personality traits)	Compared with controls, athletes were associated with: • Better sleep quality • Shorter SOL • Fewer WASO • Less tiredness • Greater daytime concentration • Fewer anxiety and depressive symptoms • More favorable personality traits Women had fewer variations in sleep than men

SOL: sleep onset latency; WASO: wakings after sleep onset

Conclusion
Chronic vigorous exercise improved sleep quality and led to better daytime functioning among adolescents.

Commentary
For adolescents, there is a bi-directional relationship between acute[1] and chronic[2] sleep disturbances and poor physical and psychological functioning. To cope with poor sleep, clinical experience indicates a growing reliance on substances, either to induce sleep (alcohol, cannabis) or to reduce daytime sleepiness (caffeine, energy drinks). By contrast, lay people, physicians and experts[3] alike regard exercise as an effective and inexpensive means of preventing and reducing sleep problems. However, the scientific basis for this assumption is weak, and with respect to adolescence, there are almost no relevant findings.

To test the hypotheses that during adolescence regular vigorous exercising is positively associated with favourable psychological functioning and favourable sleep, we assessed 434 adolescents (mean age:.17.2). Of these, 258 were high exercisers recruited from elite sports classes, reporting up to 18h/week of intense and strenuous physical activity. Participants completed self-rating questionnaires related to sleep and psychological functioning. Findings showed that compared to controls, high exercisers reported more favourable results such as an increased sleep quality, increased mood, and increased concentration and decreased tiredness during the day, as well as favourable personality traits such as increased assertiveness, a positive attitude towards life, and an increased self-confidence. Introducing gender as a further factor, the pattern of results revealed that above all male low exercisers were at increased risk to report poor sleep, increased stress, and low self-confidence.

To conclude, the pattern of results suggests that regular vigorous exercising is positively related to favourable psychological functioning and increased sleep quality. Most importantly, in adolescents, this pattern of results does not seem to be limited to vigorous exercising; rather, already moderate regular exercising (5-8h/weekly)[4] leads to very similar results. In this view, further efforts should be made to promote regular exercising and to activate male low exercisers, who seem to be at increased risk for poor sleep and poor psychological functioning.

Serge Brand
Sleep and Depression Research Unit
Psychiatric Hospital of the University of Basel

References
1. Kaneita Y et al. Association between mental health status and sleep status among adolescents in Japan. A nationwide cross-sectional survey. J Clin Psychiatry. 2007; 68:1426–35.
2. Roberts RE et al. Chronic insomnia and its negative consequences for health and functioning of adolescents: A 12-month prospective study. J Adolesc Health. 2008; 42:294–302.
3. American Academy of Sleep Medicine, ed. Sleep hygiene. Chicago, American Academy of Sleep Medicine, 2004.
4. Brand S et al. Exercising, sleep-EEG patterns, and psychological functioning are related among adolescents. World J Biol Psychiatry. 2010 Mar;11(2):129-40.

Sleep quality and motor vehicle crashes in adolescents. Pizza F, Contardi S, Antognini AB, Zagoraiou M, Borrotti M, Mostacci B, Mondini S, Cirignotta F. *J Clin Sleep Med. 2010 Feb 15;6(1):41-5.*

Does the presence of sleep-related complaints increase the risk of car crashes among adolescents?

Subjects	Methods	Outcomes
339 adolescent subjects who had driver's licenses	Assessments: • Self-administered questionnaires 1. Driving habits 2. Lifestyle habits 3. Sleep quality 4. Sleepiness 5. Car crashes	Prevalence: • Bad sleep: 19% • Daytime sleepiness: 64% • Sleepiness while driving: 40% • At least 1 car crash: 24% (76% of which were males) • Sleepiness considered as main cause of car crash: 15% Compared to those without car crashes, subjects who had ≥ 1 crash had: • More frequent driving at night* • More frequent driving while sleepy** • More frequent bad sleep*** • More frequent use of stimulants[#] • More frequent use of tobacco[##] • More frequent use of drugs[###] Factors predicting risk of car crashes: • Male gender[^] • Tobacco use[^^] • Sleepiness while driving[^^^] • Bad sleep[+]

MVA: motor vehicle accident; OR: odds ratio; *25% vs. 9%; **56% vs. 35%; ***29% vs. 16%; #32% vs. 19%; ##54% vs. 27%; ###21% vs. 7%; ^P < 0.0001; OR = 3.3; ^^P < 0.0001; OR = 3.2; ^P = 0.010; OR = 2.1; +P = 0.047; OR = 1.9

Conclusion
Sleep-related complaints increased the likelihood of car crashes among adolescents.

Commentary
Motor vehicle crashes are one of the leading causes of death in developed countries, notably the first one among young people under the age of 30 years old. In the last 15 years many researchers disclosed the role of sleepiness in the determination of car crashes: up to 20% of accidents are now considered "sleep-related" (SRA), being sleepiness either a primary cause or an important contributing factor[1,2] that is able to enhance accidents' consequences such as serious injuries and fatalities.[3] In this context, young people, especially males, display an increased SRA risk profile during the night[1,4,5], that seems to progressively shift across lifetime to early afternoon hours[4]

Puberty and adolescence are life periods with important changes in sleep physiology and habits: a progressive reduction of slow wave sleep together with an increase of daytime sleep propensity occur across puberty[6], whereas nocturnal sleep is curtailed during adolescence for a delay in bed time due to a shift towards an evening circadian preference coupled with the forced early morning awakening for school.[7] These factors lead to a condition of chronic sleep deprivation associated with increased daytime sleep propensity. Additionally, during adolescence several sleep disturbances may appear, further enhancing the intrinsic trend towards daytime sleepiness.

In our study, we explored sleep and driving habits in a population of 339 adolescents with driver's license in order to investigate the relationships between nocturnal sleep quality and car accidents risk. As expected, we confirmed the frequent occurrence of sleep complaints such as daytime sleepiness (up to 64%), chronic sleep deprivation, evening circadian preference, nocturnal bad sleep, and symptoms suggesting specific sleep disorders, with the additional association between daytime sleepiness and poor nocturnal sleep. Concerning driving habits, 135 students (40%) experienced sleepiness at wheel, with only 19% of them stopping the car, thus adopting adequate countermeasures to drowsy driving. Eighty students (24%) already crashed at least once: they were mainly males (Odd Ratio, OR: 3.3), smokers (OR: 3.2), feeling sleepiness at wheel (OR: 2.1), and complaining of bad sleep (OR: 1.9).

Our study is in line with the current knowledge concerning SRA risk, further confirmed in a recent large epidemiological French survey, showing that the 18-30 age category and the experience of sleepiness at wheel were strong predictors of accident risk.[8] Moreover, our results strongly support the need to implement interventional strategies targeting young drivers such as graduated driving licensing[9], or a delay of school start times in order to permit a longer nocturnal sleep that proved efficacy in reducing the number of car crashes.[10] Finally, an interesting association between adequate sleep and health-related behaviors further suggests that unhealthy life habits may be influenced by short sleep duration as well as by evening circadian preference.[11,12] Therefore, the development of educational programs not only on the risks associated with driving[13], but also on the sleep related issues[14], is highly warranted within school programs.

Fabio Pizza
Department of Neurological Sciences
University of Bologna

References

1. Horne JA et al. Sleep related vehicle accidents. BMJ. 1995; 310(6979):565-7.
2. Garbarino S et al. The contributing role of sleepiness in highway vehicle accidents. Sleep. 2001; 24(2):203-6.
3. Philip P et al. Fatigue, alcohol, and serious road crashes in France: factorial study of national data. BMJ. 2001; 322(7290):829-30.
4. Pack AI et al. Characteristics of crashes attributed to the driver having fallen asleep. Accid Anal Prev. 1995; 27(6):769-75.
5. Akerstedt T et al. Age, gender and early morning highway accidents. J Sleep Res. 2001; 10(2):105-10.
6. Carskadon MA et al. Pubertal changes in daytime sleepiness. Sleep. 1980; 2(4):453-60.
7. Carskadon MA et al. Regulation of sleepiness in adolescents: update, insights, and speculation. Sleep. 2002; 25(6):606-14.
8. Sagaspe P et al. Sleepiness, near-misses and driving accidents among a representative population of French drivers. J Sleep Res. 2010; 19(4):578-84.
9. Hartling L et al. Graduated driver licensing for reducing motor vehicle crashes among young drivers. Cochrane Database Syst Rev. 2004;(2):CD003300.
10. Danner F et al. Adolescent sleep, school start times, and teen motor vehicle crashes. J Clin Sleep Med. 2008; 4(6):533-5.
11. Chen MY et al. Adequate sleep among adolescents is positively associated with health status and health-related behaviors. BMC Public Health. 2006; 6:59.
12. Giannotti F et al. Circadian preference, sleep and daytime behaviour in adolescence. J Sleep Res. 2002; 11(3):191-9.
13. Senserrick T et al. Young driver education programs that build resilience have potential to reduce road crashes. Pediatrics. 2009; 124(5):1287-92.
14. Cortesi F et al. Knowledge of sleep in Italian high school students: pilot-test of a school-based sleep educational program. J Adolesc Health. 2004; 34(4):344-51.

The sleep of children with attention deficit hyperactivity disorder on and off methylphenidate: a matched case-control study. Galland BC, Tripp EG, Taylor BJ. *J Sleep Res. 2010 Jun;19(2):366-73.*

Does methylphenidate given for attention deficit hyperactivity disorder affect sleep architecture?

Subjects	Methods	Outcomes
27 children with ADHD • Age: 6-12 yrs 27 healthy controls	Subjects with ADHD were randomized to on- and 48-hr off methylphenidate protocol No medications were given to controls Assessments: • 2 PSGs	Methylphenidate administration in subjects with ADHD was associated with: • More prolonged SOL by an average of 29 min* • Reduced SE by 6.5%** • Shortened sleep by 1.2 hrs*** • Decreased REM sleep by 2.4% • No difference in N1, N2 and N3 sleep PSG parameters were comparable for ADHD subjects off-medication and controls

ADHD: attention deficit hyperactivity disorder; CI: confidence interval; N1: sleep stage 1; N2: sleep stage 2; PSG: polysomnography; REM: rapid eye movement; SE: sleep efficiency; SOL: sleep onset latency; SWS: slow wave sleep; *CI 11.6, 46.7; **CI 2.6, 10.3; ***CI 0.65, 1.9

Conclusion

Children given methylphenidate for attention deficit hyperactivity disorder had prolonged sleep onset latency, reduced sleep efficiency, and shortened sleep.

Commentary

Sleep disruption is a common finding in children diagnosed with Attention Deficit Hyperactivity Disorder (ADHD), the cause of which is unknown but may be related to: 1) sleep related breathing disorders or periodic limb movements (these have a higher prevalence in children diagnosed with ADHD); 2) the stimulant drug regime used in the management of the disorder, and/or; 3) uniquely related to the disorder itself. There is a behavioral component to sleep, and parents report difficulties getting their child to sleep. In addition, there may be comorbid conditions such as anxiety that can disrupt sleep. The sleep problems are obviously important to manage for the child, but they also have wider implications for family functioning.[1]

Although non-stimulant drugs used for symptom control of ADHD have been shown to reduce sleep side-effects[2], methylphenidate, a central nervous system stimulant, is the most widely prescribed drug to manage ADHD symptoms. Methylphenidate affects children's sleep with adverse consequences reported on both sleep quantity[3] and quality[4], but accuracy around interpretation is thwarted by studies with small sample sizes. Many compare their findings with a control group of different sample size not individually matched for age, even though participants' age ranges cover middle childhood to adolescent years. This creates a confounder for interpreting sleep architecture which shows considerable age-related changes over these years[5] including changes in sleep timing and quantity. The aim of this study was to assess the effects of methylphenidate medication in children diagnosed with ADHD, on sleep duration, timing, and architecture. By studying ADHD children on and off medication and employing a matched case-control study design, we sought to dissociate sleep problems that were ADHD-related from those that were drug-related.

Children aged 6 to 12 years meeting diagnostic criteria for DSM-IV ADHD were studied (n=27); median age = 10 y 4 mo and M/F = 21/6. Controls were recruited matching for age (± 3 months) and gender. Two nights of standard polysomnographic (PSG) recordings were conducted. ADHD children were randomly allocated to an on- or 48 h off-methylphenidate protocol for first or second recordings. Control children's recordings were matched for night, but no medication was used. Mixed modelling was employed in the analyses so that the full dataset was used to determine medication effects.

We found methylphenidate prolonged sleep onset by an average of 29 minutes (CI; 11.6, 46.7), reduced sleep efficiency by 6.5% (CI; 2.6, 10.3) and shortened sleep by 1.2 h (CI; 0.65, 1.9). Arousal indices were preserved. Relative amounts of stage 1, 2, and SWS were unchanged by medication. REM sleep was reduced (-2.4%) on the medication night, an effect that became non-significant when control data were incorporated in the analyses. PSG data from ADHD children off-medication were similar to control data. Usual practice for ADHD children at home was to go to bed 20 minutes earlier than controls, but to go to sleep significantly later, extending the "bedtime to sleep" latency to 70 minutes compared to 40 minutes in controls. We surmise this may reflect coping strategies adopted by the parent/s who consistently report bedtime resistance as a behavioral feature of ADHD.

Results from this PSG study suggest that methylphenidate reduces sleep quantity but not sleep quality (architecture) in children diagnosed with ADHD. Effects on sleep quantity could have an additional negative impact on the daytime symptoms the drug is targeted to control. Our study was not without its limitations; one of the most important being that 48 hours abstaining from methylphenidate was more than adequate for drug elimination, but drug use may incur a sleep debt resulting in rebound sleep extending into the off-medication night recording. In light of this we suggest any study intending to replicate our work take this into consideration. The ability to capture children's sleep before and after they start on a course of stimulant medication would be desirable, as would being able to study the sleep of control children on methylphenidate, but the latter would be difficult to justify for research purposes only.

Our findings emphasize the need to apply research effort into counteracting sleep side effects of medication used to control ADHD symptoms. Improving sleep by improving sleep hygiene may be worthy of pursuing, as would regular drug holidays to reduce sleep side effects. Research efforts should also be directed at optimal dosing regimens and formulations that achieve consistent duration of effects throughout the day while minimizing sleep problems. Medication for sleep problems in children with ADHD is used, with some effectiveness, but evaluation has been limited to small studies.[6-9] Clonidine, an alpha-agonist, is a common medication for sleep problems in children with ADHD, but the safety of use in children is of concern.[10] It is encouraging to note that the first known large randomized controlled trial of a behavioral intervention aiming to treat sleep problems in children with ADHD has been registered.[11]

Barbara C Galland
Department of Women's & Children's Health
University of Otago

References

1. Sung V et al. Sleep problems in children with attention-deficit/hyperactivity disorder: prevalence and the effect on the child and family. Arch Pediatr Adolesc Med. 2008; 162:336-342.

2. Owens JA. Sleep disorders and attention-deficit / hyperactivity disorder. Curr Psychiatry Rev. 2008; 10:439–444.

3. Corkum P et al. Acute impact of immediate release methylphenidate administered three times a day on sleep in children with attention-deficit/hyperactivity disorder. J Pediatr Psychol. 2008; 33:368-379.

4. Greenhill L et al. Sleep architecture and REM sleep measures in prepubertal children with attention deficit disorder with hyperactivity. Sleep. 1983; 6:91-101.

5. Sheldon SH et al. Principles and Practice of Pediatric Sleep Medicine. Elsevier Inc., Philadelphia, 2005.

6. Prince JB et al. Clonidine for sleep disturbances associated with attention-deficit hyperactivity disorder: a systematic chart review of 62 cases. J Am Acad Child Adolesc Psychiatry. 1996; 35:599-605.

7. Tjon Pian GCV et al. Melatonin for treatment of sleeping disorders in children with attention deficit/hyperactivity disorder: a preliminary open label study. Eur J Pediatr. 2003; 162:554-555.

8. Weiss MD et al. Sleep hygiene and melatonin treatment for children and adolescents with ADHD and initial insomnia. J Am Acad Child Adolesc Psychiatry. 2006; 45:512-519.

9. Van der Heijden KB et al. Effect of melatonin on sleep, behavior, and cognition in ADHD and chronic sleep-onset insomnia. Am Acad Child Adolesc Psychiatry. 2007; 46:233-241.

10. Sinha Y et al. Clonidine poisoning in children: A recent experience. J Paediatr Child Health. 2004; 40:678-680.

11. Sciberras E et al. Study protocol: the Sleeping Sound with Attention-Deficit/Hyperactivity Disorder Project. BMC Pediatrics. 2010; 10:101.

Aging

Ghrelin increases slow wave sleep and stage 2 sleep and decreases stage 1 sleep and REM sleep in elderly men but does not affect sleep in elderly women. Kluge M, Gazea M, Schüssler P, Genzel L, Dresler M, Kleyer S, Uhr M, Yassouridis A, Steiger A. *Psychoneuroendocrinology. 2010 Feb;35(2):297-304.*

Does ghrelin affect sleep of older adults?

Subjects	Methods	Outcomes
20 elderly subjects • Gender: 50% males • Age: 1. Males: 64.0 ± 2.2 yrs 2. Postmenopausal females: 63.0 ± 2.9 yrs	Single-blind, randomized, cross-over study Subjects were given either (at 2200, 2300, 0000, and 0100 h): • Ghrelin 50 mcg • Placebo Assessments: • Sleep EEG (2300-0700 h) • GH and cortisol secretion (2000-0700 h)	In men, compared to placebo, ghrelin was associated with: • More N2 sleep (221.0 ± 12.2 vs. 183.3 ± 6.1 min) • More N3 sleep (44.3 ± 7.7 vs. 33.4 ± 5.1 min) • More NREM sleep (318.2 ± 11.0 vs. 272.6 ± 12.8 min) • Less N1 sleep (50.9 ± 7.6 vs. 56.9 ± 8.7 min) • Less REM sleep (52.5 ± 5.9 vs. 71.9 ± 9.1 min) Higher delta power and lower alpha and beta power during the 1st half of the night No effects on sleep were noted in women after ghrelin administration Ghrelin increased GH and cortisol in both men and women

EEG: electroencephalography; GH: growth hormone; HPA: hypothalamic-pituitary-adrenal axis; N1: sleep stage 1; N2: sleep stage 2; NREM: non-rapid eye movement; REM: rapid eye movement; SWS: slow wave sleep

Conclusion
Ghrelin increased N2 and N3 sleep, and decreased N1 and REM sleep, in older men but not in older women.

Commentary

Ghrelin, the endogenous ligand of the growth hormone (GH) secretagogue receptor, is primarily known as an orexigenic hormone. However, ghrelin has numerous other endocrine effects.[1] For example, ghrelin very strongly stimulates the activity of the somatotropic axis and -to a somewhat less extent- of the hypothalamic-pituitary-adrenal (HPA) axis, as indicated by increased growth hormone (GH) and cortisol plasma levels.[2] These two endocrine axes are crucially involved in sleep regulation: While GH releasing hormone (GHRH) has been shown to improve sleep in men and to impair sleep in women, corticotrophin releasing hormone (CRH), the hypothalamic releasing hormone of the HPA axis, appears to impair sleep in both men and women.[3,4]

Overall, ghrelin caused an improvement of sleep in elderly men in the present study. Ghrelin administration was associated with a significant increase of stage 2 sleep, SWS, and non-REM sleep and a significant decrease of stage 1 sleep and REM sleep in elderly men. While the effects on stage 2 sleep and REM sleep predominantly occurred during the second half of night, the effect on SWS predominantly occurred during the first half. Consistently, delta power, considering slow waves between 0.5-4 Hz, was significantly higher during the first half of night. In contrast no effects on sleep were observed in elderly women,

The finding that ghrelin improves sleep in men is very consistent. It has been also made in various samples of young men[5,6] and men suffering from major depression.[7] It is also in line with reports of reduced ghrelin plasma levels in men with chronic insomnia.[8]

As in young women[9] ghrelin did not affect sleep in postmenopausal elderly women. Yet in women with major depression, ghrelin affected sleep by decreasing amount of REM sleep and increasing REM latency.[7]

Taken together, this and other studies indicate that ghrelin exerts a sexually dimorphic effect on sleep as this has been also shown for GHRH. However, while both ghrelin and GHRH improve sleep in men, sleep in healthy women is not affected by ghrelin but impaired by GHRH. In addition, the results indicate that ghrelin's effects on sleep are not age-dependent.

Ghrelin had remarkably strong sleep-improving effects in elderly men. At a descriptive level, they were relatively stronger than those seen in a previous study in young men (Kluge et al.2008): Stage 2 sleep was increased by 21% (young men: 10%) and SWS even by 33% (young men: 10%). Also the absolute mean increases of stage 2 sleep and SWS were higher in elderly (SWS: 10.9 min, stage 2 sleep: 37.7 min) than young men (SWS: 9.2 min, stage 2 sleep: 22.4 min).

Findings in rodents are inconsistent. While peripheral administration of ghrelin was associated with an increase of non-REM sleep (NREM)[10] as in humans, a decrease of NREM was found after injection in the central nervous system.[11,12] Of note, in both of the latter studies food intake was significantly stimulated. In fact, it appears likely that increased appetite and food intake impede sleep.[13] Following this concept, the sleep impairing effect after central ghrelin injection is secondary to increased appetite and is not an intrinsic effect of ghrelin. Consistently, ghrelin as given in the present[14] and previous studies of our group[6,9] (4 doses of 50 µg) was not associated with an increased appetite. The finding that ghrelin knockout mice had significantly less NREM than the wild type is another indication that ghrelin increases NREM also in rodents.[15]

While ghrelin affected sleep differently in men and women, cortisol and GH increases and secretion patterns after ghrelin injections were comparable in both sexes.

Michael Kluge
Klinik und Poliklinik für Psychiatrie
Universitätsklinikum Leipzig AöR

References

1. van der Lely AJ et al. Biological, physiological, pathophysiological, and pharmacological aspects of ghrelin. Endocr Rev. 2004; 25:426-457.
2. Takaya K et al. Ghrelin strongly stimulates growth hormone release in humans. J Clin Endocrinol Metab. 2000; 85:4908-4911.
3. Steiger A. Neurochemical regulation of sleep. J Psychiatr Res. 2007; 41:537-552.
4. Schüssler P et al. Sleep-impairing effect of intravenous corticotropin-releasing hormone on sleep EEG in young healthy women. Experimental and Clinical Endocrinology & Diabetes. 2009; 117:664.
5. Weikel JC et al. Ghrelin promotes slow-wave sleep in humans. Am J Physiol Endocrinol Metab. 2003; 284:E407-E415.
6. Kluge M et al. Ghrelin alone or co-administered with GHRH or CRH increases non-REM sleep and decreases REM sleep in young males. Psychoneuroendocrinology. 2008; 33:497-506.
7. Kluge M et al. Effects of ghrelin on psychopathology, sleep and secretion of cortisol and growth hormone in patients with major depression. J Psychiatr Res. 2010, in press.
8. Motivala SJ et al. Nocturnal levels of ghrelin and leptin and sleep in chronic insomnia. Psychoneuroendocrinology. 2009; 34:540-545.
9. Kluge M et al. Ghrelin enhances the nocturnal secretion of cortisol and growth hormone in young females without influencing sleep. Psychoneuroendocrinology. 2007; 32:1079-1085.
10. Obal F Jr et al. Sleep in mice with nonfunctional growth hormone-releasing hormone receptors. Am J Physiol Regul Integr Comp Physiol. 2003; 284:R131-R139.
11. Szentirmai E et al. Ghrelin-induced sleep responses in ad libitum fed and food-restricted rats. Brain Res. 2006; 1088:131-140.
12. Szentirmai E et al. Ghrelin microinjection into forebrain sites induces wakefulness and feeding in rats. Am J Physiol Regul Integr Comp Physiol. 2007; 292:R575-R585.
13. Steiger A. Ghrelin and sleep-wake regulation. Am J Physiol Regul Integr Comp Physiol. 2007; 292:R573-R574.
14. Kluge M et al. Ghrelin increases slow wave sleep and stage 2 sleep and decreases stage 1 sleep and REM sleep in elderly men but does not affect sleep in elderly women. Psychoneuroendocrinology. 2010; 35:297-304.
15. Szentirmai E et al. Spontaneous sleep and homeostatic sleep regulation in ghrelin knockout mice. Am J Physiol Regul Integr Comp Physiol. 2007; 293:R510-R517.

Sleep Among Women

Eszopiclone improves insomnia and depressive and anxious symptoms in perimenopausal and postmenopausal women with hot flashes: a randomized, double-blinded, placebo-controlled crossover trial. Joffe H, Petrillo L, Viguera A, Koukopoulos A, Silver-Heilman K, Farrell A, Yu G, Silver M, Cohen LS. *Am J Obstet Gynecol. 2010 Feb;202(2):171.e1-171.e11.*

What are the effects of eszopiclone on sleep and mood of peri- and post-menopausal women with hot flashes?

Subjects	Methods	Outcomes
59 peri/postmenopausal women with insomnia, hot flashes, and depression and/or anxiety • Age: 40-65 yrs Note: 46 women completed the study	Double-blind, randomized, crossover 11 week trial Subjects were randomized to either: • Eszopiclone (3 mg) • Placebo Assessments: • Depression and anxiety • Hot flashes • ISI • QOL • Sleep diary	Compared to placebo, eszopiclone was associated with: • Reduced ISI scores (by 8.7 ± 1.4)* • Improved sleep parameters** • Improved depressive and anxiety symptoms** • Improved QOL** • Improved nighttime hot flashes** • No change in daytime hot flashes

ISI: Insomnia severity index; QOL: quality of life; *$P < .0001$; **$P < .05$

Conclusion
Eszopiclone improved menopause-related insomnia, nighttime hot flashes and changes in mood.

Commentary
The menopause transition is a period of risk for insomnia in women, with the prevalence of an insomnia disorder increasing from 13% in older premenopausal women to 26% in peri- and postmenopausal women.[1] Other common symptoms of the menopause transition include hot flashes, night sweats, and depression. Peri/postmenopausal women with insomnia are highly likely to concurrently experience hot flashes[1],together with mild depressive and anxiety symptoms, that interfere with their function and quality-of-life.[2] Given that insomnia commonly co-occurs with other menopause-associated symptoms[3], therapies targeting sleep disturbance may provide an important approach to treating multiply symptomatic women and improving quality-of-life overall.

This study was a double-blinded, placebo-controlled, cross-over trial of eszopiclone 3-mg/day conducted in 59 peri/postmenopausal women with sleep-onset and/or sleep-maintenance insomnia, hot flashes, depressive and/or anxiety symptoms.[4] Women were randomly assigned to eszopiclone or placebo for 4 weeks and then crossed over to the other treatment for another 4 weeks after a 2-week wash-out period. Eszopiclone reduced insomnia scores on the Insomnia Severity Index by 8.7 ± 1.4 more points than placebo ($P < 0.0001$), and improved all diary-reported sleep parameters (wake time after sleep-onset, sleep efficiency, and total sleep time), depressive symptoms, anxiety symptoms, and quality-of-life ($P < 0.05$). Eszopiclone also reduced nighttime hot flashes ($P < 0.05$), but did not improve daytime hot flashes. The findings of this study show that use of a nonbenzodiazepine hypnotic agent to target sleep disturbance in multiply symptomatic midlife women improves insomnia and other symptom domains, resulting in improved quality-of-life.

Our results are consistent with placebo-controlled trials in adults with primary insomnia showing that eszopiclone improves sleep-onset and sleep-maintenance symptoms[5-7], daytime function, and quality-of-life.[5-8] In previous trials conducted specifically in peri/postmenopausal women with insomnia, eszopiclone has been shown to improve sleep in those with isolated *sleep-onset* insomnia[8] and zolpidem has been shown to improve sleep in those with *sleep-maintenance* insomnia and hot flashes.[9] Our study population differed from previous trials[8, 9] because they had sleep-onset and/or sleep-maintenance disturbances that co-occurred with other common menopause-associated symptoms of depressive, anxiety, and vasomotor symptoms. Taken together, this series of studies emphasizes the therapeutic value of nonbenzodiazepine hypnotic agents in the treatment of menopause-associated insomnia.

In our study, hot flashes were not an eligibility criterion; however, they were universal in our participants. Women who experience hot flashes during the menopause transition report worse sleep quality[10-13], and are more likely to meet insomnia criteria[1],than those without hot flashes. Treatment with eszopiclone reduced nocturnal, but not daytime, hot flashes relative to placebo, a selective effect which suggests that eszopiclone either suppresses hot flashes at peak serum levels (half-life 6 hours) or reduces reports of nighttime hot flashes only because women sleep through them. A direct effect of eszopiclone on hot flashes is not expected because the hypnotic modulates γ-aminobutyric acid receptors, which is not thought to be a core mechanism for other hot flash treatments. Regardless, this beneficial effect suggests that hypnotic therapies may be an important treatment consideration for women with insomnia and bothersome nighttime hot flashes.

Our findings are also consistent with other studies that have demonstrated the benefit of co-administration of eszopiclone for affective symptoms in patients with insomnia co-occurring with major depression[14] and generalized anxiety disorder.[15] In contrast to previous studies[14, 15], our participants received eszopiclone as monotherapy and had mild affective symptoms that did not meet criteria for psychiatric illness. Regardless, we observed improvement in depressive and anxiety symptoms. These findings suggest that eszopiclone may improve affective symptoms either as an indirect consequence of improving sleep or because of a direct effect of the medication on psychological symptoms.

In summary, results of this randomized, placebo-controlled, crossover study indicate that targeting sleep disturbance in peri- and postmenopausal women who present with sleep-onset and/or sleep-maintenance insomnia in combination with other menopause-associated symptoms has beneficial effects on multiple symptom domains, including sleep disturbance, mood, anxiety, and nighttime hot flashes. Because insomnia is highly prevalent in midlife women and other bothersome symptoms commonly co-occur with insomnia in this population, our findings suggest that nonbenzodiazepine hypnotic agents may serve an important therapeutic role in the management of women with sleep problems and other menopause-related symptoms that impact quality-of-life during the menopause transition.

Hadine Joffe
Center for Women's Mental Health
Massachusetts General Hospital
Harvard Medical School

Stephanie Connors
Center for Women's Mental Health
Massachusetts General Hospital
Harvard Medical School

References

1. Ohayon MM. Severe hot flashes are associated with chronic insomnia. Arch Intern Med. 2006; 166:1262-8.
2. Joffe H et al. Depression is associated with worse objectively and subjectively measured sleep, but not more frequent awakenings, in women with vasomotor symptoms. Menopause. 2009; 16:671-9.
3. Reed SD et al. Night sweats, sleep disturbance, and depression associated with diminished libido in late menopausal transition and early postmenopause: baseline data from the Herbal Alternatives for Menopause Trial (HALT). Am J Obstet Gynecol. 2007; 196:593 e1-7.
4. Joffe H et al. Eszopiclone improves insomnia, depressive and anxious symptoms in perimenopausal and postmenopausal women with hot flashes: a randomized, double-blinded, placebo-controlled cross-over trial. Am J Obstet Gynecol. 2010; in press.
5. Walsh JK et al. Nightly treatment of primary insomnia with eszopiclone for six months: effect on sleep, quality of life, and work limitations. Sleep. 2007; 30:959-68.
6. Krystal AD et al. Sustained efficacy of eszopiclone over 6 months of nightly treatment: results of a randomized, double-blind, placebo-controlled study in adults with chronic insomnia. Sleep. 2003; 26:793-9.
7. Rosenberg R et al. An assessment of the efficacy and safety of eszopiclone in the treatment of transient insomnia in healthy adults. Sleep Med. 2005; 6:15-22.
8. Soares CN et al. Eszopiclone in patients with insomnia during perimenopause and early postmenopause: a randomized controlled trial. Obstet Gynecol. 2006; 108:1402-10.
9. Dorsey CM et al. Effect of zolpidem on sleep in women with perimenopausal and postmenopausal insomnia: a 4-week, randomized, multicenter, double-blind, placebo-controlled study. Clin Ther. 2004; 26:1578-86.
10. Kravitz HM et al. Sleep difficulty in women at midlife: a community survey of sleep and the menopausal transition. Menopause. 2003; 10:19-28.
11. Young T et al. Objective and subjective sleep quality in premenopausal, perimenopausal, and postmenopausal women in the Wisconsin Sleep Cohort Study. Sleep. 2003; 26:667-72.

12. Dennerstein L et al. A prospective population-based study of menopausal symptoms. Obstet Gynecol. 2000; 96:351-8.
13. Thurston RC et al. Association between hot flashes, sleep complaints, and psychological functioning among healthy menopausal women. Int J Behav Med. 2006; 13:163-72.
14. Fava M et al. Eszopiclone co-administered with fluoxetine in patients with insomnia coexisting with major depressive disorder. Biol Psychiatry. 2006; 59:1052-60.
15. Pollack M et al. Eszopiclone coadministered with escitalopram in patients with insomnia and comorbid generalized anxiety disorder. Arch Gen Psychiatry. 2008; 65:551-62.

Miscellaneous

An automated sleep-analysis system operated through a standard hospital monitor. Amir O, Barak-Shinar D, Amos Y, MacDonald M, Pittman S, White DP. *J Clin Sleep Med. 2010 Feb 15;6(1):59-63.*

Can sleep disordered breathing events be accurately identified using a computerized analysis system of signals obtained from standard hospital monitors, and how does this method compare to polysomnography?

Subjects	Methods	Outcomes
53 subjects with suspected SDB • Gender: 68% males • Age (mean): 48 yrs • BMI (median): 31	Detection of SDB events were analyzed by simultaneous PSG and a computerized analysis system (CAS) using signals (ECG, RI, ETCO$_2$ and SaO$_2$) from standard hospital monitors*	The following values derived from CAS and PSG were highly correlated: • AHI** 1. Mean values were 15.5 ± 20.0 for CAS and 15.4 ± 24.0 for PSG • TST***

AHI: apnea hypopnea index; BMI: body mass index; CAS: computerized analysis system; ECG: electrocardiography; ETCO$_2$: end-tidal carbon dioxide; PSG: polysomnography; RI: respiratory impedance; SaO$_2$: arterial oxygen saturation; SDB: sleep disordered breathing; TST: total sleep time; * Morpheus Hx, WideMed, Ltd., Herzliya, Israel; ** linear regression values R = 0.96; *** linear regression values R = 0.82

Conclusion
Computerized analysis of electrocardiographic, respiratory impedance, oxygen saturation and end-tidal carbon dioxide data obtained from standard hospital monitors accurately identified sleep disordered breathing events.

Commentary
SDB may have clinical importance to cardiovascular morbidity and is commonly under diagnosed.[1-3] Sleep apnea occurs in approximately 30% to 50% of Heart Failure (HF) patients, mainly due to systolic dysfunction. Whether SDB contributes to mortality independently of other risk factors is still a matter of debate. Some authors suggest that mortality does appear to be increased in HF patients with nocturnal SDB and Cheyne Stokes Breathing compared to those without it.[4-6] A major limitation in assessing the true prevalence and significance of SDB in patients with heart failure (HF) is the need for a full-night polysomnographic test. Polysomnography, the gold-standard diagnostic test for this condition, requires a complex apparatus of equipment and personnel. It is not uncommon for sick patients to refuse participation in sleep studies because of the need either to travel or to spend the night in a sleep laboratory. To overcome these difficulties, research studies in recent years have examined the feasibility of using portable monitoring systems and the accuracy of such systems compared with full polysomnography. In most of these studies the equipment has been tested in a

laboratory setting concomitantly with a full polysomnography monitoring. In some cases, the patients have used the devices at their homes. The majority of reports indicate good correlation in SDB parameters between portable recordings and full polysomnography and a fair reproducibility of the method.

In different with the above studies, we used an existing monitor which is commonly used to detect routine vital signs in already hospitalized patients. Albeit some limitations of this study; i.e. small sample size, diverse severity of OSA, and the setting of sleep laboratory rather than hospital one, our results do confirm both the accuracy and the practicality of this kind of sleep monitoring; leading to the potential use of an automated bedside system in hospitalized patients who require an overnight hospital monitoring due to their illness. Moreover, this mode of data may avert the need for further more complex sleep-lab evaluation. Considering the lack of any significant additional cost, the CAS may have a significant advantage in providing data related to the coexistence and the severity of SDB over other conventional modalities, as bedside automatic scoring by the Morpheus Hx system was shown to be both feasible and accurate when compared with the manual procedure of gold-standard polysomnography. Further studies are needed to provide definitive evidence of the usefulness of this method in selected hospitalized patients and, in particular, those with cardiovascular disease.

Offer Amir
WideMed Ltd.

Deganit Barak-Shinar
WideMed Ltd.

References

1. Amir O et al. Implications of Cheyne-Stokes Breathing in Advanced Systolic Heart Failure. Clinical Cardiology. 2010; 33(3):E8–E12.
2. Amir O et al. Prediction of death and hospital admissions via innovative detection of cheyne-stokes breathing in heart failure patients. Cardiovascular Engineering and Technology. 2010;1(2): 132–137.
3. Amir O et al. Long term assessment of Nocturnal Cheyne-Stokes Respiration in Patients with Heart Failure. Sleep and Breathing, 2010; in press.
4. Hanly PJ et al. Increased mortality associated with Cheyne-stokes respiration in patients with congestive heart failure. Am J Respir Crit Care Med. 1996; 153:272-276.
5. Lanfranchi PA et al. Prognostic Value of Nocturnal Cheyne-Stokes Respiration in Chronic Heart Failure. Circulation. 1999; 99:1435-1440.
6. Javaheri S et al. Central sleep apnea, right ventricular dysfunction, and low diastolic blood pressure are predictors of mortality in systolic heart failure. J Am Coll Cardiol. 2007; 49:2028-2034.

Hypoxemia and hypoventilation syndrome improvement after laparoscopic bariatric surgery in patients with morbid obesity. Lumachi F, Marzano B, Fanti G, Basso SM, Mazza F, Chiara GB. *In Vivo. 2010 May-Jun;24(3):329-31.*

In persons with severe obesity and hypoxemia, what are the effects of laparoscopic Roux-en-Y gastric bypass surgery on body mass index, PaO_2 and SaO_2?

Subjects	Methods	Outcomes
11 obese subjects with hypoxemia • Age: 41.2 ± 10.2 yrs • Gender: 36% male • BMI (median): 52.3 • Baseline spirometry 1. SaO_2: 88.3 ± 3.9% 2. FVC: 84.5 ± 8.3% 3. FEV_1: 79.9 ± 10.1%	Prospective study Assessments (before and 6 and 12 months after laparoscopic Roux-en-Y gastric bypass surgery): • ABG • BMI • EWL • FEV_1 • FVC • PaO_2 • $PaCO_2$ • Awake SaO_2	No correlation between BMI, SaO_2, and FEV_1* Significant correlation noted: • Between SaO_2 and PaO_2** • Between SaO_2 and EWL*** Changes in EWL[#]: • 3 months after sugery: 18.9% • 6 months after surgery: 26.4% • 12 months after surgery: 39.6% Spirometry at 1-yr follow-up: • SaO_2: 96.2 ± 3.2%[##] • FVC: 112.3 ± 9.9%[###] • FEV_1: 101.6 ± 18.8%[^]

ABG: arterial blood gas measurement; BMI: body mass index; EWL: excess weight loss; FEV_1: forced expiratory volume exhaled in one second; FVC: forced vital capacity; $PaCO_2$: partial pressure of carbon dioxide; PaO_2: partial pressure of oxygen; SaO_2: arterial oxygen saturation; *$P > 0.01$; **$R = 0.74$, $P = 0.009$; ***$R = -0.75$, $P = 0.008$; [#]$P < 0.001$; [##]$P < 0.001$; [###]$P < 0.001$; [^]$P = 0.003$

Conclusion
Weight reduction following laparoscopic bariatric surgery in persons with severe obesity and hypoxemia improved SaO_2, FVC and FEV_1.

Commentary
Obesity is a multifactorial disorder which produces a number of complications and metabolic sequelae, including risk of severe cardiovascular diseases and respiratory diseases.[1] Morbid obesity is frequently accompanied by serious co-morbidity, enclosed obstructive sleep apnea and obesity-hypoventilation syndrome (OHS), and thus many morbidly obese patients require

surgical interventions.[2] Obese patients with hypoventilation display blunted respiratory responses to hypoxia, developing hypoxemia due to decreased ventilation, and weight loss obtained by bariatric surgery is associated with significant long-term improvements in obstructive respiratory syndrome and oxygenation.[3] Patients with OHS should have daytime hypoxia ($PO_2 < 70$ mm Hg) and hypercapnia ($PCO_2 > 45$ mm Hg), and the associated changes in lung function play an important role in the pathogenesis of pulmonary hypertension.[4] In our series, all patients had hypoxemia, and reduced FVC and FEV1.

Leptin is a hormone produced in adipose cells, and its interaction with specific hypothalamic receptors suppresses appetite. It is also a respiratory modulator, and hypoxic suppression of leptin production or central nervous system (CNS) resistance has been observed in patients with OHS.[5]

Several studies showed that weight loss is associated with marked improvement in pulmonary function, decreasing pCO_2, and expanding lung volume.[6] In our patients, the main pre- and postoperative parameters were: $SpO_2 = 88.3 \pm 3.9\%$ vs. $96.2 \pm 3.2\%$ (< 0.001), FVC = $84.5 \pm 8.3\%$ vs. $112.3 \pm 9.9\%$ ($P < 0.001$), and FEV1 = $79.9 \pm 10.1\%$ vs. $101.6 \pm 18.8\%$ ($P = 0.003$). However, we did not find any relationship ($P = NS$) between SpO_2 and BMI nor between pCO_2 and BMI. The figure resumes the mechanism of hypoxemia and hypercapnia in obese patients with OHS.

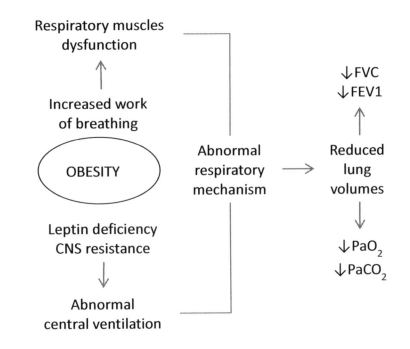

Franco Lumachi
Department of Surgical & Gastroenterological Sciences
School of Medicine
University of Padua

References

1. Hellerstein MK et al. Obesity & Overweight. In: Basic and Clinical Endocrinology. Greenspan FS et al (eds.). New York, NY, Lange Medical Books/McGraw-Hill, 2001; pp. 745-761.
2. Lumachi F et al. Relationship between body mass index, age and hypoxemia in patients with extremely severe obesity undergoing bariatric surgery. In Vivo. 2010; 24:775-777.
3. Fritscher LG et al. Bariatric surgery in the treatment of obstructive sleep apnea in morbidly obese patients. Respiration. 2007; 74:647-652.
4. Powers MA. The obesity hypoventilatory syndrome. Respir Care. 2008; 53:1723-1730.
5. Redolfi S et al. Long-term noninvasive ventilation increases chemosensitivity and leptin in obesity-hypoventilation syndrome. Respir Med. 2007; 101:1191-1195.
6. Scheuller M et al. Bariatric surgery for treatment of sleep apnea syndrome in 15 morbidly obese patients: long-term results. Otolayngol Head Neck Surg. 2001; 125:299-302.

Normalizing effects of modafinil on sleep in chronic cocaine users. Morgan PT, Pace-Schott E, Pittman B, Stickgold R, Malison RT. *Am J Psychiatry. 2010 Mar;167(3):331-40.*

Does modafinil affect sleep and daytime sleepiness in chronic cocaine users?

Subjects	Methods	Outcomes
20 subjects • Cocaine dependent 12 healthy controls	Double-blind randomized trial Subjects were randomized (at 7:30 am for 16 days) to: • Modafinil (n = 10): 400 mg • Placebo (n = 10) Assessments: • Subjects 1. PSG (days 1 to 3, 7 to 9, and 14 to 16) 2. MSLT at 11:30 am, 2:00 pm, and 4:30 pm on days 2, 8, and 15 • Controls 1. 1 experimental PSG after 1 accommodation PSG	Cocaine abstinence was associated with worse PSG parameters Among subjects, compared with placebo, modafinil was associated with: • Decreased nighttime SL • Increased SWS • Longer TST • Shorter REM SL • Increased daytime SL (MSLT) • Decrease in subjective daytime sleepiness

MSLT: Multiple sleep latency test; PSG: polysomnography; REM: rapid eye movement; SL: sleep latency; SWS: slow wave sleep; TST: total sleep time

Conclusion
During cocaine abstinence, morning administration of modafinil improved nighttime sleep and daytime alertness.

Commentary
Co-morbid sleep problems are rampant in psychiatric illness, including substance abuse.[1] More than just symptoms to be treated, disturbances in sleep may be integral to the underlying disease processes.[2] If so, then treatment of the sleep disturbance may be important for recovery from illness. For cocaine dependence, this may be particularly important, as there is no FDA approved medication for its treatment. We have shown that abstinence from chronic cocaine use is associated with marked abnormalities in sleep that worsen rather than improve over 3 weeks of abstinence.[3-6] These abnormalities include increases in sleep latency, decreases in total sleep time and slow-wave sleep time, and alterations in REM sleep that are associated with sleep-related cognitive deficits.

In this study, we examined the effect of modafinil on sleep architecture in chronic cocaine users. Modafinil is a stimulant that appears to function largely as a dopamine reuptake inhibitor.[7] Dosed in the morning, we hypothesized that modafinil would improve daytime sleepiness while decreasing nocturnal sleep latency and increasing total sleep time. Potential participants were heavy, chronic cocaine users who did not meet criteria for dependence on any drugs besides cocaine with the exception of nicotine. All participants used cocaine within 3 days of beginning the 16-day, inpatient study. 20 participants completed the study of which 10 received 400 mg modafinil daily at 7:30 AM and 10 received matching placebo. Sleep was restricted to 11 PM to 7 AM, and polysomnographic sleep recording was performed on study days 1-3, 7-9, and 14-16 (i.e. the first, second and third week of abstinence). Modified multiple sleep latency testing was performed on days 2, 8 and 15.

We found that modafinil decreased subjective daytime sleepiness in the afternoon during the second and third weeks of abstinence. Evening sleepiness was indistinguishable between the modafinil and placebo groups, suggesting that the stimulant effects of modafinil had worn off. Objective sleepiness as measured by MSLT was less in the modafinil group, but only during the first week of abstinence. Evening sleepiness across the study was greater in the modafinil group, as noted by decreased nocturnal sleep latency. In addition, modafinil increased total sleep time and slow-wave sleep time. Compared to age-matched healthy participants studied in the same setting, modafinil was associated with the normalization of slow-wave sleep time and improvements in total sleep time, REM sleep time, and sleep onset latency.

Controlled trials of modafinil in the treatment of cocaine dependence indicate positive effects on abstinence from cocaine.[8,9] Human laboratory work indicates that modafinil decreases cocaine intake.[10] The present work ties the clinical promise of modafinil in the treatment of cocaine dependence by identifying a biological marker of cocaine dependence whose responsiveness to pharmacological intervention may not only parallel[11] but also contribute to positive clinical outcomes. Ongoing work is exploring this as yet unanswered question.

Peter T. Morgan
Department of Psychiatry
Yale University

References

1. Breslau N et al. Sleep disturbance and psychiatric disorders: a longitudinal epidemiological study of young adults. Biol Psychiatry. 1996; 39:411-418.
2. Krystal A. Sleep and psychiatric disorders: future directions. Psychiatr Clin North Am. 2006; 29:1115-1130.
3. Morgan PT et al. Sleep, sleep-dependent procedural learning and vigilance in chronic cocaine users: evidence for occult insomnia. Drug Alcohol Depend. 2006; 82:238-249.
4. Morgan PT et al. Sleep architecture, cocaine and visual learning. Addiction. 2008; 103:1344-1352.
5. Morgan PT et al. Sex differences in sleep and sleep-dependent learning in abstinent cocaine users. Pharmacol Biochem Behav. 2009; 93:54-58.
6. Matuskey D et al. A multistudy analysis of the effects of early cocaine abstinence on sleep. Drug and Alcohol Depend. 2010; Epub ahead of print.
7. Volkow ND et al. Effects of modafinil on dopamine and dopamine transporters in the male human brain. JAMA. 2009; 301:1148-1154.
8. Dackis CA et al. A double-blind, placebo-controlled trial of modafinil for cocaine dependence. Neuropsychopharmacology. 2005; 30:205-211.

9.   Anderson AL et al. Modafinil for the treatment of cocaine dependence. Drug and Alcohol Depend. 2009; 104:133-139.
10. Hart CL et al. Smoked cocaine self-administration is decreased by modafinil. Neuropsychopharmacology. 2008; 33(4):761-8.
11. Dackis C et al. Normalizing effects of modafinil on cocaine-induced sleep abnormalities. Comment. Am J Psychiatry. 2010; 167(3):248-249.

Made in the USA
Charleston, SC
29 April 2011